Gene-Based Therapies for Pediatric Blood Diseases

Editors

NIRALI N. SHAH
SUNG-YUN PAI

HEMATOLOGY/ONCOLOGY CLINICS OF NORTH AMERICA

www.hemonc.theclinics.com

Consulting Editors
GEORGE P. CANELLOS
EDWARD J. BENZ Jr

August 2022 • Volume 36 • Number 4

ELSEVIER

1600 John F. Kennedy Boulevard • Suite 1800 • Philadelphia, Pennsylvania, 19103-2899

http://www.theclinics.com

HEMATOLOGY/ONCOLOGY CLINICS OF NORTH AMERICA Volume 36, Number 4
August 2022 ISSN 0889-8588, ISBN 13: 978-0-323-98775-2

Editor: Stacy Eastman
Developmental Editor: Ann Gielou M. Posedio

Hematology/Oncology Clinics (ISSN 0889-8588) is published bimonthly by Elsevier Inc., 360 Park Avenue South, New York, NY 10010-1710. Months of issue are February, April, June, August, October, and December. Business and Editorial Offices: 1600 John F. Kennedy Blvd., Ste. 1800, Philadelphia, PA 19103–2899. Customer Service Office: 3251 Riverport Lane, Maryland Heights, MO 63043. Periodicals postage paid at New York, NY and at additional mailing offices. Subscription prices are $470.00 per year (domestic individuals), $1190.00 per year (domestic institutions), $100.00 per year (domestic students/residents), $495.00 per year (Canadian individuals), $100.00 per year (Canadian students/residents), $1232.00 per year (Canadian institutions) $563.00 per year (international individuals), $1232.00 per year (international institutions), and $255.00 per year (international students/residents). International air speed delivery is included in all *Clinics* subscription prices. All prices are subject to change without notice. **POSTMASTER:** Send address changes to *Hematology/Oncology Clinics of North America*, Elsevier Health Sciences Division, Subscription Customer Service, 3251 Riverport Lane, Maryland Heights, MO 63043. Customer Service (orders, claims, online, change of address): Elsevier Health Sciences Division, Subscription **Customer Service, 3251 Riverport Lane, Maryland Heights, MO 63043. Tel: 1-800-654-2452 (U.S. and Canada); 314-447-8871 (outside U.S. and Canada). Fax: 314-447-8029. E-mail: journalscustomerservice-usa@elsevier.com (for print support); journalsonlinesupport-usa@elsevier.com (for online support).**

Reprints. For copies of 100 or more, of articles in this publication, please contact the Commercial Reprints Department, Elsevier Inc., 360 Park Avenue South, New York, New York 10010-1710; Tel.: 212-633-3874, Fax: 212-633-3820, E-mail: reprints@elsevier.com.

Hematology/Oncology Clinics of North America is covered in *MEDLINE/PubMed (Index Medicus), EMBASE/ Excerpta Medica, and BIOSIS.*

Contributors

CONSULTING EDITORS

GEORGE P. CANELLOS, MD
William Rosenberg Professor of Medicine, Department of Medical Oncology, Dana-Farber
Cancer Institute, Boston, Massachusetts, USA

EDWARD J. BENZ Jr, MD
Professor, Pediatrics, Richard and Susan Smith Professor, Medicine, Professor, Genetics,
Harvard Medical School, President and CEO Emeritus, Office of the President,
Dana-Farber Cancer Institute, Boston, Massachusetts, USA

EDITORS

NIRALI N. SHAH, MD, MHSc
Pediatric Oncology Branch, Center for Cancer Research, National Cancer Institute,
National Institutes of Health, Bethesda, Maryland, USA

SUNG-YUN PAI, MD
Senior Investigator, Immune Deficiency Cellular Therapy Program, Center for Cancer
Research, National Cancer Institute, National Institutes of Health, Bethesda, Maryland,
USA

AUTHORS

ALESSANDRO AIUTI, MD, PhD
Pediatric Immunohematology and Bone Marrow Transplantation Unit, San Raffaele
Telethon Institute for Gene Therapy (SR-Tiget), IRCSS San Raffaele Scientific Institute,
Vita-Salute San Raffaele University, Milan, Italy

COLLEEN ANNESLEY, MD
Seattle Children's Research Institute, Seattle Children's Hospital, Seattle, Washington,
USA

KRISTIN BAIRD, MD
Office of Tissue and Advanced Therapies, Center for Biologics Evaluation and Research,
US Food and Drug Administration, Silver Spring, Maryland, USA

MARIA ESTER BERNARDO, MD, PhD
Pediatric Immunohematology and Bone Marrow Transplantation Unit, San Raffaele
Telethon Institute for Gene Therapy (SR-Tiget), IRCSS San Raffaele Scientific Institute,
Vita-Salute San Raffaele University, Milan, Italy

CHALLICE L. BONIFANT, MD, PhD
The Sidney Kimmel Comprehensive Cancer Center, Department of Pediatrics,
Johns Hopkins School of Medicine, Baltimore, Maryland, USA

MELISSA BONNER, PhD
bluebird bio, Inc, Cambridge, Massachusetts, USA

CLAIRE BOOTH, MBBS, PhD
Professor, Department of Paediatric Immunology and Gene Therapy, Great Ormond
Street Hospital, UCL Great Ormond Street Institute of Child Health, London, United
Kingdom

NAJAT BOUCHKOUJ, MD
Office of Tissue and Advanced Therapies, Center for Biologics Evaluation and Research,
US Food and Drug Administration, Silver Spring, Maryland, USA

NICOLA BRUNETTI-PIERRI, MD
Department of Translational Medicine, Federico II University, Scuola Superiore
Meridionale, School for Advanced Studies, Naples, Italy; Telethon Institute of Genetics
and Medicine, Pozzuoli, Naples, Italy

HILDEGARD BÜNING, PhD
Institute of Experimental Hematology, REBIRTH Research Center for Translational
Regenerative Medicine, Hannover Medical School, German Center for Infection
Research, Partner Site Hannover-Braunschweig

KRITIKA CHETTY, MBBS
Department of Paediatric Immunology and Gene Therapy, Great Ormond Street Hospital,
London, United Kingdom

ILIAS CHRISTODOULOU, MD
The Sidney Kimmel Comprehensive Cancer Center, Johns Hopkins School of Medicine,
Baltimore, Maryland, USA

GIULIA CONSIGLIERI, MD
Pediatric Immunohematology and Bone Marrow Transplantation Unit, San Raffaele
Telethon Institute for Gene Therapy (SR-Tiget), IRCSS San Raffaele Scientific Institute,
Milan, Italy; Department of Biomedicine and Prevention, University of Rome Tor Vergata,
Rome

STACY E. CROTEAU, MD, MMS
Boston Children's Hospital, Boston Hemophilia Center, Boston, Massachusetts, USA

CHRISTINE N. DUNCAN, MD
Department of Pediatric Hematology and Oncology, Boston Children's Hospital,
Department of Pediatric Oncology, Dana-Farber Cancer Institute, Boston,
Massachusetts, USA

ELIZABETH K. GARABEDIAN, RN, MSLS
Office of the Clinical Director, National Human Genome Research Institute, National
Institutes of Health, Bethesda, Maryland, USA

BEN C. HOUGHTON, BSc, PhD
UCL Great Ormond Street Institute of Child Health, London, United Kingdom

MATTHEW M. HSIEH, MD
Cellular and Molecular Therapeutics Branch, National Heart, Lung, and Blood Institute,
National Institutes of Health, Bethesda, Maryland, USA

LAUREN JIMENEZ-KURLANDER, MD
Department of Pediatric Hematology and Oncology, Boston Children's Hospital, Department of Pediatric Oncology, Dana-Farber Cancer Institute, Boston, Massachusetts, USA

NICO JÄSCHKE, PhD
Institute of Experimental Hematology, Hannover Medical School, Hannover, Germany

MEGHA KAUSHAL, MD
Office of Tissue and Advanced Therapies, Center for Biologics Evaluation and Research, US Food and Drug Administration, Silver Spring, Maryland, USA

CAROLINE Y. KUO, MD
Division of Allergy and Immunology, Department of Pediatrics, David Geffen School of Medicine, University of California, Los Angeles, Los Angeles, California, USA

ALEXIS LEONARD, MD
Cellular and Molecular Therapeutics Branch, National Heart, Lung, and Blood Institute, National Institutes of Health, Bethesda, Maryland, USA

JOSEPH D. LONG, MS
Division of Allergy and Immunology, Department of Pediatrics, David Geffen School of Medicine, University of California, Los Angeles, Los Angeles, California, USA

HARRY L. MALECH, MD
Genetic Immunotherapy Section, Laboratory of Clinical Immunology and Microbiology, National Institute of Allergy and Infectious Diseases, National Institutes of Health, Bethesda, Maryland, USA

REGINA MYERS, MD
Division of Oncology, Children's Hospital of Philadelphia, Philadelphia, Pennsylvania, USA

GIORGIO OTTAVIANO, MD
Senior Clinical Research Fellow, Infection, Immunity and Inflammation Department, UCL Great Ormond Street Institute of Child Health, London, United Kingdom

SUNG-YUN PAI, MD
Senior Investigator, Immune Deficiency Cellular Therapy Program, Center for Cancer Research, National Cancer Institute, National Institutes of Health, Bethesda, Maryland, USA

MARA PAVEL-DINU, PhD
Instructor, Department of Pediatrics, Division of Stem Cell Transplantation and Regenerative Medicine, Stanford Medical School, Stanford, California, USA

MATTHEW H. PORTEUS, MD, PhD
Professor, Department of Pediatrics, Division of Stem Cell Transplantation and Regenerative Medicine, Stanford Medical School, Stanford, California, USA

WASEEM QASIM, BMedSci, MBBS, PhD
Professor of Cell and Gene Therapy, Infection, Immunity and Inflammation Department, UCL Great Ormond Street Institute of Child Health, London, United Kingdom

RUYAN RAHNAMA, MD, MSc
The Sidney Kimmel Comprehensive Cancer Center, Department of Pediatrics, Johns Hopkins School of Medicine, Baltimore, Maryland, USA

KRISTEN RECTOR, MS

HANEEN SHALABI, DO
Pediatric Oncology Branch, Center for Cancer Research, National Cancer Institute, National Institutes of Health, Bethesda, Maryland, USA

POORNIMA SHARMA, MD
Office of Tissue and Advanced Therapies, Center for Biologics Evaluation and Research, US Food and Drug Administration, Silver Spring, Maryland, USA

AIMEE C. TALLEUR, MD
Department of Bone Marrow Transplantation and Cellular Therapy, St. Jude Children's Research Hospital, Memphis, Tennessee, USA

JOHN F. TISDALE, MD
Cellular and Molecular Therapeutics Branch, National Heart, Lung, and Blood Institute, National Institutes of Health, Bethesda, Maryland, USA

EDWARD C. TROPE, MS
Division of Allergy and Immunology, Department of Pediatrics, David Geffen School of Medicine, University of California, Los Angeles, Los Angeles, California, USA

JENNIFER YANG, BS
Department of Psychology, University of California, Los Angeles, Los Angeles, California, USA

Contents

The earliest conceptual history of gene therapy began with the recognition of DNA as the transforming substance capable of changing the phenotypic character of a bacterium and then as the carrier of the genomic code. Early studies of oncogenic viruses that could insert into the mammalian genome led to the concept that these same viruses might be engineered to carry new genetic material into mammalian cells, including human hematopoietic stem cells (HSC). In addition to properly engineered vectors capable of efficient safe transduction of HSC, successful gene therapy required the development of efficient materials, methods, and equipment to procure, purify, and culture HSC. Increased understanding of the preparative conditioning of patients was needed to optimize the engraftment of genetically modified HSC. Testing concepts in pivotal clinical trials to assess the efficacy and determine the cause of adverse events has advanced the efficiency and safety of gene therapy. This article is a historical overview of the separate threads of discovery that joined together to comprise our current state of gene therapy targeting HSC.

Innovations in programmable nucleases have expanded genetic engineering capabilities, raising the possibility of a new approach to curing monogenic hematological diseases. Feasibility studies using ex vivo targeted genome-editing, and nonintegrating viral vectors show outstanding potential for correcting genetic conditions at their root cause. This article reviews the latest technological advances in the CRISPR/Cas9 system alone and combined with engineered viruses as editing tools for human hematopoietic stem and progenitor cells (HSPCs). We discuss the early phase in human trials of genome editing-based therapies for hemoglobinopathies.

Although the number of market-approved gene therapies is still low, this new class of therapeutics has become an integral part of modern medicine. The success and safety of gene therapy depend on the vectors used to deliver the therapeutic material. Adeno-associated virus (AAV) vectors have emerged as the most frequently used delivery system for in vivo gene therapy. This success was achieved with first-generation vectors, using capsids derived from natural AAV serotypes. Their broad tropism, the high seroprevalence for many of the AAV serotypes in the human population, and the high vector doses needed to transduce a sufficient number of therapy-relevant target cells are challenges that are addressed by engineering the capsid and the vector genome, improving the efficacy of these biological nanoparticles.

The recent progress in gene and gene-modified cellular therapies has shown great promise for numerous pediatric diseases. Nevertheless, the development of these products is complicated, and the regulatory pathway is rigorous. There are, however, several opportunities for programmatic support within the Food and Drug Administration. This article highlights the life cycle of product development through approval and many of the available resources and programs to support product development.

Chimeric antigen receptor T-cell (CART) therapy has transformed the treatment paradigm for pediatric patients with relapsed/refractory B-cell acute lymphoblastic leukemia (B-ALL), with complete remission rates in key pivotal CD19-CART trials ranging from 65% to 90%. Alongside this new therapy, new toxicity profiles and treatment limitations have emerged, necessitating toxicity consensus grading systems, cooperative group trials, and novel management approaches. This review highlights the results of key clinical trials of CART for pediatric hematologic malignancies, discusses the most common toxicities seen to date, and elucidates challenges, opportunities, and areas of active research to optimize this therapy.

Chimeric antigen receptor (CAR) T-cells are widely being investigated against malignancies, and allogeneic 'universal donor' CAR-T cells offer the possibility of widened access to pre-manufactured, off-the-shelf therapies. Different genome-editing platforms have been used to address human leukocyte antigen (HLA) barriers to generate universal CAR-T cell therapy and early applications have been reported in children and adults against B cell malignancies. Recently developed Clustered Regularly Interspaced Short Palindromic Repeats (CRISPR)-based systems and related technologies offer the prospect of enhanced cellular immunotherapies for a wider range of hematological malignancies.

Pediatric blood cancers are among the most common malignancies that afflict children. Intensive chemotherapy is not curative in many cases, and novel therapies are urgently needed. NK cells hold promise for use as immunotherapeutic effectors due to their favorable safety profile, intrinsic cytotoxic properties, and potential for genetic modification that can enhance specificity and killing potential. NK cells can be engineered to express CARs targeting tumor-specific antigens, to downregulate inhibitory and regulatory signals, to secrete cytokine, and to optimize interaction with small molecule engagers. Understanding NK cell biology is key to designing immunotherapy for clinical translation.

β-thalassemia and sickle cell disease (SCD) are the most common monogenic diseases in the world and are potentially curable after allogeneic hematopoietic stem cell transplantation (HSCT) or autologous HSCT after genetic modification. Autologous gene therapy has the potential to offer a universal cure that overcomes many limitations of allogeneic HSCT including the lack of available donors, graft-vs-host disease, and graft rejection. Significant progress in gene therapy for the hemoglobinopathies has been made over the last several decades, now with multiple ongoing clinical trials investigating both gene addition and gene-editing strategies. Available results from a small number of patients, some with relatively short follow-up, are promising, with current efforts focused on continuing to improve the efficacy, durability, and safety of gene therapies for the cure of hemoglobin disorders.

Adeno-associated virus (AAV)-mediated gene transfer has successfully raised, and in some cases transiently normalized, FVIII or FIX activity levels in adults with severe hemophilia. Raising FVIII/IX levels, particularly greater than ~ 15 IU/dL (mild deficiency), corresponds to a marked decrease in spontaneous and provoked bleeding, dramatic reduction in factor concentrate use, and improved quality of life (QoL). Limited understanding of innate and adaptive immune system responses and hepatocyte transgene expression and stress responses to AAV-mediated gene transfer contribute to the variability in initial and long-term factor protein expression. Lentiviral (LV) and CRISPR/Cas-9 gene therapy approaches may further bolster the range of eligible participants and improve transgene expression and durability.

Severe combined immune deficiency (SCID) causes profound deficiency in T cells and variable deficiencies in B and NK cells. Untreated, the condition is fatal within the first 2 years of life. HSCT has traditionally been the only curative approach; however, success rates are suboptimal in those lacking an HLA-matched donor and conditioning regimens can cause significant toxicity. Gene therapy was pioneered for adenosine deaminase (ADA-SCID) over 3 decades ago and has produced highly successful results. Encouraging data for X-SCID and preclinical work for Artemis-SCID and RAG1-SCID are paving the way for the therapy to become a viable curative treatment option.

Joseph D. Long, Edward C. Trope, Jennifer Yang, Kristen Rector, and
Caroline Y. Kuo

The field of gene therapy has experienced tremendous growth in the last
decade ranging from improvements in the design of viral vectors for
gene addition of therapeutic gene cassettes to the discovery of site-
specific nucleases targeting transgenes to desired locations in the
genome. Such advancements have not only enabled the development of
disease models but also created opportunities for the development of
tailored therapeutic approaches. There are 3 main methods of gene modification that can be used for the prevention or treatment of disease. This
includes viral vector-mediated gene therapy to supply or bypass a
missing/defective gene, gene editing enabled by programmable nucleases
to create sequence-specific alterations in the genome, and gene silencing
to reduce the expression of a gene or genes. These gene-modification
platforms can be delivered either in vivo, for which the therapy is injected
directed into a patient's body, or ex vivo, in which cells are harvested from
a patient and modified in a laboratory setting, and then returned to the
patient.

Lauren Jimenez-Kurlander and Christine N. Duncan

Pediatric lysosomal and peroxisomal storage disorders, leukodystrophies,
and motor neuron diseases can have devastating neurologic manifestations. Despite efforts to exploit cross-correction to treat these monogenic
disorders for several decades, definitive treatment has yet to be identified.
This review explores recent attempts to transduce autologous hematopoietic stem cells with functional gene or provide therapeutic gene in vivo.
Specifically, we discuss the rationale behind efforts to treat pediatric
neurologic disorders with gene therapy, outline the specific disorders
that have been targeted at this time, and review recent and current clinical
investigations with attention to the future direction of therapy efforts.

Giulia Consiglieri, Maria Ester Bernardo, Nicola Brunetti-Pierri, and
Alessandro Aiuti

Enzyme replacement therapy (ERT) and allogeneic hematopoietic stem
cell transplantation (HSCT) are standard treatments for some mucopolysaccharidoses. Nevertheless, ERT is not curative, and HSCT is associated
with significant mortality and morbidity, leaving a substantial disease
burden of brain and skeletal manifestations. To overcome these limitations, different gene therapy (GT) strategies are under preclinical and clinical development. Data from ex-vivo GT clinical trials have demonstrated
encouraging biochemical and early clinical outcomes. In-vivo GT, based
on local brain delivery or systemic intravenous injections, resulted in
biochemical and clinical stabilization of the disease.

HEMATOLOGY/ONCOLOGY CLINICS OF NORTH AMERICA

SERIES OF RELATED INTEREST

Surgical Oncology Clinics of North America
https://www.surgonc.theclinics.com/

THE CLINICS ARE AVAILABLE ONLINE!
Access your subscription at:
www.theclinics.com

Preface

Current Status and Future Directions of Gene-Based Therapy for Pediatric Blood Diseases

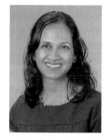 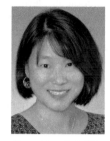

Nirali N. Shah, MD, MHSc   Sung-Yun Pai, MD
Editors

Tremendous advances in the clinical application of gene therapy in hematologic disease have transformed the field, particularly over the past 5 years. This explosion of novel approaches has had an important role in the treatment of inherited conditions and other childhood diseases—particularly in areas where current standard-of-care approaches are insufficient. Impressively, the very first approved gene-based therapy in the United States was in the treatment of children and young adults with relapsed/refractory leukemia—illustrating the potential of gene therapy and how it may change our current and future treatment paradigms for children with life-threatening illnesses and other chronic conditions.

In this issue of *Hematology/Oncology Clinics of North America*, we summarize current applications of gene-based therapy in pediatric blood diseases, highlight pivotal advances in the field, and outline future directions. The series of articles in this issue cover a full spectrum from nonmalignant to malignant hematologic and other conditions, illustrating the depth and breadth of the field. Comprehensive in its scope with a contemporary vantage point, we anticipate that the readership will deeply value this issue and realize that we are at an inflection point in the evolution of these groundbreaking therapies.

The first several sections in this issue are devoted to establishing the foundation and history upon which the current and future applications of gene-therapy are based. Understanding this foundation is of critical importance, to reflect upon both how far we have come as a field and what challenges have been overcome. These earlier sections also facilitate establishing the basic definitions used in gene-based therapy and highlight the available tools and strategies that are being used to propel the field forward. The clinical translation cannot occur without an understanding of the regulatory

Hematol Oncol Clin N Am 36 (2022) xiii–xiv
https://doi.org/10.1016/j.hoc.2022.06.001
0889-8588/22/© 2022 Published by Elsevier Inc.

aspects that provide the framework to bring these therapies to the clinic—and thus a section devoted to this infrastructure serves as a transition to the more clinically oriented sections in this issue.

The subsequent sections then focus on gene-based modification of specific cell types to target individual diseases. Starting with adoptive cellular therapy-based approaches using genetically modified T cells and NK cells to direct immune-effector cell-based cytotoxicity and eradicate underlying hematologic malignancies, several articles serve to summarize the status of the field and anticipate the changes we are likely to see in the forthcoming years. Shifting gears to therapeutic strategies based on genetic manipulation of hematopoietic stem cells, the remaining articles focus on benign hematologic conditions, inborn errors of immunity, and inherited metabolic and neurologic diseases, providing the full scope of the potential of these novel approaches, particularly when standard therapies are limited.

As you will see, the authors comprise a range of experts who are actively advancing the field, devoted to the care of children and young adults with life-threatening illness, and brilliant scientists. We wish to express our deep gratitude to our colleagues who have authored the articles within this issue, and we are honored to have them lead this issue and share their expertise with us all.

Nirali N. Shah, MD, MHSc
Pediatric Oncology Branch
Center for Cancer Research
National Cancer Institute
National Institutes of Health
9000 Rockville Pike
Building 10, 1W-5750
Bethesda, MD 20892, USA

Sung-Yun Pai, MD
Immune Deficiency Cellular Therapy Program
Center for Cancer Research
National Cancer Institute
National Institutes of Health
10 Center Drive, Building 10
1E-5142, MSC 1102
Bethesda, MD 20892, USA

E-mail addresses:
nirali.shah@nih.gov (N.N. Shah)
sung-yun.pai@nih.gov (S.-Y. Pai)

Evolution of Gene Therapy, Historical Perspective

Harry L. Malech, MD[a],*, Elizabeth K. Garabedian, RN, MSLS[b], Matthew M. Hsieh, MD[c]

KEYWORDS

- Gamma retrovirus vector • Lentiviral vector • Gene editing
- Hematopoietic stem cells • Transduction • Apheresis • CD34+ HSC
- Insertional mutagenesis

KEY POINTS

- Gene therapy by the genetic modification of hematopoietic stem cells (HSC) has reached a stage of development that has resulted in substantial clinical benefits.
- This article explores the separate threads of knowledge, conceptual design, materials, and equipment required to reach our current era of clinically beneficial gene therapy.
- The history of gene therapy targeting hematopoietic stem cells include improvements in integrating vectors such as lentivectors and improvements in gene editing methods such as CRISPR/Cas9.
- Understanding the pathophysiology of adverse events such as insertional mutagenesis is important for seeking improvements in vector design that may enhance the safety of gene therapy.

INTRODUCTION TO THEORETIC CONCEPTS AND EARLY BACKGROUND HISTORY IMPACTING HEMATOPOIETIC STEM CELL GENE THERAPY

The history of gene therapy comprises the advance of theoretic concepts, understanding of the human genome, availability of critical materials and instruments, design of vectors and chemical tools to manipulate and change genomic DNA, improvements in the procurement and culture/maintenance of stemness of HSC in culture, improvements in myeloid conditioning, the outcomes of conduct of clinical trials, observing successes and problems occurring in clinical trials, and deep study and

Conflict of Interest: The authors declare no conflicts.

[a] Genetic Immunotherapy Section, Laboratory of Clinical Immunology and Microbiology, National Institute of Allergy and Infectious Diseases, National Institutes of Health, 10 Center Drive, MSC1456, Bldg 10, Rm 5-3750, Bethesda, MD 20892-1456, USA; [b] National Human Genome Research Institute, NIH, 10 Center Dr, MSC1611, Bldg 10, Rm 10C-103, Bethesda, MD 20892-1611, USA; [c] National Heart, Lung, and Blood Institute, NIH, 10 Center Drive, MSC1812, Bldg 10, Rm 9N119, Bethesda, MD 20892-1812, USA

* Corresponding author.

E-mail address: hmalech@niaid.nih.gov

Hematol Oncol Clin N Am 36 (2022) 627–645
https://doi.org/10.1016/j.hoc.2022.05.001   hemonc.theclinics.com
0889-8588/22/Published by Elsevier Inc.

elucidation of the mechanisms of problems that arise in clinical trials to seek and incorporate corrective measures. The evolution of our understanding of ethical issues impacting gene therapy, and the logistics of access to and cost of successful gene therapy treatments are also important elements of this history.[1]

In this broad brush and somewhat unconventional view of the history of gene therapy, we address general principles; key experiments, basic science, and clinical trials that illustrate some general principle; and the evolution of materials and instrumentation that make current clinical approaches to gene therapy of HSC possible. We aim to complement rather than duplicate the extensive discussion of the background studies of gene therapy and the march of the many published clinical trials in specific disorders or categories of disorders that are the subject of the other chapters in this series, as well as excellent recent reviews.[2]

The earliest experiments that laid the foundation for gene therapy began with experiments on the transforming properties of bacteria.[3] Alloway reported in 1932 that nonvirulent (R type) pneumococci became lethal by adding cell-free extracts from virulent (S type) pneumococci. When injected with these "transformed" pneumococci, the mice developed pneumonia and died.

In our view, the key conceptual background to all gene therapy emerged in the 1940s with the seminal work by Avery and colleagues on bacterial transformation (which one could perhaps very loosely call gene therapy of bacteria). They identified DNA as the transforming factor that could change the physiology of a bacterial strain,[4] and more specifically, showed that the "transforming substance" was precipitated out by alcohol and later confirmed to be DNA. This was one of the key background elements to Watson and Crick in identifying the structure of DNA,[5] postulating its role as the genomic code of all prokaryotic and eukaryotic organisms, and thus demonstrating that nucleic acid sequences, rather than proteins, carry genetic information. The next critical discovery was that of Marshall Nirenberg, who in 1961 discovered the "triplet" code by which DNA encodes for the assembly of the 20 amino acids that serve as the building blocks of proteins.[6]

In parallel with this elucidation of the biochemical basis of heredity, were emerging concepts from early transformation studies in mammalian cells, for example, the early reports that the transformation of 8-azaguanine sensitive cells with nuclei and chromosomes from 8-azaguanine resistant cells rendered the transformants resistant due to transfer of a mutated hypoxanthine-guanine phosphoribosyltransferase gene.[7,8] An early review of mammalian cell transformation studies conducted over the following 18 years was reviewed in 1980 by Shows and Sakaguchi.[9] This body of work further established that newly acquired biochemical traits from DNA transformation experiments in mammalian cells can be heritable.

Many other key concepts that evolved into current methods of viral vector-mediated gene therapy were developed in the 1970s, during a period of the active investigation of viruses capable of transforming normal tissues into cancers. From this work, the concept emerged that perhaps these DNA and RNA tumor viruses known to insert into the genome of target cells could be modified in some way to remove the tumor causing elements, but retain their genome insertion capabilities to deliver a therapeutic payload. Some of the earliest published reviews of the history of gene therapy incorporating these essential concepts were those written in a series of reports over time by Theodore Friedmann[10–13] who shared the 2015 Japan Prize with Alain Fischer for "For the Proposal of the Concept of Gene Therapy and its Clinical Applications."

More generally, the term "gene therapy" now broadly includes the introduction or manipulation of DNA or RNA sequences in human cells to treat disease. There is a general consensus among the US Food and Drug Administration (FDA),[14] the European Medicines Agency (EMA),[15] and the American Society of Gene and Cell Therapy (ASGCT)[16] defining gene therapy as changes in gene expression, achieved by replacing or correcting a disease-causing gene, inactivating a target gene, or inserting a new or modified gene, using a vector or delivery system of genetic sequence or gene, genetically modified microorganisms, viruses, or cells.

By the late 1970s, while our understanding of the molecular basis of human diseases was advancing through cloning and sequencing of genes, there were major technical challenges to implement gene transfer. Exogenous DNA could be introduced to target cells by transformation or transfection, but the overall efficiency was low. Additionally, if the introduced gene(s) did not provide a survival advantage, the durability of gene transfer was also low. The resulting gene transfer efficiency at that time was about one in 100,000 cells, but nonetheless was proposed as a method to achieve genetic correction.[17]

Intense interest in inherited hemoglobinopathies such as sickle cell disease and beta-thalassemia fueled work on beta-globin, one of the first genes to be cloned and then studied with the intent of gene transfer for clinical application. Mulligan and colleagues replaced the viral capsid protein (VP1) of the SV40 genome with complementary DNA of rabbit beta-globin in a monkey kidney cell line, which produced large quantities of rabbit beta-globin mRNA and protein.[18] As there was no inherent advantage for beta-globin gene transformed cells, several laboratories worked on selectable genes to be cotransferred. Pellicer and colleagues successfully inserted beta-globin and thymidine kinase (TK) genes into murine teratocarcinoma cells.[19] The Cline laboratory inserted dihydrofolate reductase (DHFR) or TK in murine marrow cells.[20]

Cline and colleagues from UCLA then applied these results and tested them clinically.[21–23] An experimental protocol to insert genetically modified marrow cells from patients with beta-thalassemia, inject the cells in the femur after local irradiation, and treat with a selecting agent was submitted to the human research review committee at their home institution. Because the first 2 patients to be treated were receiving their care in other countries (in a hospital in Naples, Italy and at Hadassah Hospital, Jerusalem, Israel), not covered by the UCLA review committee, the team sought in parallel and secured permission in Naples and Hadassah for the clinical study. Both patients were informed of the experimental nature and the low likelihood of success in this approach. After femur irradiation and infusion of modified marrow cells, the patients reported no adverse events, and selective agents were not used. Three months later, there was no demonstrable clinical benefit in both patients. Although safety of this clinical gene transfer was undebated, many controversial issues were brought forth.[24–26] Can a clinical protocol proceed with permission from some but not all institutions? How many preclinical experiments (in vitro or animal), and what degree of "success" are needed to garner approval? While the responses to these issues are much more straightforward today, various review committees at that time were caught off guard and the consensus was that this was a rather premature and in retrospect problematic initial attempt at the clinical application of gene therapy.[27]

These first 2 attempts at human gene therapy generated much media attention and scrutiny by regulatory committees. The remainder of the decade into the early 1990s, scientists was quietly working on recombinant DNA methods, in vitro and animal models for testing, and strategies to enhance transgene expression. It quickly became clear that using viral vectors was more efficient in gene transfer than the previous methods of physical entry by transfection, fusion, or even electroporation. Much of the gene transfer experiments then focused on vector optimization and design, and brought this background discussion into the early modern era of gene therapy.

The following sections of this review will provide a historical background of a number of parallel developments that provided the laboratory and clinical tools and materials that facilitate our current approaches to gene therapy targeting blood cells including HSC.

DESIGN OF INTEGRATING VECTORS USED FOR HEMATOPOIETIC STEM CELLS GENE THERAPY

Vectors engineered from gamma retroviruses,[28] long under study as the cause of a variety of cancers in mice, had the desired property of efficient insertion into the genome of target cells. Murine gamma retroviruses and their derivatives were the first of the genome integrating vectors to be applied to T lymphocytes and HSC in the clinical setting.

Gamma retroviruses are RNA viruses, that on entry into a cell, are "reverse transcribed" (hence "retro"virus) into a DNA sequence. It is the DNA virus sequence that ultimately inserts itself into the host cell's genomic DNA, becoming a "provirus" that in turn generates RNA virus sequences and viral mRNAs encoding virus proteins required for the replication phase of the virus life cycle. The critical issue was how to turn these viruses that efficiently insert provirus DNA genomic sequence into mammalian cell genomes, but are also efficient at causing tumors, into safe tools for gene therapy. The solution was to remove and/or inactivate as many elements of the virus genome as possible, while still retaining the ability of the highly engineered provirus sequence to insert efficiently into the mammalian cell genome. The goal was a functioning single-cycle virus capable of cell entry, uncoating, reverse transcription into provirus DNA, and insertion into the genome, but incapable of generating infectious virus. The solution involved separating the key elements required to generate replication-incompetent viral vector into 3 separate "production plasmids": (1) an envelope (env) producing element (the vector virus coat also serving the purpose of binding to target cell and facilitating virus payload entry); (2) a gag-pol producing element (gag protein important for vector RNA packaging and polymerase for reverse transcribing the RNA); and (3) the vector sequence (retaining the psi element needed for packaging and the long terminal repeat (LTR) sequences at both ends of the vector sequence, which serves both as the internal strong promoter driving the production of a therapeutic protein and containing initiation elements binding the 2 ends of the vector for the circle formation required for reverse transcription). Where possible the env and gag-pol codons were changed to avoid recombination events that could reconstruct a replication-competent virus. To simplify the process of making different gamma retrovirus vectors, permanent packaging lines were devised that constitutively produce env and gag-pol, and when a specific vector sequence is added, clones could be assessed and chosen that constitutively produced vector in adequate titers. Many laboratories contributed to this technology and created a large array of different "flavors" of therapeutic gene therapy gamma retrovirus vectors. Many of these continue to be used for the production of some CAR-T lymphocytes or therapeutic cloned T cell receptors. This tour-de-force of engineering involving the contribution of many laboratories has served as the core technology used in the first generation of gene therapy targeting HSC or lymphocytes.

The LTRs of gamma retroviruses were retained in the engineered vectors as convenient, very strong promoters to drive high levels of production of downstream inserted therapeutic protein-coding sequences. However, these same LTR elements contain strong enhancer elements that can activate nearby genes. The engineered vectors by design retained the insertion targeting elements of the parent virus required to insert the DNA provirus into the mammalian genome. While the insertion of vector seems to be random, it is actually stochastic in that the mechanism used by the vector couples to cellular elements, resulting in preferred sites of insertion into the genome. These preferred sites (also known as integration sites) are often located near the start of genes and in enhancer elements, and may in turn strongly interact with enhancer elements in the LTR.[29,30] While the odds of any one insert occurring in a sensitive site are very low, gene therapy for a human subject may involve tens to hundreds of millions of insertions. Depending on the vector, the LTR and the host human subject disease substrate, we now know from adverse leukemic insertional mutagenesis events occurring in a number of clinical trials, that gamma retroviral vectors can transactivate oncogenes such as *LMO2*, the *MECOM* complex, and other oncogene targets to initiate the development of leukemia. These insertional mutagenesis events will be further discussed in greater detail in the last section of this historical review. Curiously, insertional mutagenesis leading to leukemic events has not been observed when the target of gamma retroviral vector gene therapy is T lymphocytes.

Well before the first insertional mutagenesis, oncogenic events were observed in clinical trials of gene therapy using gamma retroviral vectors, certain limitations of this class of vectors (eg, limits of therapeutic payload size, limits on the use of alternate promoter elements instead of the LTR, absolute requirement for cell division for vector insertion into the genome) encouraged the development of gene therapy vectors derived from human immunodeficiency virus (HIV). HIV is part of a different group of retroviruses called lentiviruses and the vectors engineered from HIV are referred to here as "lentivectors." HIV and other lentiviruses have a more complex structure, and have a number of required functional elements not present in gamma retroviruses, such as rev, that needed to be considered while engineering HIV into a safe gene therapy tool.[31,32] As with gamma retroviruses, determining how much could be removed from the virus and whether the addition of elements from other viruses might enhance function and efficiency of the vector was an iterative discovery process. From a historical perspective, some key advantages of lentivector function and engineering, and the insertional mutagenesis oncogenic events noted above have resulted for the most part in the abandonment of gamma retroviral vectors for the transduction of HSC for clinical trials.

As with gamma retrovirus vectors, the production of lentivectors that are functional, but replication incompetent, required the separation of packaging elements into plasmids separate from the transfer vector. Almost all lentivector production for clinical application uses the membrane fusion G protein derived from vesicular stomatitis virus (VSV-G) as the vector envelope element, rather than the natural env component of HIV. The cell membrane target of the VSV-G protein is ubiquitous to all cells with high efficiency of binding and vector membrane fusion. Almost from the start, lentivector engineering strategies incorporated a self-inactivating (SIN) feature, modifying the LTR element that contains strong enhancers with transactivating potential and using safer promotors with little enhancer activity instead. This was accomplished by creating a deletion in the 3' LTR of the vector production plasmid. During vector production, the intact 5' LTR assists in the important packaging biochemistry needed to produce infective but replication-incompetent lentivirus vector. During transduction, the SIN 3' LTR binds to the 5' LTR in the circularization and priming step that retrotranscribes the insertional provirus DNA from the lentivector RNA, and is incorporated into the 5' end of the provirus DNA, thus "self-inactivating" the 5' LTR. This safety feature removes enhancer and activator elements, and allows the therapeutic payload transgene(s) to be transcribed from a promoter of choice. The use of the SIN feature with an alternate internal promoter is not limited to lentivectors. A group of investigators incorporated the SIN feature into the gamma retroviral vector that was efficacious in a clinical trial targeting hematopoietic stem cells (HSC) to treat infants with X-linked severe combined immunodeficiency (X-SCID). This SIN gamma retroviral vector showed clinical efficacy,[33] with no insertional oncogenesis after median of 9 years of follow-up (personal communication S.-Y. Pai, 2022). Importantly, this maneuver does not alter the pattern of insertion characteristic of gamma retroviruses that tends to target enhancer elements and the 5′ end of genes.[33]

The larger payload capacity of lentivectors, SIN design, and potential to incorporate tissue-specific promoters and enhancers catalyzed concerted efforts by several investigators to develop lentivectors that would drive high-level beta-globin expression at specific stages of erythroid precursor development. In the 1990s, the locus control region of beta-globin was discovered to contain hypersensitive sites (HS) that were important for high-level expression. After a series of in vitro experiments, a lentivector containing optimized regulatory elements, the TNS9 vector, was shown to drive high-level erythroid-specific expression of adult beta-globin in transduced murine HSC, successfully correcting a murine model of beta-thalassemia.[34] This seminal work was followed shortly by the same group to correct another more severe phenotype of beta-thalassemia in Berkeley mice.[35]

In parallel, another group designed a modified adult beta-globin for which the 87th amino acid was switched from threonine to glutamine, to mimic the antisickling effect of gamma-globin. This T87Q version successfully corrected 2 sickle mouse models[36] and was expressed at high levels when transduced human sickle cord blood stem cells were transplanted into immunodeficient mice.[37] These reassuring preclinical studies ultimately led to the treatment of a patient with compound beta-E/beta-0 thalassemia, who achieved transfusion independence.[38]

From those early efforts, an increasing number of successful clinical trials have emerged to treat thalassemia and sickle cell disease, described in significant detail in other chapters in this series. Some of these studies will be revisited later in this article in comments relating to transduction enhancers and certain types of adverse events associated with gene therapy.

GENE EDITING OF HEMATOPOIETIC STEM CELLS

Gene editing is the most recently evolving technology to be applied to gene therapy for HSCs, having the capability of targeting a specific sequence within the genome, in contrast to the stochastic semirandom insertion of integrating viruses throughout the genome. The 4 main types of gene editing systems are meganucleases, zinc finger nucleases, transcription activator-like effector nucleases (TALENs),[39] and clustered regularly interspaced short palindromic repeats-Cas (CRISPR-Cas).[40] Of particular near term historical note are recent clinical reports of unequivocal clinical benefit from successful application of the CRISPR technology applied to HSCs for the correction of hemoglobinopathies.[41,42]

CRISPR is derived from an antivirus system that evolved in bacteria to "copy and memorize" virus sequence, thereby allowing the bacterium to target that same virus sequence for cleavage when subsequently infected by a similar virus.[43] The discovery of the use of the CRISPR system for gene editing was the basis for the 2020 Nobel Prize in Chemistry (https://www.nobelprize.org/prizes/chemistry/2020/press-release/). The CRISPR system has revolutionized the field, due to its ease of application and versatility. CRISPR-based derivative methods such as base editing and prime editing use the core element of the CRISPR system to find the genome target sequence to enzymatically convert a single base pair or reverse transcribe a short sequence change into the genome, respectively.[44]

Most current approaches to editing use electroporation to introduce the editing elements (CRISPR-Cas9 mRNA or protein, guide RNA, and any additional factors to augment editing) into HSC. There have been a number of small scale non-GMP research-grade electroporation instruments available for gene editing development work. Fortuitously, clinical scale and high throughput GMP compliant commercial instruments in development in the past few years have become available just in time for the current initiatives in gene editing of HSC.

HEMATOPOIETIC STEM CELLS: SOURCING, SELECTING, CULTURING, AND TRANSDUCING

Parallel to the development of vectors and editing tools for gene modifying HSC, advances in the procurement, culture, transduction, and engraftment of HSC have had an important impact on the field.

HSC occupy niches in the marrow that facilitate the retention of pluripotent potential to give rise to all hematopoietic lineages and asymmetric proliferation of some progeny into lineage-specific progenitors.[45] Sourcing HSC for gene therapy or conventional allogeneic transplants initially was restricted to the harvesting of bone marrow with needles. That HSC are constantly translocating at a slow rate from marrow to the circulation and back to the marrow was a key discovery that ultimately led to alternate sourcing of HSC.[46] There is a steady state presence of CD34+ HSC or progenitors in the peripheral blood of healthy humans of about 1400 cells per ml (1.4 per μl). This low baseline frequency of CD34+ HSC and progenitors in the circulation can be increased by daily injections of granulocyte colony-stimulating factor (G-CSF or filgrastim), which induces a transient release of CD34+ HSC and progenitors from the marrow into the peripheral blood, peaking at 5 to 6 days at an average of 76 per μl (a 50-fold increase), then declining, even with additional daily injections.[47,48] Subsequent studies indicated that CXCR4 (the receptor for stromal cell-derived factor-1 [SDF-1], also known as CXCL12) tethers HSC within the marrow and that G-CSF breaks that tether by increasing granulocyte proliferation and release of granule enzymes in the marrow, thereby enhancing the release of HSC into the circulation. More recently a small molecule inhibitor of the binding site of CXCR4, plerixafor (previously called AMD3100), was also shown to release HSC from the marrow to the circulation,[49] and when administered in the combination with G-CSF results in a synergistic mobilization of HSC to the peripheral blood.[50]

The ease of apheresis collection of stem cells using continuous flow instruments following mobilization has resulted in this method becoming the preferred sourcing of HSC for many gene therapy clinical studies. Some patients with some inherited blood disorders that impair marrow proliferation (Fanconi anemia for example) will not mobilize, and infants who are too small for standard apheresis procedures still require bone marrow aspiration for sourcing HSC for gene therapy. Patients with sickle cell disease are at high risk of adverse events including vaso-occlusive crises when treated with G-CSF. Fortunately, several groups have shown that efficient and safe mobilization of HSC from marrow to peripheral blood can be accomplished using plerixafor alone as the mobilization agent in patients with sickle cell.[51–54]

Apheresis

The first apheresis device for separating blood components was developed in a collaboration between the National Cancer Institute and IBM,[55] and was appreciated at the time as a critical breakthrough in instrumentation for the separation and collection of blood components.[56] A number of companies developed a series of progressively efficient continuous flow instruments to harvest of fractions enriched in HSC from G-CSF and/or plerixafor mobilized donors. Without this instrumentation now commonplace in blood collection centers, and simply viewed by the gene therapy community as "background" standard banking technology, much of the current progress in gene therapy would not have been possible.

Selection of Hematopoietic Stem Cells from Marrow or Apheresis Products

Multipotent permanently repopulating HSC express the CD34 surface antigen that was originally called My-10 as detected by a murine monoclonal antibody, raised against the KG-1a human tumor cell line.[57] Studies later demonstrated that immunomagnetic beads coated with anti-CD34 antibody could form complexes with HSC in a marrow or apheresis product, which in turn could be purified with magnets. These initial studies used incubation with chymopapain to release HSC from the beads.[58] This magnetic bead selection approach became the basis for the commercial development of instruments for selective enrichment of HSC, 2 of which reached the late commercialization phase.

Baxter International, Inc (then called Baxter Healthcare Corporation) together with its "spin-off" subsidiary Nexell, Inc was the first to develop a fully automated instrument called the Isolex 300i that relied on the binding of HSC to magnetic beads coated with the anti-CD34 antibody. Following magnetic separation, the washed product was exposed to an octapeptide that directly competed for the binding site of the anti-CD34 antibody to the CD34 antigen, thus removing the antibody complexed magnetic beads from the cells. This allowed the beads to be retained by a second pass through the magnetic field, yielding a cell product free of the beads and antibody.[59] A precommercial manual version of the Isolex system was used in one of the earliest clinical studies of gene therapy for CGD.[60]

A very similar system developed in parallel by Miltenyi Biotec GmbH became their CliniMACS CD34 Reagent System. This system uses anti-CD34 antibody chemically conjugated to dextran beads with an iron oxide/hydroxide core. A binding column with a magnetic gradient is used to separate the HSC bound to the anti-CD34 magnetic dextran bead from marrow or apheresis product. Unlike the Isolex system, there is no maneuver to separate the cells from the antibody-conjugated beads, which are presumably degraded in culture or *in vivo* following transplantation. In October 2003 exclusive rights to market, the Isolex system was acquired by Miltenyi and not further developed by them leaving only the CliniMACS and its derivative devices available currently for the clinical selection of HSC for gene therapies.[61]

Culture and Transduction of Hematopoietic Stem Cells

As noted previously, successful gamma retrovirus vector transduction requires 1 cell division cycle to complete integration into the genome of a cell. While lentivector transduction does not absolutely require cell division, HSC must enter at least the G1 phase of the cell cycle, and exposure of HSC to growth factors for a period of time in culture seems to enhance transduction efficiency. While it was initially hoped that gene editing methods might not require the activation of HSC, a similar improvement of gene editing when HSC are cultured with growth factors has been observed by many investigators. Defining *ex vivo* culture conditions and growth factor combinations that enhance transduction or editing while minimizing loss of long-term marrow repopulating potential has been intensely studied. The discovery of each of the many critical HSC growth factors important for both efficient vector transduction and gene editing approaches will not be reviewed here; suffice it to say that without the work to identify, clone, and provide GMP compliant growth factors, gene therapy for HSC could not have advanced. While there is no consensus about "best" conditions, the minimum combination of three growth factors, stem cell factor (SCF), FLT3-L, and thrombopoietin (TPO) is used by most of the investigators for clinical gene therapy for HSC applications. Additional factors used by some investigators include interleukin (IL)-3 and/or IL-6. A key limiting issue is that culture in these growth conditions beyond 3 to 4 days results in a significant loss of long-term repopulating potential. Outside the scope of this review is the discovery of other biochemical factors and conditions that may prolong the period during which HSC can be maintained in culture while delaying the loss of long-term engraftment potential. This is an important emerging field for the future impact on HSC gene therapy.

While culture and transduction of HSC may be performed in standard tissue culture flasks, gas permeable flexible plastic culture bags are increasingly used to achieve more "closed system" handling. The earliest application of such systems in gene therapy clinical trials suggests better gas exchange, more consistent high viability and yield, and transduction efficiency.[60,62]

Transduction Enhancers

Maneuvers to achieve the highest efficiency transduction by gamma retroviral and lentiviral vectors have been an important aspect of the history of gene therapy. Quite early on, it was shown that the addition of certain charged polymers to the transduction culture, such as polybrene or protamine sulfate, would enhance transduction by gamma retrovirus vectors; of the 2, protamine sulfate continues to be used to enhance the transduction of lentivectors.[63] Physical maneuvers such as centrifuging the culture plate or gas permeable bag have also been shown to enhance transduction,[64] but the practicalities of application at clinical scale have limited the translation of this maneuver into the clinic. It has been presumed but not proven that ionic polymers and centrifugation worked in part by enhancing the binding of vector to cells. A major advance was achieved when David Williams discovered that a fragment of fibronectin, when bound to the surface of a culture vessel, would greatly enhance transduction by gamma retrovirus vectors, likely both by binding vector and via some signaling effect on the target cells.[65] This fragment was commercialized as RetroNectin and became a standard element applied into the clinic for gamma retroviral gene therapy transductions at clinical scale.[66,67] While RetroNectin is used by some for lentivector transduction, it may not have a strong effect in enhancing lentivector transduction as it does for gamma retroviral transduction.

Several very potent enhancers of lentivector transduction have been described recently and are an area of very active investigation. A group of related poloxamers,[68] the first of which has been developed into a commercial product available GMP compliant called LentiBOOST, can enhance transduction efficiency 2- to 5-fold. Prostaglandin E2 (PG-E2) alone enhances transduction by lentivectors several folds,[69] and in combination with LentiBOOST or other poloxymer enhances lentivector transduction 10- to 20-fold.[70,71] The combination of LentiBOOST plus low dose (1 uM) PG-E2 has been applied to a clinical trial of lentivector gene therapy for X-linked SCID with more than 10-fold increase in efficiency of the transduction of HSC.[72] Another recently discovered transduction enhancer is cyclosporin H.[73] The use of transduction enhancers has had a dramatic impact on the success of gene therapy using lentivectors to treat sickle cell disease; the ability to consistently achieve vector copy numbers greater than 3 in autologous transduced HSC of patients with sickle cell greatly enhanced the degree of clinical benefit and durability of disease correction[74] (and as reviewed in greater detail in other chapters in this series).

Conditioning Regimens

Choice and intensity of marrow ablative conditioning for HSC targeted ex vivo gene therapy and determining in which situations it may also be appropriate to target T, B, and/or NK cells remains as contentious a topic with as little broad consensus as to the choice of conditioning for allogeneic bone marrow transplantation. Much has been "borrowed" from studies and experience with what is needed to achieve multi-lineage engraftment in the allogeneic transplant setting, including the concept that for transplant of some disorders, very modest nonmyeloablative conditioning may be sufficient to achieve the desired clinical goal. There is emerging evidence that busulfan may be a better conditioning agent for targeting long-term repopulating HSC than melphalan, but the comparative toxicity profiles of these 2 agents have influenced some investigators to use melphalan over busulfan in some HSC gene therapy settings.

Many of the earliest trials of HSC gene therapy for the treatment of immune deficiencies with gamma retrovirus transduced HSC did not use any conditioning, assuming that the infused autologous transduced HSC or T lymphocytes would have "advantage" and therefore conditioning was not needed. The contrast between outcomes observed when no conditioning was used in trials for different diseases is striking. In early trials of gene therapy for chronic granulomatous disease (CGD), a disorder in which gene-corrected HSC or differentiated progeny have no survival or growth advantage over unmodified cells, engraftment of transduced myeloid cells was very low and transient, despite the infusion of high numbers of transduced cells.[60] In severe combined immunodeficiency caused by deficiency of adenosine deaminase (ADA-SCID), a survival and growth advantage was known to result in the reconstitution of T cells in the setting of allogeneic transplant in infancy without conditioning. The very first study of retroviral gene therapy for ADA-SCID targeting only T lymphocytes did result in long-term persistence and even some expansion of gene-corrected T cells. But the production of adenosine deaminase was insufficient to achieve adequate detoxification of deoxyATP metabolites and there was no correction of B cell function.[75] The initial study and similar studies of gamma retrovirus transduced HSC gene therapy for ADA-SCID[76] did not use any conditioning. Though low-level correction of T lymphocytes was seen, the gene marked HSC did not persist in the marrow and the clinical benefit overall was very modest.[77] In contrast, the landmark first gamma retrovirus HSC gene therapy treatment of infants with X-SCID caused by mutations in the *IL2RG* gene conducted in Paris by Alain Fischer and Marina Cavazzana in 2000[78] was extraordinarily successful at restoring T cell immunity to almost all of the infants treated without conditioning. Myeloid and HSC gene marking was very low and did not persist, and for the most part, these patients had modest to nil long-term restoration of B and NK cell function.

A critical conceptual breakthrough was achieved by Alessandro Aiuti and colleagues who prepared pediatric patients with ADA-SCID with very modest doses of busulfan conditioning before infusing autologous gamma retrovirus transduced HSC.[79] The outcome of this maneuver was the achievement of robust T and B cell function in the majority of patients and associated significant detoxification of deoxy-ATP metabolites, in the face of low levels of gene marking of bone marrow HSC and myeloid cells. Other investigators began and have continued to use busulfan conditioning to enhance the engraftment of transduced autologous HSC gene therapy for a number of other disorders. Of note was the first use of low dose busulfan to condition older children and young adults with X-SCID before infusion of corrective lentivector transduced autologous HSC. This resulted for the first time in significant long-term restoration of B cell function and production of NK cells in addition to the production of functional T cells.[80] This was followed by the demonstration of robust restoration of functional T, B, and NK cells in newly diagnosed infants with X-SCID undergoing autologous gene therapy with the same vector after conditioning with low dose busulfan.[81] Thus low dose busulfan seems necessary and sufficient to achieve immune reconstitution in forms of SCID whereby lymphocytes have a selective survival and growth advantage. However, for the treatment of disorders affecting myeloid cells or platelets, or for the correction of metabolic disorders requiring substantial production of the detoxifying enzyme, higher levels of myeloid engraftment of gene-corrected HSCs are required. For that reason, higher doses of busulfan into the submyeloablative level were applied in both the early studies using gamma retroviruses and more recent studies using lentivector transduced HSC gene therapy of X-linked CGD and Wiskott–Aldrich syndrome.[82–87]

Alessandra Biffi conducted seminal studies defining the optimal conditioning agent for transduced HSC gene therapy in early-onset metachromatic leukodystrophy, whereby the delivery of the corrective gene and enzyme production in the brain by microglia seems critical to therapeutic corrective benefit.[88] In preclinical studies, she showed unequivocally that high dose busulfan was uniquely capable of targeting and clearing brain microglia, which was an essential maneuver to achieving rapid replacement of this compartment by incoming gene-corrected microglia precursors.[89] Other conditioning agents such as melphalan were not capable to achieve this goal of detoxification of harmful metabolites in the brain of patients with metabolic and storage disease disorders.

Beyond the scope of this historical review, but likely to have a significant impact in the near future for gene therapy for HSC are the emerging developments in monoclonal antibodies directly targeting HSC. At least one of these antibodies targeting cKit (CD117) is already in the clinic for allogeneic transplant (ClinicalTrials.gov identifier: NCT04429191 and NCT02963064), and likely will be used for HSC gene therapy in the near future.

LEARNING FROM ADVERSE EVENTS IN GENE THERAPY

In this last section, we review adverse events observed in clinical trials of gene therapy. These important events, while unfortunate for the participants and sobering to the field, have informed the science of gene therapy and have resulted in corrective measures going forward.

Early discussions about the potential hazards of gene therapy mostly centered around the possibility that recombination events during vector production or after transduction could result in the restoration of replication competence to the vector. Much of the engineering of both the transfer plasmid that is the core element of the treatment vector and the packaging elements (separating these elements into different plasmids and altering codons to avoid recombination) for both gamma retroviral and lentiviral vectors was intended to prevent recombination events. Molecular and virus replication assays were developed to high sensitivity that could detect very small numbers of replication-competent virus in the final vector production product, in transduced target cells and their culture media, and in the patients treated with gene therapy. The US FDA and European regulatory agencies established strict criteria for steps in the process and for when and how such testing for replication-competent virus should be conducted.[90] Perhaps because of these strict testing criteria and careful engineering, no case of replication competent vector has been reported to occur in any patient treated with either gamma retroviral or lentiviral vector gene therapy.

As the integrating retrovirus vectors insert throughout the genome of HSC, which are long-lived with differentiating progeny that is highly proliferative, it was surmised that an insertional event could activate an oncogene or growth program, or inhibit a cancer protection gene or other gene critical for cell function. Because vector-related oncogenesis was rarely if ever seen in preclinical animal studies, insertional mutagenesis was presumed to be unlikely. It was thus both surprising and concerning when first cancer, a T lymphocytic leukemia, was detected about 3 years after treatment in one of the patients in the otherwise clinically very beneficial trial in Paris of gamma retrovirus gene therapy in infants with X-SCID.[78] The T lymphocytic leukemia cells had vector insertion within the first intron of the LMO2 proto-oncogene such that the enhancer elements in the LTR of the vector activated the LMO2 promoter driving aberrant overexpression.[91,92] Through the examination of stored blood samples, the investigators showed that this insertion was followed by other oncogenic events as this clone evolved progeny clones, eventually giving rise to cancer. Subsequent studies of other patients demonstrated that the activation of protooncogenes other than LMO2 could give rise to the same clonal evolution process in cancer. Of the first 18 infants with X-SCID treated with gamma retrovirus gene therapy who achieved long-term gene marking correction of T lymphocytes in clinical trials at sites in Paris and London, 5 developed insertional mutagenesis related leukemia in the first 5 years. A 6th patient developed leukemia at about 15 years after treatment, indicating that while the greatest risk occurs in the first few years after treatment, there remains a long-term risk of oncogenesis as well.

These insertional mutagenesis oncogenic events led to the exploration of SIN modifications to gamma retroviruses, and accelerated the ongoing development of SIN lentivectors. It also led to development of specialized cell lines that could be used to assess the potential of any candidate vectors to activate the LMO2 gene.[93] While initially, recipients of gamma retrovirus transduced HSC gene therapy for ADA-SCID seemed to be spared, very recently the first case of insertional mutagenesis mediated cancer was observed to occur in a patient with ADA-SCID treated with the commercialized gamma retrovirus (Strimvelis) (See: https://ir.orchard-tx.com/news-releases/news-release-details/orchard-statement-strimvelisr-gammaretroviral-vector-based-gene).

Gamma retrovirus insertional mutagenesis induced cancers were subsequently in patients undergoing autologous HSC gene therapy for X-linked CGD[94] and Wiskott–Aldrich syndrome.[95] In these patients' insertions in or near the MECOM oncogene complex or other oncogenes more associated with the development of myelodysplastic syndrome (MDS) and myeloid leukemias was often the instigating event, followed by clonal evolution involving additional oncogenic events leading to the oncogenic clone. As with the development of a preclinical test to assess the potential of activation of the LMO2 gene, a specific test assessing the potential of a given vector to activate MECOM and related protocol oncogenes in mouse bone marrow cells and drive immortalization was developed by Ute Modlich and Christopher Baum.[96] This in vitro immortalization preclinical assay assessing genotoxicity has become a standard component of the testing required by the US FDA and the European regulatory agencies for insertional gene therapy vectors.

While insertional mutagenesis had not been observed with SIN lentivectors, very recently, a patient with adrenoleukodystrophy treated with corrective SIN lentivector transduced autologous HSC in an otherwise clinically beneficial clinical trial[97] was reported to have leukemia.[98,99] Of note, the internal promoter of this SIN lentivector

(MND) was originally derived from a murine gamma-retrovirus vector. The MND LTR had been modified to reduce enhancer activity,[100] but no insulator was added to the vector to reduce any "cross-talk" of this gamma retrovirus-derived promoter to nearby genes. While studies are still ongoing to understand this event, the vector insertional event likely responsible for the oncologic transformation is in or near the *MECOM* proto-oncogene complex, invoking an oncogenic process similar to that observed in patients with X-linked CGD or Wiskott–Aldrich syndrome after gamma retrovirus-based gene therapy described above.

Two patients from the otherwise very successful clinical trial of lentivector trans-duced HSC gene therapy for sickle cell disease[74] have also developed acute myeloid leukemia.[101] In the first patient, the leukemic clone did not have any vector insert, indi-cating that the leukemic process was not driven by vector insertion. In the second pa-tient, the leukemic clone had a vector insert within intron 4 of the *VAMP4* gene, which has never been implicated in oncogenesis.[102] There was no effect on *VAMP4* gene expression and very low expression of the beta-globin transgene in the leukemic blast cells. Over 70% of the blast cells had monosomy 7 with partial loss of chromosome, with other genetic changes associated with the evolution of the original clone into the leukemic clone. The investigators concluded that the insert was a passive passenger with respect to the initiation and clonal evolution of the oncogenic process leading to this patient's leukemia. As leukemia is increasingly recognized in patients with sickle cell who receive myeloid conditioning with an allogeneic HSC transplant who either have mixed chimerism or loss of donor graft with the recovery of host marrow, the au-thors also speculated that marrow stress from their disease may place patients with sickle cell with preexisting higher risk of leukemic transformation.

One of the first patients to be treated with lentivector gene therapy for β-thalassemia had a dominant clonal expansion with vector insert into the *HMGA2* gene primarily in the myeloid lineage to greater than 10% of the lineage.[38] High mobility group A2 (HMGA2) protein is a nonhistone architectural transcription factor that may serve as a growth element in HSC and primitive myeloid progenitors. In this patient, the insert seemed to result in the production of a truncated HMGA2 protein lacking sequence responsive to LET-7, which normally enhances the degradation of HMGA2. In this setting the clone, while persistent, seemed to be benign, not affecting hematopoiesis nor with any evi-dence for oncologic evolution, and slow decreased in the clonal dominance over a 10-year follow-up. In a clinical study of lentivector transduced HSC gene therapy for X-SCID,[80] a very significant overall increase in lentivector inserts within *HMGA2* relative to what would have been expected from "random" insertion, particularly in the myeloid lineage has been seen. The clonal expansions observed in these patients seem to be caused by a cryptic splice acceptor in the cHS4 insulator element of the vector, which generates an aberrant transcript encoding a functional but truncated HMGA2 protein when the vector inserts into intron 3 of the *HMGA2* gene. A study in primates showed that forced expression of 3' truncated *HMGA2* using lentivector resulted in the expan-sion of transduced HSCs and myeloid progenitors likely through the growth effect of this factor, but did not affect normal hematopoiesis nor result in any malignant transforma-tion.[103] While to date this seems to be benign and does not affect hematopoiesis, it bears watching for the long term. These observations point out the importance of testing lentivectors for cryptic splice sites as part of the screening and design process.

SUMMARY

Decades of discovery and invention of critical theories, materials, molecular engineer-ing, and devices have led to the current emerging era of clinical benefit from gene therapy.[104] We are likely only beginning to reap the full clinical benefit of our current technology, and the field is in a rapid phase of new discovery of methods that will enhance our ability to efficiently make desired changes in HSC to treat and cure disease. All current HSC gene therapy in the clinic is performed *ex vivo* requiring collection, purification, and culture of HSC, but future developments may allow *in vivo* delivery of gene modification materials that will gene alter HSC *in situ* for disease treatment. There also will almost certainly also be unexpected adverse events, which will enhance future safety and efficacy of gene therapy if these are properly studied.

CLINICS CARE POINTS

- Gene therapy is the change in gene expression, achieved by replacing or correcting a disease-causing gene, inactivating a target gene, or inserting a new or modified gene, using a vector or delivery system.
- Gene therapy clinical trials are benefitting a growing number of patients with immunodeficiency, beta-globin disorders, and brain disorders.

ACKNOWLEDGEMENT

This work is supported in part by the intramural programs of the NIH institutes which employ each of these authors including the National Institute of Allergy and Infectious Diseases, the National Human Genome Research Institute, and the National Heart, Lung, and Blood Institute.

REFERENCES

1. Salzman R, Cook F, Hunt T, et al. Addressing the Value of Gene Therapy and Enhancing Patient Access to Transformative Treatments. Mol Ther 2018; 26(12):2717–26.
2. Kohn DB. Historical Perspective on the Current Renaissance for Hematopoietic Stem Cell Gene Therapy. Hematol Oncol Clin North Am 2017;31(5):721–35.
3. Alloway JL. The Transformation in Vitro of R Pneumococci into S Forms of Different Specific Types by the Use of Filtered Pneumococcus Extracts. J Exp Med 1932;55(1):91–9.
4. Avery OT, Macleod CM, McCarty M. Studies on the Chemical Nature of the Substance Inducing Transformation of Pneumococcal Types : Induction of Transformation by a Desoxyribonucleic Acid Fraction Isolated from Pneumococcus Type Iii. J Exp Med 1944;79(2):137–58.
5. Watson JD, Crick FH. Genetical implications of the structure of deoxyribonucleic acid. Nature 1953;171(4361):964–7.
6. Matthaei JH, Jones OW, Martin RG, et al. Characteristics and composition of RNA coding units. Proc Natl Acad Sci U S A 1962;48:666–77.
7. Szybalska EH, Szybalski W. Genetics of human cell line. IV. DNA-mediated heritable transformation of a biochemical trait. Proc Natl Acad Sci U S A 1962;48: 2026–34.
8. Degnen GE, Miller IL, Eisenstadt JM, et al. Chromosome-mediated gene transfer between closely realted strains of cultured mouse cells. Proc Natl Acad Sci U S A 1976;73(8):2838–42.
9. Shows TB, Sakaguchi AY. Gene transfer and gene mapping in mammalian cells in culture. In Vitro 1980;16(1):55–76.

10. Friedmann T, Roblin R. Gene therapy for human genetic disease? Science 1972; 175(4025):949–55.
11. Friedmann T, Xu L, Wolff J, et al. Retrovirus vector-mediated gene transfer into hepatocytes. Mol Biol Med 1989;6(2):117–25.
12. Friedmann T. A brief history of gene therapy. Nat Genet 1992;2(2):93–8.
13. Friedmann T. Human gene therapy–an immature genie, but certainly out of the bottle. Nat Med 1996;2(2):144–7.
14. US Food and Drug Administration. What is gene therapy?. Available at: https://www.fda.gov/vaccines-blood-biologics/cellular-gene-therapy-products/what-gene-therapy. Accessed July 25, 2018.
15. European Medicines Agency. Multidisciplinary: Gene Therapy. Available at: https://www.ema.europa.eu/en/human-regulatory/research-development/scientific-guidelines/multidisciplinary/multidisciplinary-gene-therapy. Accessed April 29, 2022.
16. American Society of Gene and Cell Therapy. Gene Therapy 101: Different Approaches. Available at: https://patienteducation.asgct.org/gene-therapy-101/different-approaches. Accessed April 29, 2022.
17. Mercola KE, Cline MJ. Sounding boards. The potentials of inserting new genetic information. N Engl J Med 1980;303(22):1297–300.
18. Mulligan RC, Howard BH, Berg P. Synthesis of rabbit beta-globin in cultured monkey kidney cells following infection with a SV40 beta-globin recombinant genome. Nature 1979;277(5692):108–14.
19. Pellicer A, Wagner EF, el-Kareh A, et al. Introduction of a viral thymidine kinase gene and the human beta-globin gene into developmentally multipotential mouse teratocarcinoma cells. Proc Natl Acad Sci U S A 1980;77(4):2098–102.
20. Mercola KE, Bar-Eli M, Stang HD, et al. Insertion of new genetic information into bone marrow cells of mice: comparison of two selectable genes. Ann N Y Acad Sci 1982;397:272–80.
21. Dickson D. Cline stripped of research grants. Nature 1981;294(5840):391–2.
22. Dickson D. NIH censure for Dr Martin Cline: tighter rules for future research plans. Nature 1981;291(5814):369.
23. Sun M. Cline loses two NIH grants. Science 1981;214(4526):1220.
24. Wade N. UCLA gene therapy racked by friendly fire. Science 1980;210(4469):509–11.
25. Wade N. Gene therapy pioneer draws Mikadoesque rap. Science 1981;212(4500):1253.
26. Wade N. Gene therapy caught in more entanglements. Science 1981;212(4490):24–5.
27. Human Gene Therapy - A Background Paper (Washington, DC: U.S. Congress, Office of Technology Assessment, OTA-BP-BA-32). 1984. Available at: https://www.princeton.edu/~ota/disk3/1984/8415/8415.PDF.
28. Cone RD, Mulligan RC. High-efficiency gene transfer into mammalian cells: generation of helper-free recombinant retrovirus with broad mammalian host range. Proc Natl Acad Sci U S A 1984;81(20):6349–53.
29. De Ravin SS, Su L, Theobald N, et al. Enhancers are major targets for murine leukemia virus vector integration. J Virol 2014;88(8):4504–13.
30. Deichmann A, Brugman MH, Bartholomae CC, et al. Insertion sites in engrafted cells cluster within a limited repertoire of genomic areas after gammaretroviral vector gene therapy. Mol Ther 2011;19(11):2031–9.
31. Dull T, Zufferey R, Kelly M, et al. A third-generation lentivirus vector with a conditional packaging system. J Virol 1998;72(11):8463–71.

32. Zufferey R, Dull T, Mandel RJ, et al. Self-inactivating lentivirus vector for safe and efficient in vivo gene delivery. J Virol 1998;72(12):9873–80.

33. Hacein-Bey-Abina S, Pai SY, Gaspar HB, et al. A modified gamma-retrovirus vector for X-linked severe combined immunodeficiency. N Engl J Med 2014; 371(15):1407–17.

34. May C, Rivella S, Callegari J, et al. Therapeutic haemoglobin synthesis in beta-thalassaemic mice expressing lentivirus-encoded human beta-globin. Nature 2000;406(6791):82–6.

35. Rivella S, May C, Chadburn A, et al. A novel murine model of Cooley anemia and its rescue by lentiviral-mediated human beta-globin gene transfer. Blood 2003; 101(8):2932–9.

36. Pawliuk R, Westerman KA, Fabry ME, et al. Correction of sickle cell disease in transgenic mouse models by gene therapy. Science 2001;294(5550):2368–71.

37. Imren S, Fabry ME, Westerman KA, et al. High-level beta-globin expression and preferred intragenic integration after lentiviral transduction of human cord blood stem cells. J Clin Invest 2004;114(7):953–62.

38. Cavazzana-Calvo M, Payen E, Negre O, et al. Transfusion independence and HMGA2 activation after gene therapy of human beta-thalassaemia. Nature 2010;467(7313):318–22.

39. Urnov FD, Rebar EJ, Holmes MC, et al. Genome editing with engineered zinc finger nucleases. Nat Rev Genet 2010;11(9):636–46.

40. Sander JD, Joung JK. CRISPR-Cas systems for editing, regulating and targeting genomes. Nat Biotechnol 2014;32(4):347–55.

41. Esrick EB, Lehmann LE, Biffi A, et al. Post-Transcriptional Genetic Silencing of BCL11A to Treat Sickle Cell Disease. N Engl J Med 2021;384(3):205–15.

42. Frangoul H, Altshuler D, Cappellini MD, et al. CRISPR-Cas9 Gene Editing for Sickle Cell Disease and beta-Thalassemia. N Engl J Med 2021;384(3):252–60.

43. Le Rhun A, Escalera-Maurer A, Bratovic M, et al. CRISPR-Cas in Streptococcus pyogenes. RNA Biol 2019;16(4):380–9.

44. Anzalone AV, Koblan LW, Liu DR. Genome editing with CRISPR-Cas nucleases, base editors, transposases and prime editors. Nat Biotechnol 2020;38(7): 824–44.

45. Scadden DT. The stem-cell niche as an entity of action. Nature 2006;441(7097): 1075–9.

46. McCredie KB, Hersh EM, Freireich EJ. Cells capable of colony formation in the peripheral blood of man. Science 1971;171(3968):293–4.

47. Hohaus S, Goldschmidt H, Ehrhardt R, et al. Successful autografting following myeloablative conditioning therapy with blood stem cells mobilized by chemotherapy plus rhG-CSF. Exp Hematol 1993;21(4):508–14.

48. Sekhsaria S, Fleisher TA, Vowells S, et al. Granulocyte colony-stimulating factor recruitment of CD34+ progenitors to peripheral blood: impaired mobilization in chronic granulomatous disease and adenosine deaminase–deficient severe combined immunodeficiency disease patients. Blood 1996;88(3):1104–12.

49. Liles WC, Broxmeyer HE, Rodger E, et al. Mobilization of hematopoietic progenitor cells in healthy volunteers by AMD3100, a CXCR4 antagonist. Blood 2003; 102(8):2728–30.

50. Flomenberg N, Devine SM, Dipersio JF, et al. The use of AMD3100 plus G-CSF for autologous hematopoietic progenitor cell mobilization is superior to G-CSF alone. Blood 2005;106(5):1867–74.

51. Uchida N, Leonard A, Stroncek D, et al. Safe and efficient peripheral blood stem cell collection in patients with sickle cell disease using plerixafor. Haematologica 2020;105(10):e497.
52. Boulad F, Shore T, van Besien K, et al. Safety and efficacy of plerixafor dose escalation for the mobilization of CD34(+) hematopoietic progenitor cells in patients with sickle cell disease: interim results. Haematologica 2018;103(5): 770–7.
53. Esrick EB, Manis JP, Daley H, et al. Successful hematopoietic stem cell mobilization and apheresis collection using plerixafor alone in sickle cell patients. Blood Adv 2018;2(19):2505–12.
54. Lagresle-Peyrou C, Lefrere F, Magrin E, et al. Plerixafor enables safe, rapid, efficient mobilization of hematopoietic stem cells in sickle cell disease patients after exchange transfusion. Haematologica 2018;103(5):778–86.
55. Freireich EJ, Judson G, Levin RH. Separation and collection of leukocytes. Cancer Res 1965;25(9):1516–20.
56. Continuous Flow Blood Cell Separator. JAMA 1965;194(4):27–9.
57. Civin CI, Strauss LC, Brovall C, et al. Antigenic analysis of hematopoiesis. III. A hematopoietic progenitor cell surface antigen defined by a monoclonal antibody raised against KG-1a cells. J Immunol 1984;133(1):157–65.
58. Strauss LC, Trischmann TM, Rowley SD, et al. Selection of normal human hematopoietic stem cells for bone marrow transplantation using immunomagnetic microspheres and CD34 antibody. Am J Pediatr Hematol Oncol 1991;13(2): 217–21.
59. Rowley SD, Loken M, Radich J, et al. Isolation of CD34+ cells from blood stem cell components using the Baxter Isolex system. Bone Marrow Transplant 1998; 21(12):1253–62.
60. Malech HL, Maples PB, Whiting-Theobald N, et al. Prolonged production of NADPH oxidase-corrected granulocytes after gene therapy of chronic granulomatous disease. Proc Natl Acad Sci U S A 1997;94(22):12133–8.
61. Avecilla ST, Goss C, Bleau S, et al. How do I perform hematopoietic progenitor cell selection? Transfusion 2016;56(5):1008–12.
62. Malech HL. Use of serum-free medium with fibronectin fragment enhanced transduction in a system of gas permeable plastic containers to achieve high levels of retrovirus transduction at clinical scale. Stem Cells 2000;18(2):155–6.
63. Coelen RJ, Jose DG, May JT. The effect of hexadimethrine bromide (polybrene) on the infection of the primate retroviruses SSV 1/SSAV 1 and BaEV. Arch Virol 1983;75(4):307–11.
64. Kotani H, Newton PB 3rd, Zhang S, et al. Improved methods of retroviral vector transduction and production for gene therapy. Hum Gene Ther 1994;5(1):19–28.
65. Moritz T, Dutt P, Xiao X, et al. Fibronectin improves transduction of reconstituting hematopoietic stem cells by retroviral vectors: evidence of direct viral binding to chymotryptic carboxy-terminal fragments. Blood 1996;88(3):855–62.
66. Pollok KE, Hanenberg H, Noblitt TW, et al. High-efficiency gene transfer into normal and adenosine deaminase-deficient T lymphocytes is mediated by transduction on recombinant fibronectin fragments. J Virol 1998;72(6):4882–92.
67. Dao MA, Hashino K, Kato I, et al. Adhesion to fibronectin maintains regenerative capacity during ex vivo culture and transduction of human hematopoietic stem and progenitor cells. Blood 1998;92(12):4612–21.
68. Hofig I, Atkinson MJ, Mall S, et al. Poloxamer synperonic F108 improves cellular transduction with lentiviral vectors. J Gene Med 2012;14(8):549–60.

69. Heffner GC, Bonner M, Christiansen L, et al. Prostaglandin E2 Increases Lentiviral Vector Transduction Efficiency of Adult Human Hematopoietic Stem and Progenitor Cells. Mol Ther 2018;26(1):320–8.

70. Masiuk KE, Zhang R, Osborne K, et al. PGE2 and Poloxamer Synperonic F108 Enhance Transduction of Human HSPCs with a beta-Globin Lentiviral Vector. Mol Ther Methods Clin Dev 2019;13:390–8.

71. Uchida N, Nassehi T, Drysdale CM, et al. High-Efficiency Lentiviral Transduction of Human CD34(+) Cells in High-Density Culture with Poloxamer and Prostaglandin E2. Mol Ther Methods Clin Dev 2019;13:187–96.

72. De Ravin SS, Anaya O'Bien S, Kwatemaa N, et al. Enhanced Transduction Lentivector Gene Therapy for Treatment of Older Patients with X-Linked Severe Combined Immunodeficiency. Blood 2019;134(Suppl 1):608. https://doi.org/10.1182/blood-2019-127439.

73. Petrillo C, Thorne LG, Unali G, et al. Cyclosporine H Overcomes Innate Immune Restrictions to Improve Lentiviral Transduction and Gene Editing In Human Hematopoietic Stem Cells. Cell Stem Cell 2018;23(6):820–32.e9.

74. Kanter J, Walters MC, Krishnamurti L, et al. Biologic and Clinical Efficacy of LentiGlobin for Sickle Cell Disease. N Engl J Med 2022;386(7):617–28.

75. Blaese RM, Culver KW, Miller AD, et al. T lymphocyte-directed gene therapy for ADA- SCID: initial trial results after 4 years. Science 1995;270(5235):475–80.

76. Bordignon C, Notarangelo LD, Nobili N, et al. Gene therapy in peripheral blood lymphocytes and bone marrow for ADA- immunodeficient patients. Science 1995;270(5235):470–5.

77. Ferrua F, Aiuti A. Twenty-Five Years of Gene Therapy for ADA-SCID: From Bubble Babies to an Approved Drug. Hum Gene Ther 2017;28(11):972–81.

78. Cavazzana-Calvo M, Hacein-Bey S, de Saint Basile G, et al. Gene therapy of human severe combined immunodeficiency (SCID)-X1 disease. Science 2000;288(5466):669–72.

79. Aiuti A, Slavin S, Aker M, et al. Correction of ADA-SCID by stem cell gene therapy combined with nonmyeloablative conditioning. Science 2002;296(5577):2410–3.

80. De Ravin SS, Wu X, Moir S, et al. Lentiviral hematopoietic stem cell gene therapy for X-linked severe combined immunodeficiency. Sci Transl Med 2016;8(335):335ra357.

81. Mamcarz E, Zhou S, Lockey T, et al. Lentiviral Gene Therapy Combined with Low-Dose Busulfan in Infants with SCID-X1. N Engl J Med 2019;380(16):1525–34.

82. Ott MG, Schmidt M, Schwarzwaelder K, et al. Correction of X-linked chronic granulomatous disease by gene therapy, augmented by insertional activation of MDS1-EVI1, PRDM16 or SETBP1. Nat Med 2006;12(4):401–9.

83. Kang EM, Choi U, Theobald N, et al. Retrovirus gene therapy for X-linked chronic granulomatous disease can achieve stable long-term correction of oxidase activity in peripheral blood neutrophils. Blood 2010;115(4):783–91.

84. Boztug K, Schmidt M, Schwarzer A, et al. Stem-cell gene therapy for the Wiskott-Aldrich syndrome. N Engl J Med 2010;363(20):1918–27.

85. Aiuti A, Biasco L, Scaramuzza S, et al. Lentiviral hematopoietic stem cell gene therapy in patients with Wiskott-Aldrich syndrome. Science 2013;341(6148):1233151.

86. Hacein-Bey Abina S, Gaspar HB, Blondeau J, et al. Outcomes following gene therapy in patients with severe Wiskott-Aldrich syndrome. JAMA 2015;313(15):1550–63.

87. Kohn DB, Booth C, Kang EM, et al. Lentiviral gene therapy for X-linked chronic granulomatous disease. Nat Med 2020;26(2):200–6.
88. Sessa M, Lorioli L, Fumagalli F, et al. Lentiviral haemopoietic stem-cell gene therapy in early-onset metachromatic leukodystrophy: an ad-hoc analysis of a non-randomised, open-label, phase 1/2 trial. Lancet 2016;388(10043):476–87.
89. Capotondo A, Milazzo R, Politi LS, et al. Brain conditioning is instrumental for successful microglia reconstitution following hematopoietic stem cell transplantation. Proc Natl Acad Sci U S A 2012;109(37):15018–23.
90. Wilson CA, Cichutek K. The US and EU regulatory perspectives on the clinical use of hematopoietic stem/progenitor cells genetically modified ex vivo by retroviral vectors. Methods Mol Biol 2009;506:477–88.
91. Hacein-Bey-Abina S, von Kalle C, Schmidt M, et al. A serious adverse event after successful gene therapy for X-linked severe combined immunodeficiency. N Engl J Med 2003;348(3):255–6.
92. Hacein-Bey-Abina S, Von Kalle C, Schmidt M, et al. LMO2-associated clonal T cell proliferation in two patients after gene therapy for SCID-X1. Science 2003;302(5644):415–9.
93. Zhou S, Mody D, DeRavin SS, et al. A self-inactivating lentiviral vector for SCID-X1 gene therapy that does not activate LMO2 expression in human T cells. Blood 2010;116(6):900–8.
94. Stein S, Ott MG, Schultze-Strasser S, et al. Genomic instability and myelodysplasia with monosomy 7 consequent to EVI1 activation after gene therapy for chronic granulomatous disease. Nat Med 2010;16(2):198–204.
95. Braun CJ, Boztug K, Paruzynski A, et al. Gene therapy for Wiskott-Aldrich syndrome–long-term efficacy and genotoxicity. Sci Transl Med 2014;6(227): 227ra233.
96. Baum C, Modlich U, Gohring G, et al. Concise review: managing genotoxicity in the therapeutic modification of stem cells. Stem Cells 2011;29(10):1479–84.
97. Eichler F, Duncan C, Musolino PL, et al. Hematopoietic Stem-Cell Gene Therapy for Cerebral Adrenoleukodystrophy. N Engl J Med 2017;377(17):1630–8.
98. First gene therapy for adrenoleukodystrophy. Nat Biotechnol 2021;39(11):1319.
99. Servick K. Gene therapy clinical trial halted as cancer risk surfaces. Science News. 2021. Available at: https://www.science.org/content/article/gene-therapy-clinical-trial-halted-cancer-risk-surfaces. Accessed April 29, 2022.
100. Halene S, Wang L, Cooper RM, et al. Improved expression in hematopoietic and lymphoid cells in mice after transplantation of bone marrow transduced with a modified retroviral vector. Blood 1999;94(10):3349–57.
101. Hsieh MM, Bonner M, Pierciey FJ, et al. Myelodysplastic syndrome unrelated to lentiviral vector in a patient treated with gene therapy for sickle cell disease. Blood Adv 2020;4(9):2058–63.
102. Goyal S, Tisdale J, Schmidt M, et al. Acute Myeloid Leukemia Case after Gene Therapy for Sickle Cell Disease. N Engl J Med 2022;386(2):138–47.
103. Bonner MA, Morales-Hernandez A, Zhou S, et al. 3' UTR-truncated HMGA2 overexpression induces non-malignant in vivo expansion of hematopoietic stem cells in non-human primates. Mol Ther Methods Clin Dev 2021;21: 693–701.
104. Malech HL, Ochs HD. An emerging era of clinical benefit from gene therapy. JAMA 2015;313(15):1522–3.

A Curative DNA Code for Hematopoietic Defects
Novel Cell Therapies for Monogenic Diseases of the Blood and Immune System

Matthew H. Porteus, MD, PhD[a],*, Mara Pavel-Dinu, PhD[b],*,
Sung-Yun Pai, MD[c]

KEYWORDS

- Hematopoietic stem cells • CRISPR/Cas9 • DNA repair • Engineered viruses
- Gene correction • Prime editing • Base editing • Hematological diseases

KEY POINTS

- Precise gene correction, using programmable nucleases, enables an era of personalized medicine to treat incurable monogenic hematological and immunologic conditions.
- Direct changes to the DNA sequence of a cell are based on a growing genome editing toolset that can be applied to the hematopoietic system and extends beyond semirandom integrating viruses: nonhomologous end joining (NHEJ)-dependent gene editing, base editing, primer editing, and homology-direct repair (HDR)-mediated gene correction.
- Targeted correction of the hematopoietic system holds great promises and unique challenges on its path to a safe and effective clinical translation.
- Manufacturing advances of ex vivo gene correction therapies will be needed to reduce costs and enable cures of a broad array of ultra-rare and rare hematological disorders.

INTRODUCTION

Hematopoietic stem cell transplantation (HSCT)[1,2] is the most advanced treatment strategy for life-threatening conditions caused by developmental and functional defects of the mature hematopoietic lineages. The highest success rates for allogeneic

[a] Department of Pediatrics, Division of Stem Cell Transplantation and Regenerative Medicine, Stanford Medical School, Lokey Stem Cell Research Building, G3040B, MC 5462, 265 Campus Drive, Stanford, CA 94305, USA; [b] Department of Pediatrics, Division of Stem Cell Transplantation and Regenerative Medicine, Stanford Medical School, Lokey Stem Cell Research Building, G3045, MC 5175, 265 Campus Drive, Stanford, CA 94305, USA; [c] Immune Deficiency Cellular Therapy Program, Center for Cancer Research, National Cancer Institute, 10 Center Drive, MSC 1102, Bethesda, MD 20892, USA
* Corresponding authors.
E-mail addresses: mporteus@stanford.edu (M.H.P.); marahd@stanford.edu (M.P.-D.)

Hematol Oncol Clin N Am 36 (2022) 647–665
https://doi.org/10.1016/j.hoc.2022.05.002   hemonc.theclinics.com

(allo-) HSCT is associated with using a matched human leukocyte antigen (HLA)-identical donor graft.[2] However, as the demand for matched donors outweighs the supply, 75% of patients in need of a transplant rely on HLA-mismatched stem cells. Allo-HSCT confers a considerable risk of morbidity (eg, incomplete immune reconstitution, graft-versus-host disease, graft rejection) when the source of stem cells is derived from HLA-mismatched individuals.

Autologous stem cell-based gene therapy offers the greatest immunologic compatibility, delivering an ideal solution for genetic diseases of the blood and immune system while avoiding the allogeneic complications of standard treatment. This cutting-edge restorative therapy for untreatable diseases is leading to the development of regenerative medicine. The evolution from a treatment that introduces a new copy of the "healthy" gene (gene addition)[3] to a treatment that corrects the "mutated gene" (genome editing),[4] marks a critical turning point in modern medicine. Hematopoietic stem cells (HSCs) are the prototypical cells used in gene therapy due to their lifelong regenerative potential.[5] They are defined by 2 fundamental properties–self-renewal and differentiation–with a multipotent and narrow spectrum of differentiation potential restricted to blood cells and immune lineages.[6] These unique biological properties allow HSCs to form and replenish the hematopoietic system and act as an internal repair process during injury. These cellular attributes of HSCs give great potential for developing innovative, safer, and durable therapies.

Inherited and acquired genetic alterations originating in HSCs disrupt the output of the hematopoietic system resulting in hematological conditions whereby mature blood or immune cells fail to develop or function properly. Experiments of nature have shown that genetic somatic reversion from a pathogenic to a wild-type sequence can lead to a curative outcome,[7] a concept that is the cornerstone of the modern era of gene therapy. In the early days of gene therapy trials, the adverse effect of a malfunctioning gene was counteracted by integrating viral vector-mediated gene transfer.[8] This approach demonstrated clear benefits in patients with selected hematological conditions.[9–12] However, the "gene addition" approach does not achieve the spatiotemporal gene regulation and expression that many blood and immune-related genes depend on. Clinical correction was not a consistent outcome in these gene therapy trials due to transient and low-level transgene expression unable to support robust hematopoiesis; safety was also compromised by leukemic events caused by insertional mutagenesis, reported during long-term follow-up.[13–16]

Technological innovations in the genome engineering field through the development of genome editing tools usher in a new era of gene therapy.[17–19] Genome engineering through editing relies on a "hit-and-run" approach to permanently modify a specific genomic sequence. Conceptually, genome editing is achieved through transient expression of an engineered nuclease that works in conjunction with the DNA repair machinery with or without a predesigned repair template to modify a sequence of DNA permanently. When a donor/repair template is used, targeted transgene integration to achieve in situ reconstitution of a mutated gene while preserving robust and predictable expression can be achieved, thus abrogating the limitations previously associated with gene addition. The successful transfer of the bench to bedside gene-correction approach is contingent on overcoming cellular barriers, escaping immunologic surveillance, sustaining a physiologic gene expression, correcting abundant stem and progenitor cells to reverse the condition, and assuring that the hematopoietic system is robustly reprogrammed to maintain long-term benefits.

Genome engineering of human HSCs generates a "live biological" therapeutic drug of unparalleled complexity with potential unknown and unintended effects on patients. Combining genome editing with gene therapy, a patient's hematopoietic system can be restored to achieve disease correction at its root cause–directly correcting the pathologic mutation at the DNA level. Preclinical data, using animal models, provided the first evidence of the efficacy, specificity, and safety of this approach in support of its advancement to first-in-human clinical trials. Early phase trials of gene editing, including direct gene correction-based approaches, have already received FDA clearance for patients with severe forms of sickle cell disease (**Table 1**). While this therapy is in its pioneering stage, precautionary measurements and long-term surveillance will be necessary to determine whether the safety, efficacy, and durability of disease correction have been achieved at an acceptable risk/benefit ratio. Nonetheless, there is optimism that the curative strategy will result in the benefits outweighing the risks for patients. This article reviews the progress in advancing genome-editing technology and its application to regenerative medicine, the biological processes underpinning these innovations, and addresses the challenges and triumphs in transferring genome-editing-based gene therapies from bench to bedside. We highlight throughout examples of the key accomplishments in genome editing in blood and immune diseases, with particular emphasis on inborn errors of immunity (IEI) and severe hemoglobinopathies such as sickle cell disease (SCD) and beta-thalassemia (see also Alexis Leonard and colleagues' article, "Gene Therapy for Hemoglobinopathies: Beta-Thalassemia, Sickle Cell Disease"; Kritika Chetty and colleagues' article, "Gene Therapy for Inborn Errors of Immunity: Severe Combined Immunodeficiencies"; and Joseph D. Long and colleagues' article-Genes as Medicine: The Development of Gene Therapies for Inborn Errors of Immunity," in this issue).

MOLECULAR INTERVENTIONS FOR CORRECTING A GENE

Gene therapy relies on modifying the patient own human hematopoietic system to achieve disease correction. The approach is confined to a defined subset of cells ($CD34^+$ hematopoietic stem and progenitor cells, ie, HSPCs) of patient origin, transduced by viral vectors to deliver a therapeutic payload into the cell's genome before infusion back into the patient. Until a decade ago, "gene addition" gene therapy leveraged the biology of semi-randomly integrated retro- (RV) and lenti- (LV) viruses[8] to offset a faulty gene within a cell, which adversely affected its fitness. However, *stochastic genomic integration* of a functional gene copy did not always produce reliable clinical outcomes, with results varying among patients and trials. The rationale for redesigning the clinical vectors[20–22] to alleviate previously reported genotoxicity decreased but did not eliminate the oncogenic risk of large numbers of semi-random integrations in the clinical setting.

Advances in genome engineering technology are transforming the field of gene therapy. Rather than relying on uncontrolled vectors to deliver an exogenous therapeutic gene, *genome editing directly modifies the defective endogenous gene* using a "cut" and "paste" approach to restore the target gene's function. The ability to identify one incorrect nucleotide out of 6 billion that make up the human diploid genome and modify it precisely is an astonishing accomplishment made possible by discovering nucleases that can stimulate DNA repair responses by 1000-fold.[23–26] As exciting as it is for translational medicine, genome editing is also a fundamental biological process crucial to developing the human adaptive immune system. For example, in the absence of our natural genome editing system, lymphocytes cannot generate a

Table 1
Clinical-stage (phase I/II) gene editing candidate therapies for sickle cell disease

Product ID/Company	Clinical Trial ID	Disease	Gene Editing Approach	Description	Preclinical Data
GPH101 *Graphite Bio*	CEDAR NCT04819841	SCD	CRISPR/Cas9-AAV6 beta-globin	• Ex vivo-edited autologous HSPC • Correction of beta-globin mutation • Adult and adolescents • Adult and adolescents	46
CRISPR_SCD001	NCT04774536	SCD	CRISPR-Cas9 beta-globin	• Ex vivo-edited autologous HSPC • Correction of beta-globin mutation • 9 participants, 12–35 y old • Sponsor: Dr. Mark Walters (UCSF) Benioff Children Hospital, UCLA and UC Berkeley	
CTX001 *Vertex Pharm CRISPR Therap*	CLIMB-121 NCT03745287	SCD	CRISPR-Cas9 Ablating *BCL11A* enhancer	• Ex vivo-edited autologous HSPC • Restore fetal hemoglobin (HbF) • 7 adult participants • Sponsor: US-based companies	109,110
BIVV003 *Sangamo Therapeutics*	PRECIZN-1 NCT03653247	SCD	ZFN mRNA Ablating *BCL11A* enhancer	• Ex vivo-edited autologous HSPC • Restore fetal hemoglobin (HbF) • 8 adult participants • Sponsor: Sanofi, France	61

				[59,60]
OTQ923 HIX763 Novartis Pharm	NCT04443907	SCD	CRISPR-Cas9 Ablating *BCL11A* enhancer	• Ex vivo-edited autologous HSPC • Restore fetal hemoglobin (HbF) • Section 1: OTQ923 tested in adults • Section 2: HIX763 tested in adults • Section 3: HIX763 or OTQ923 • 30 participants 2–17 y old and 18–40 y old • Sponsor: Novartis and Intellia Therap.
EDIT-301 *Editas Medicine*	RUBY NCT04853576	SCD	CRISPR-Cas12a Enhance *HBG1/2* promoter region in beta-globin locus	• Ex vivo-edited autologous HSPC • Restore fetal hemoglobin (HbF) • Tested in 0–18 y old • Sponsor: US-based company
BEAM-101 *Beam Therapeutics*	BEACON-101 Not yet recruiting	SCD	Base-editing *HBG1* and *HBG2*	• Ex vivo-edited autologous HSPC • A to G-based editing in the *HBG1* and *HBG2* promoter region • Mimics HbF natural mutation to increase HbF • Sponsor: US-based company

Currently, no gene-editing clinical trials are opened for PIDs.
Abbreviations: BCL11A, BAF chromatin remodeling complex subunit; HbF, fetal hemoglobin; HBG1/2, hemoglobin subunit gamma 1/2; HSPC, hematopoietic stem and progenitor cell; SCD, sickle cell disease.

pool of receptors with a diverse repertoire required to sustain a robust immune response against infections.[27–29]

GENOME EDITING MEDIATED BY DNA DOUBLE-STRANDED BREAKS

The genome-editing process may be catalyzed by a nuclease designed to recognize, bind, and cut a predetermined DNA sequence.[30] The double-strand breaks (DSBs) generated by the nuclease mark the region for the DNA repair enzymes to insert, delete or replace a sequence while repairing the breaks. Earlier genome editing platforms relied on homing endonucleases[23] and chimeric proteins–zinc finger nucleases (ZFNs)[31–34] and transcription activator-like effectors (TALENs)[35,36]–to introduce DSBs at precise genomic locations. These breaks prompt the recruitment of DNA repair enzymes that are steered by adeno-associated virus (AAV), a nonintegrating viral vector, to introduce the desired nucleotide sequence. The cellular choice of DNA repair–nonhomologous end-joining (NHEJ) or homologous recombination (HR) (see later in discussion)—determines the outcome of nuclease-based genome editing. While these earlier nuclease platforms are still being used in translational clinical trials, in the last 7 years, the Clustered Regulatory Interspaced Short Palindromic Repeats Cas9 nuclease (CRISPR/Cas9) has transformed the field[17,18] because of its ease of use, remarkable activity in a variety of human cells (including HSPCs), and its surprising specificity.

While ZFNs and TALENs use proteins engineered to recognize predefined 9 to 18 or 11 to 12 nucleotides, respectively, as docking sites for DSBs generation, the CRISPR/Cas9 platform is an RNA-guided DNA endonuclease. Originally part of the bacterial adaptive immune system,[17] whereby the CRISPR locus was used as an information storage mechanism for past viral infections, CRISPR/Cas9's role was to recognize and destroy viral genomes through sequence-specific DNA–RNA base pairing. The system was repurposed for genome editing applications in the biomedical field, offering significant advantages over previous platforms. Though the CRISPR locus itself is unique to the bacterial immune system[18] features from the CRISPR array were used in the human genome. First, the guide RNA (gRNA), which is transcribed from the CRISPR locus to recognize incoming viral sequences in the bacterial system, was redesigned to recognize the unique 20-nucleotide human genome sequence. The gRNA complexes to the Cas9 protein and directs the Cas9 protein (which contains the nuclease activity to make a break) to the correct site in the genome. These breaks are created 3 base pairs (bp) away from the adjacent protospacer motif (PAM), marking the genomic site complementary to the gRNA. Second, the dual RNA system of bacteria (crRNA and trRNA) was replaced by a single gRNA system (sgRNA), thus reducing the complexity of the system from 3 components (Cas9, trRNA, crRNA) to 2 components (Cas9 and sgRNA). The CRISPR Cas9/sgRNA system's ease of design, combined with high activity and specificity, has democratized and transformed the genome-editing field and has made it the most used nuclease platform to enable the development of preclinical "gene correction" therapies.

DOUBLE-STRAND BREAKS REPAIR PATHWAYS AND THE EFFECT OF CELL CYCLE AND CHROMATIN STRUCTURE ON GENOME EDITING

The outcome of a Cas9-mediated genome editing depends on the DNA repair pathway being used. The classical nonhomologous end joining (cNHEJ) repair pathway is active across all cell cycle stages. The Cas9/sgRNA ribonucleoprotein complex (RNA protein enzyme) cuts the target strand 3 bp upstream of the PAM site and 3 bp, 4 bp, or 5 bp on the nontarget strand, thus generating DSBs with blunt or staggered ends.[37,38] cNHEJ ligates the blunt ends with high fidelity, but the stagger ends are processed in an error-prone way, resulting in 1 to 2 bp insertions or deletions (INDELs).[39] *NHEJ-based genome editing* can, therefore, be used to (i) silence pathogenic forms of a gene, such as a dominant active gene, (ii) restore the correcting reading frame, or (iii) introduce targeted deletions of exons or enhancers. It is important to note that the nature of INDELs is highly variable between different sgRNA guides.

During the S/G$_2$ phase of the cell cycle, 3 repair pathways are active and in competition to resolve the DSBs: *cNHEJ*, microhomology-mediated end joining (*MMEJ*), and homologous recombination (homologous direct repair (*HDR*)). Short 3′ end ssDNA overhangs can be routed into MMEJ-dependent repair by resetting and filling the gaps via DNA synthesis. Like cNHEJ, MMEJ does not require a DNA repair template and results in loss of sequence information. The repair outcome usually generates larger deletions than the deletions created by cNHEJ (>3 bp).[39] Inhibition of the DNA ligase (Lig I and III) active in the final step of MMEJ, using small molecule inhibitors, can bias the repair mechanism toward using a homologous repair (HR) pathway, an error-free repair approach.

HDR describes using a donor DNA molecule as a template for repairing the break to generate precise nucleotide changes in the genome (not INDELs). HDR can be harnessed using double-stranded DNA (*classic HR*) or single-stranded DNA template repair (*SSTR*).[40] The presence of either repair template will result in template-dependent, high-fidelity repair outcomes driven by different repair mechanisms. Exogenously provided double-stranded DNA donor template bearing homology arms (~400 base pairs) to the target site is incorporated into the genome by an *HR mechanism*.[41] This genome-editing approach provides the flexibility of (i) changing a pathogenic single-nucleotide polymorphism (SNP) and (ii) inserting a full-length cDNA or open reading frame of a gene in-frame with the endogenous start site or at a safe-harbor locus if constitutive overexpression of the gene could provide a therapeutic benefit without inducing adverse events. Safeguarding the endogenous levels of gene expression and regulation while eliminating the risk of insertional mutagenesis is the most sought-after genome-editing outcome that would benefit larger classes of monogenic diseases (**Fig. 1**). HR-mediated targeted correction of point mutations has been successfully used for correcting single point mutation both for SCD[42–46] and IEI, for example, X-linked chronic granulomatous disease.[47] The use of a full-length cDNA for *in situ* gene correction has the advantage of establishing a *"universal gene correction"* therapeutic strategy for conditions not caused by recurrent mutations but by a broader array of mutations scattered throughout the gene. The feasibility of this latter approach has been demonstrated most extensively by using adenovirus-associated viruses to deliver the cDNA, as discussed later.

SSTR-mediated genome editing can achieve small genomic changes (single to tens of base pairs), and it also occurs with high efficiency in mammalian cells, though through a mechanism that is not via the classic HR repair machinery (SSTR is Rad51 independent). In SSTR, a synthesized single-stranded oligonucleotide (ssODN) of length 70 to 150 base pairs (bps) is used, making it more accessible to investigators than classic HR donor templates. The range of changes engineered by SSTR is substantially more limited than what can be achieved by classic HR[43,47] though it does offer a viable approach for introducing limited genetic edits.

Although genome editing varies considerably between different genomic sites, the nucleotides next to the Cas9 cutting site can influence the repair outcome.[38,39,48,49] The most common outcomes observed in HSCs are small INDELs (1–2 bp), products of cNHEJ, and controlled by the nucleotide at the fourth position upstream of the PAM

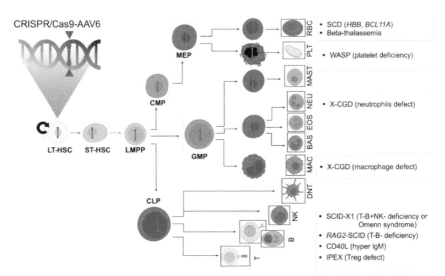

Fig. 1. Preclinical studies using a gene-editing approach for Primary Immunodeficiencies. Schematic of the human hematopoietic system and cell lineages. Gray boxes denote the hematopoietic defect causing the PID. B, B cell; BAS, basophil; CLP, common lymphoid progenitor; CMP, common myeloid progenitor; DNT, dendritic cell; EOS, eosinophil; GMP, granulocyte-monocyte progenitor; HSC, hematopoietic stem cells; LMPP, lymphoid multipotent progenitor; LT-HSCs, long-term HSC; MAC, macrophage; MAST, mast cell; MEP, megakaryocyte-erythroid progenitor; NEU, neutrophil; NK, NK cell; PLT, platelet cell; RBC, red blood cell; ST-HSC, short-term HSC; T, T cell; Treg, T regulatory cell. The image was designed using BioRender software.

site. Cas9 cutting efficiency and the choice of DNA repair pathways are affected by changes in nucleosome architecture caused by chromatin remodeling. Post-translational modifications control the recruitment of DNA repair proteins such as 53BP1 and BRCA1. For example, the ubiquitylation of histone 2A (H2A) and di-methylation of histone 4 at lysine 20 (H4K20me2) recruit 53BP1 to chromatin sites next to the DSBs. These modification states (H2A and H4) were proposed to have an antagonistic effect on the recruitment of 53BP1 and BRCA1 to define cell cycle phases, affecting the choice of DSB repair pathway. A compacted chromatin (heterochromatic) structure marked by histone 3 lysine 9 trimethylation (H3K9me2/3) promotes HR and MMEJ while open chromatin (euchromatin) state stimulates the cNHEJ repair pathway.[50,51] Although the mechanisms by which chromatin architecture promotes one repair pathway over another remain to be elucidated, fundamental insights into the genome structure can inform the development of better genome-editing strategies. Nonetheless, high frequencies of all types of editing can be achieved at loci that are transcriptionally silent in HSPCs.

NON-BREAK MEDIATED EDITING: BASE AND PRIMER EDITING

The generation of DSBs does not directly induce genome editing. It is the cellular response to the breaks that modify the DNA. DNA damage responses are intricate and tightly regulated processes. Although HR-mediated targeted correction is a highly versatile genome editing approach that corrects the DNA sequence at nucleotide resolution, it is restricted to dividing cells (the S/G_2 phase of the cell cycle). It also competes with the highly efficient NHEJ repair enzymes. This generates a heterozygous population of genome-edited alleles: some precisely corrected and others marked by INDELs. The unintended presence of INDELs as a byproduct of targeted genome editing could negatively impact the therapeutic outcome by reducing its effectiveness or generating unwanted disease-permissive genotypes. This outcome can be best exemplified by disorders of β-globin, SCD, and β-thalassemia. HR-mediated targeted genome correction of the SCD genotype (HbS/HbS) results in a large portion of the SCD patient's alleles being corrected (HbA/HbA). However, since HR-mediated genome editing cannot reach 100% efficiency, some SCD alleles will acquire INDELs that generate β-thalassemia or sickle/β-thalassemia genotypes (INDEL/INDEL; HbS/INDEL).

To eliminate "by-product events" at the targeted locus, 2 variations to the targeted genome editing approach have been described that bypass the need for introducing DSBs: base editing and prime editing. *Base editing (BE)* uses the CRISPR-Cas9 platform to modify the chemical sequence of the DNA directly and introduce any of the 4 nucleotide transitions: C to T, T to C, A to G, and G to A.[52–55] This is achieved by using an inactive nuclease form of Cas9 that retains nicking activity along with base-modification enzymes (*cytosine base editors, CBEs*, and *adenine base editors, ABEs*) active only on ssDNA. The base pairing between a DNA and an RNA molecule induces a "DNA bubble (R-loop)," allowing the deaminase enzyme to modify the DNA bases within the loop. The DNA nick created on the nonedited strand by the catalytically disabled nuclease will be repaired using the edited strand as a template. Innovative as it is, this approach is limited to a predefined window of genomic sequences that it can act on and has a limited number of genetic changes that can be engineered.

Prime editing (PE) was developed to overcome this limitation by introducing all 12 possible base conservations (transitions and transversions) without DSBs.[56,57] This genome editing platform is based on a prime editing guide RNA (pegRNA), containing both the primer binding site (PBS), the sequence to introduce the edit, and the Cas9 nickase (H840) carrying a reverse transcriptase (RT). RT is an RNA-dependent DNA polymerase that uses the pegRNA as a template to copy the desired genomic edit into the target DNA sequence. PE requires the expression of a foreign RT for editing, and the consequences (including genotoxicity) of expressing such an RT in cells are not fully understood.

The use of DNA base editors as a therapeutic tool has been demonstrated by efficiently correcting mutated genes (eg, *HBB* in β-thalassemia)[58,59] and by introducing targeted deletion in gene enhancers (eg, *BCL11 A*)[59–61] or in the promoter regions (eg, *HBG1* and *HBG2*)[62–65] to stimulate fetal hemoglobin (HbF) upregulation. Though the latter 2 approaches are not a disease correction strategy *per se*, it alleviates the symptoms associated with β-globin-related blood conditions.

Base and prime editing technologies are exciting new tools in genome editing, but they remain less developed than nuclease-based methods in translating to patients.[66–68] Addressing limitations concerning their restricted targetable sites, unintended off-target effects in both DNA and RNA, and bystander mutation events remain active areas of investigation as the BE, and PE tools are translated. Furthermore, in contrast to classic HR-based editing, neither BE nor PE can provide a one-shot universal approach to a genetic disease with disease-causing mutations scattered throughout the gene.

THE SCIENCE OF GENOME EDITING THE HEMATOPOIETIC SYSTEM

The unlimited self-renewal potential of HSC has always made these cells the preferred choice for gene therapy. To ensure that the genome editing modification is propagated indefinitely throughout the hematopoietic system, optimizing the *ex vivo* genome editing protocols must meet the highest specificity, efficiency, and safety standards without obstructing the cells' regenerative potential. The technological toolbox for genome editing must, therefore, be tailored to the biological properties of HSC to achieve optimal results.

Ex vivo Culturing Conditions

CD34[+] HSPCs are purified from the bone marrow or the peripheral blood of the recipient and cultured for 2 to 3 days in the presence of growth-stimulating cytokines.[69,70] Long-term repopulating HSCs (LT-HSCs) exit quiescence and enter the S/G_2 cell cycle phase. Under these conditions that enable genome editing, the cells are exposed to the engineered nucleases and the vector carrying the repair template. HDR-based genome editing has a limited window of action–the S/G_2 cell cycle phase–permissive to highly cycling committed progenitors but constrained in the quiescent primitive HSCs population.[71,72] Fine-tuning the culturing conditions,[73,74] incorporating stemness-preserving compounds,[74,75] and shortening the overall editing time are steps implemented to preserve the long-term multilineage repopulating capacity of the "therapeutic drug product."[76] Achieving a balance between efficient editing and maintenance of the stemness potential of human HSPCs is vital to sustaining the long-term fitness of genome-edited HSPCs and the therapeutic benefit.

Optimizing and Delivering Engineered Nucleases and Homology-Direct Repair-Mediated DNA Repair Template

The goal of the engineered nuclease platform is to deliver the highest frequencies of genome editing while minimizing the treatment toxicity. Both the DSBs and the DNA repair template can trigger cellular responses that could adversely affect the cell fitness and the competence of the DNA repair mechanisms. Primary cells, such as HSCs, have developed heightened immune responses (eg, pathogen-associated molecular patterns, PAMPs; type I interferons, IFNs; overexpression of interferon-stimulated genes, ISG, and other cytokines) to exogenous nucleic acids and proteins by inducing exit from quiescence, promoting differentiation, reducing cellular viability, and decreasing clonogenic potential.[77–80]

To dampen the immune responses against the genome-editing machinery, the sgRNAs are synthesized as RNA, purified using high-pressure liquid chromatography (HPLC), and cloaked with chemical modifications.[81] Electroporation-based delivery of the sgRNA molecule precomplexed with Cas9 protein (ribonucleoprotein, RNP, including a high-fidelity form of Cas9)[82,83] further shields the genome-editing molecules from inducing cellular responses against it. Studies have further shown that a pro-inflammatory transcriptional program[72] with a subsequence decrease in the genome-edited HSPCs' clonogenic potential is generated in response to the DNA damage evoked by the nucleases. Transient p53 inhibition is one mechanism shown to enhance HR efficiency[84] and tolerability to the genome-editing process, a treatment that restores the polyclonal composition of the grafted HSPCs.[72,74]

Nonintegrating Viral Vectors for Genome Editing

Integration deficiency lentivirus (IDLV) has been developed for different lentiviral platforms. A mutation (D116) in the catalytic domain of the integrase prevents the genomic incorporation of the viral DNA, resulting in an episomal IDLV vector that can be used as an HDR- DNA repair donor.[85] These free-ended dsDNA vectors can deliver a cargo of 10 kb[86] and are amenable to genome-editing of primary cells.[42,87,88] Although the system avoids the risk associated with insertional mutagenesis and exhibits reduced toxicity, it does result in concatemer formation: IDLV recombines with the target site before HR occurs. While IDLV-HDR donors demonstrated reasonable HR frequencies, there seemed to be an upper limit on what could be achieved.

Adeno-associated virus type 6 (AAV6) has the best tropism for transducing the human hematopoietic system ex vivo.[89] The vector has a 4.7 to 4.9 kb transgene capacity, accommodating full-length cDNAs flanked by ~400 bp homology arms. *AAV6-HDR donor* has been reported to deliver highly efficient (20%–80%) HR-based correction in ex vivo and support long-term hematopoietic engraftment.[69] Many groups have demonstrated the feasibility of using AAV6 to deliver a wild-type cDNA to be integrated into the endogenous locus upstream of all known pathogenic mutations, as a "universal correction" genome editing strategy for various hematological and immunologic disorders. Examples of IEI shown to be correctable in preclinical studies include X-linked SCID,[76,90] X-linked chronic granulomatous disease,[91] X-linked hyper-IgM syndrome,[92–94] Wiskott–Aldrich syndrome,[95] X-linked agammaglobulinemia,[96] and RAG2-SCID.[97] For severe hemoglobinopathies, this approach was also successful in replacing the SCD mutation with wild-type *HBB*,[98] and replacing *HBB* in beta-thalassemia cells with *HBA*.[99]

ssODN-HDR donors are short (<200 bp) oligos with even shorter homology arms (~30–60 bp) flanking the nucleotide change. The targeted correction in HSPCs delivered by this vector type is within the range of 5% to 40% and decreases by half following transplantation into immunodeficient mice.[43,44,47] In direct comparison to AAV6-HDR donors,[42] the HR frequencies have generally been higher (20%–80%).[76,91,95] ssODN holds certain features (eg, simple design, short production time, and low cost) that make them useful for specific applications but cannot be used to insert a large transgene in HSPCs.

PERSISTENCE OF THE THERAPEUTIC STEM CELL PRODUCT

Genome-editing-based gene therapies are entering the clinical arena. The emerging Phase I/II first-in-human clinical trials (see **Table 1**) have and will continue to generate a wealth of information on the short- and long-term safety (eg, genomic integrity, nuclease specificity) and efficacy (eg, long-term durability of the edited HSPCs both at the intended locus and spanning the hematopoietic lineages) of this pioneering therapy. These endpoint readouts will inform the treatment's risk/benefit ratio. Still, molecular analyses can be performed at the manufacturing stage, before its infusion into the patient, to inform the safety and efficacy of a "therapeutic drug product." Efforts have been made to monitor the clonal composition, as a safety profile of the genome-edited HSPCs, before and after engraftment into immunodeficient mice. Studies have quantified the INDEL diversity within the genome-edited alleles[100–103] as a surrogate readout for clonal diversity or have developed unique molecular identifiers (UMI) embedded in the HDR-corrective DNA template[74,104] to track the HDR-modified alleles. These studies have demonstrated that human hematopoiesis, established in the immunodeficient mouse models and originated from the edited HSPCs, has an oligoclonal composition signature with multi-lineage and self-renewal potential retained in the engrafted clones. The observed loss in clonal diversity can be attributed to the suboptimal manufacturing process of edited HSPCs or the inefficiency of the murine bone marrow microenvironment to support polyclonal human hematopoiesis. These preclinical studies on edited-HSPC-derived clonal composition suggest that long-term persistence can be achieved and supports advancement in clinical testing.

VALUES AND LIMITATIONS IN EVALUATING THE THERAPEUTIC PRODUCT IN MOUSE MODELS

Immunocompetent mouse models have been used as preclinical models to assess the novel gene and cell therapies' efficacy, toxicity, safety, and stability. The humanized murine system offers great value for the gene and cell therapy field because it bridges the proof-of-concept of novel gene therapy and their translation into the clinic as part of IND-enabling studies. Murine models have been used to study normal and leukemic stem cells, human hematopoietic hierarchy, human immune function, autoimmune diseases, and organ and tissue transplantation. The most common immunodeficient mouse model used for human HSPC cell engraftment is the nonobese diabetic (NOD)/severe combined immunodeficiency (SCID) $\gamma c^{-/-}$, referred to as NSG,[105] was engineered to lack murine T, B, and NK cells but are not fully humanized. NSG mice are less efficient in supporting human myeloid and erythroid lineage development, making it a suboptimal system for testing genetic diseases that disrupt the myeloid function and differentiation. Newer and related immunodeficient mouse models were designed–NOG, NRG, NSG-SGM3, BRGS, and MISTRG–to support better human HSPCs engraftment, and human myeloid lineage differentiation, in addition to lymphoid lineage development. These immunodeficient mice can be transplanted with human HSPCs purified from umbilical cord blood, bone marrow, fetal liver, or adult mobilized peripheral blood, allowing the cells to home to murine bone marrow, whereby they engraft, expand, differentiate, and establish a long-term human hematopoietic system.

Evaluating the potency and safety of gene-modified HSPCs, following engraftment into conditioned immunodeficient mice is a benchmark required by the FDA before approving a new medicine (eg, gene therapy) to treat monogenic blood disease. Often these xenotransplantation studies are carried out using healthy donor stem cells since obtaining patient-derived HSPCs to transplant a full human dose into an immunodeficient mouse cohort is often not feasible due to the low prevalence of the disease, as is the case for IEIs (eg, ADA-SCID, SCID-X1, RAG1/2-SCID, IPEX, X-CGD).[106] For SCD and some forms of thalassemia, the c-Kit mutant NSG mouse model, for the first time, allowed the therapeutic efficacy to be assessed by supporting mature red blood cells development in the murine bone marrow.[107,108] With this advancement, both toxicity and efficacy of SCD or thalassemia patient-derived and corrected HSPCs can now be evaluated using clinical-grade reagents to support initiating a clinical trial.

The data and insights generated from in vivo mouse models are essential in developing novel therapies to cure human diseases. However, humanized mouse models remain only a model, and many of them have limitations: xeno-reactive graft-versus-host disease, limited lifespan, incomplete immune function, only oligoclonal reconstitution, underdeveloped lymphoid organs, and lymphoid architecture, which require careful considerations when interpreting experimental results.

ADVANCING THIS NEW CLASS OF MEDICINE TO THE CLINIC

The Food and Drug Administration (FDA) evaluates novel therapies for safety and efficacy through clinical trials open to patients who have no available treatment or for whom current therapies are not effective. Clinical trials using CRISPR/Cas9-based gene therapies in blood disorders (see **Table 1**), cancer, eye disease, protein-folding disorders, and chronic infections have received FDA approval.

Recent reports of the investigational use of the first in human ex vivo CRISPR/Cas9-modified autologous HSPCs product provided therapeutic benefits that a single treatment can offer to patients with SCD, a severely disabling condition.[109] In the clinical trial (CLIM SCD-121) sponsored by CRISPR Therapeutics and Vertex Pharmaceuticals, patients between the age of 18 and 35 who were diagnosed with SCD (genotypes ßS/ßS or ßS/ß⁰) and experienced more than 2 severe vaso-occlusion (VOC) episodes

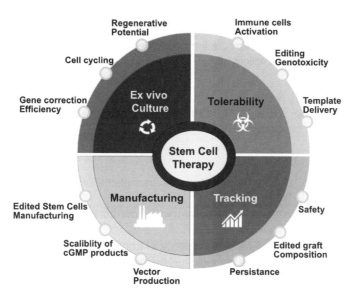

Fig. 2. Challenges in stem cell therapy. Schematic challenges toward the clinical translation of gene-editing-based stem cell therapies.

per year were eligible to participate for enrollment in the trial. Plerixafor mobilized patient's CD34$^+$ HSPCs expressing less than 30% of sickle hemoglobin following 8 weeks of transfusion were genome-edited ex vivo using sgRNA that directed CRISPR/Cas9 nuclease to the erythroid-specific enhancer region of BCL11A. Although this approach does not correct the root cause of SCD, it increases fetal hemoglobin (HbF) levels to compensate for the lack of adult hemoglobin in red blood cells. After the administration of CTX001, all 7 patients infused with the therapeutic product showed stable engraftment, which resulted in increased HbF and no VOC, 2 months postinfusion.[109,110]

Genome editing-based gene therapy is emerging as a curative therapy that reaches beyond conventional drugs. Precision medicine enables patient-specific disease correction by delivering a stable, precise, and durable therapeutic drug. As genome-based correction therapies will progress through clinical trials and demonstrate safety, efficacy, and curative potential, pharmaceutical and regulatory sectors will have to work together to build a suitable manufacturing and product release pipeline to assure that a continued supply of these highly personalized "live biological drugs" is achieved and that all patients will benefit from these innovative therapies (**Fig. 2**).

CLINICS CARE POINTS

- Genome editing of autologous hematopoietic stem cells shows great promise because of the pre-clinical data on safety and efficacy.

- Nonetheless, the clinical outcomes for patients using genome edited cells is still largely unknown, especially long term outcomes.

- Thus, clinicians should be preparted for both successes better than expected and unanticipated toxicities.

ACKNOWLEDGMENTS

This work was funded in part by the Intramural Research Program, Center for Cancer Research, National Cancer Institute.

DISCLOSURE

M.H. Porteus serves on the SAB for CRISPR Tx and Allogene Tx and is cofounder and Board of Director for Graphite Bio.

REFERENCES

1. Copelan EA. Hematopoietic stem-cell transplantation. N Engl J Med 2006; 354(17):1813–26.
2. Parkman R, Weinberg KI. Immunological reconstitution following bone marrow transplantation. Immunol Rev 1997;157:73–8.
3. High KA, Roncarolo MG. Gene therapy. N Engl J Med 2019;381(5):455–64.
4. Porteus MH. A new class of medicines through DNA editing. N Engl J Med 2019; 380(10):947–59.
5. Naldini L. Ex vivo gene transfer and correction for cell-based therapies. Nat Rev Genet 2011;12(5):301–15.
6. Notta F, Doulatov S, Laurenti E, et al. Isolation of single human hematopoietic stem cells capable of long-term multilineage engraftment. Science 2011; 333(6039):218–21.
7. Stephan V, Wahn V, Le Deist F, et al. Atypical X-linked severe combined immunodeficiency due to possible spontaneous reversion of the genetic defect in T cells. N Engl J Med 1996;335(21):1563–7.
8. Kay MA, Glorioso JC, Naldini L. Viral vectors for gene therapy: the art of turning infectious agents into vehicles of therapeutics. Nat Med 2001;7(1):33–40.
9. Aiuti A, Cattaneo F, Galimberti S, et al. Gene therapy for immunodeficiency due to adenosine deaminase deficiency. N Engl J Med 2009;360(5):447–58.
10. Gaspar HB, Cooray S, Gilmour KC, et al. Hematopoietic stem cell gene therapy for adenosine deaminase-deficient severe combined immunodeficiency leads to long-term immunological recovery and metabolic correction. Sci Transl Med 2011;3(97):97ra80.
11. Aiuti A, Biasco L, Scaramuzza S, et al. Lentiviral hematopoietic stem cell gene therapy in patients with wiskott-aldrich syndrome. Science 2013;341(6148): 1233151.
12. Hacein-Bey Abina S, Gaspar HB, Blondeau J, et al. Outcomes following gene therapy in patients with severe Wiskott-Aldrich syndrome. JAMA 2015; 313(15):1550–63.
13. Braun CJ, Boztug K, Paruzynski A, et al. Gene therapy for Wiskott-Aldrich syndrome–long-term efficacy and genotoxicity. Sci Transl Med 2014;6(227): 227ra233.
14. Hacein-Bey-Abina S, Von Kalle C, Schmidt M, et al. LMO2-associated clonal T cell proliferation in two patients after gene therapy for SCID-X1. Science 2003;302(5644):415–9.
15. Howe SJ, Mansour MR, Schwarzwaelder K, et al. Insertional mutagenesis combined with acquired somatic mutations causes leukemogenesis following gene therapy of SCID-X1 patients. J Clin Invest 2008;118(9):3143–50.

16. Stein S, Ott MG, Schultze-Strasser S, et al. Genomic instability and myelodys-plasia with monosomy 7 consequent to EVI1 activation after gene therapy for chronic granulomatous disease. Nat Med 2010;16(2):198–204.
17. Jinek M, Chylinski K, Fonfara I, et al. A programmable dual-RNA-guided DNA endonuclease in adaptive bacterial immunity. Science 2012;337(6096):816–21.
18. Mali P, Yang L, Esvelt KM, et al. RNA-guided human genome engineering via Cas9. Science 2013;339(6121):823–6.
19. Pellagatti A, Dolatshad H, Yip BH, et al. Application of genome editing technol-ogies to the study and treatment of hematological disease. Adv Biol Regul 2016; 60:122–34.
20. Hacein-Bey-Abina S, Pai SY, Gaspar HB, et al. A modified gamma-retrovirus vector for X-linked severe combined immunodeficiency. N Engl J Med 2014; 371(15):1407–17.
21. Milone MC, O'Doherty U. Clinical use of lentiviral vectors. Leukemia 2018;32(7): 1529–41.
22. Zufferey R, Dull T, Mandel RJ, et al. Self-inactivating lentivirus vector for safe and efficient in vivo gene delivery. J Virol 1998;72(12):9873–80.
23. Choulika A, Perrin A, Dujon B, et al. Induction of homologous recombination in mammalian chromosomes by using the I-SceI system of Saccharomyces cere-visiae. Mol Cell Biol 1995;15(4):1968–73.
24. Porteus MH, Baltimore D. Chimeric nucleases stimulate gene targeting in human cells. Science 2003;300(5620):763.
25. Rouet P, Smih F, Jasin M. Expression of a site-specific endonuclease stimulates homologous recombination in mammalian cells. Proc Natl Acad Sci U S A 1994; 91(13):6064–8.
26. Smithies O, Gregg RG, Boggs SS, et al. Insertion of DNA sequences into the hu-man chromosomal beta-globin locus by homologous recombination. Nature 1985;317(6034):230–4.
27. Delmonte OM, Schuetz C, Notarangelo LD. RAG Deficiency: Two Genes, Many Diseases. J Clin Immunol 2018;38(6):646–55.
28. Delmonte OM, Villa A, Notarangelo LD. Immune dysregulation in patients with RAG deficiency and other forms of combined immune deficiency. Blood 2020; 135(9):610–9.
29. Notarangelo LD, Kim MS, Walter JE, et al. Human RAG mutations: biochemistry and clinical implications. Nat Rev Immunol 2016;16(4):234–46.
30. Carroll D. Genome engineering with targetable nucleases. Annu Rev Biochem 2014;83:409–39.
31. Bibikova M, Beumer K, Trautman JK, et al. Enhancing gene targeting with de-signed zinc finger nucleases. Science 2003;300(5620):764.
32. Porteus MH, Carroll D. Gene targeting using zinc finger nucleases. Nat Bio-technol 2005;23(8):967–73.
33. Urnov FD, Miller JC, Lee YL, et al. Highly efficient endogenous human gene correction using designed zinc-finger nucleases. Nature 2005;435(7042): 646–51.
34. Kim YG, Cha J, Chandrasegaran S. Hybrid restriction enzymes: zinc finger fu-sions to Fok I cleavage domain. Proc Natl Acad Sci U S A 1996;93(3):1156–60.
35. Bogdanove AJ, Voytas DF. TAL effectors: customizable proteins for DNA target-ing. Science 2011;333(6051):1843–6.
36. Miller JC, Tan S, Qiao G, et al. A TALE nuclease architecture for efficient genome editing. Nat Biotechnol 2011;29(2):143–8.

37. Shi X, Shou J, Mehryar MM, et al. Cas9 has no exonuclease activity resulting in staggered cleavage with overhangs and predictable di- and tri-nucleotide CRISPR insertions without template donor. Cell Discov 2019;5:53.

38. Allen F, Crepaldi L, Alsinet C, et al. Predicting the mutations generated by repair of Cas9-induced double-strand breaks. Nat Biotechnol 2018. https://doi.org/10.1038/nbt.4317.

39. Shen MW, Arbab M, Hsu JY, et al. Predictable and precise template-free CRISPR editing of pathogenic variants. Nature 2018;563(7733):646–51.

40. Yeh CD, Richardson CD, Corn JE. Advances in genome editing through control of DNA repair pathways. Nat Cell Biol 2019;21(12):1468–78.

41. Jasin M, Rothstein R. Repair of strand breaks by homologous recombination. Cold Spring Harb Perspect Biol 2013;5(11):a012740.

42. Romero Z, Lomova A, Said S, et al. Editing the Sickle Cell Disease Mutation in Human Hematopoietic Stem Cells: Comparison of Endonucleases and Homologous Donor Templates. Mol Ther 2019;27(8):1389–406.

43. DeWitt MA, Magis W, Bray NL, et al. Selection-free genome editing of the sickle mutation in human adult hematopoietic stem/progenitor cells. Sci Transl Med 2016;8(360):360ra134.

44. Pattabhi S, Lotti SN, Berger MP, et al. In Vivo Outcome of Homology-Directed Repair at the HBB Gene in HSC Using Alternative Donor Template Delivery Methods. Mol Ther Nucleic Acids 2019;17:277–88.

45. Voit RA, Hendel A, Pruett-Miller SM, et al. Nuclease-mediated gene editing by homologous recombination of the human globin locus. Nucleic Acids Res 2014;42(2):1365–78.

46. Lattanzi A, Camarena J, Lahiri P, et al. Development of β-globin gene correction in human hematopoietic stem cells as a potential durable treatment for sickle cell disease. Sci Transl Med 2021;13(598):eabf2444.

47. De Ravin SS, Li L, Wu X, et al. CRISPR-Cas9 gene repair of hematopoietic stem cells from patients with X-linked chronic granulomatous disease. Sci Transl Med 2017;9(372):eaah3480.

48. Shou J, Li J, Liu Y, et al. Precise and Predictable CRISPR Chromosomal Rearrangements Reveal Principles of Cas9-Mediated Nucleotide Insertion. Mol Cell 2018;71(4):498–509.e494.

49. Chakrabarti AM, Henser-Brownhill T, Monserrat J, et al. Target-Specific Precision of CRISPR-Mediated Genome Editing. Mol Cell 2019;73(4):699–713.e696.

50. Schep R, Brinkman EK, Leemans C, et al. Impact of chromatin context on Cas9-induced DNA double-strand break repair pathway balance. Mol Cell 2021;81(10):2216–30.e2210.

51. Clouaire T, Legube G. A snapshot on the cis chromatin response to DNA double-strand breaks. Trends Genet 2019;35(5):330–45.

52. Komor AC, Kim YB, Packer MS, et al. Programmable editing of a target base in genomic DNA without double-stranded DNA cleavage. Nature 2016;533(7603):420–4.

53. Rees HA, Liu DR. Base editing: precision chemistry on the genome and transcriptome of living cells. Nat Rev Genet 2018;19(12):770–88.

54. Sakata RC, Ishiguro S, Mori H, et al. Base editors for simultaneous introduction of C-to-T and A-to-G mutations. Nat Biotechnol 2020;38(7):865–9.

55. Urnov FD. Prime Time for Genome Editing? N Engl J Med 2020;382(5):481–4.

56. Anzalone AV, Randolph PB, Davis JR, et al. Search-and-replace genome editing without double-strand breaks or donor DNA. Nature 2019;576(7785):149–57.

57. Sharon E, Chen SA, Khosla NM, et al. Functional Genetic Variants Revealed by Massively Parallel Precise Genome Editing. Cell 2018;175(2):544–57.e516.
58. Liang P, Ding C, Sun H, et al. Correction of β-thalassemia mutant by base editor in human embryos. Protein Cell 2017;8(11):811–22.
59. Zeng J, Wu Y, Ren C, et al. Therapeutic base editing of human hematopoietic stem cells. Nat Med 2020;26(4):535–41.
60. Bauer DE, Kamran SC, Lessard S, et al. An erythroid enhancer of BCL11 subject to genetic variation determines fetal hemoglobin level. Science 2013;342(6155): 253–7.
61. Bjurström CF, Mojadidi M, Phillips J, et al. Reactivating Fetal Hemoglobin Expression in Human Adult Erythroblasts Through BCL11A Knockdown Using Targeted Endonucleases. Mol Ther Nucleic Acids 2016;5(8):e351.
62. Gaudelli NM, Komor AC, Rees HA, et al. Programmable base editing of A•T to G•C in genomic DNA without DNA cleavage. Nature 2017;551(7681):464–71.
63. Koblan LW, Doman JL, Wilson C, et al. Improving cytidine and adenine base editors by expression optimization and ancestral reconstruction. Nat Biotechnol 2018;36(9):843–6.
64. Zafra MP, Schatoff EM, Katti A, et al. Optimized base editors enable efficient editing in cells, organoids and mice. Nat Biotechnol 2018;36(9):888–93.
65. Métais JY, Doerfler PA, Mayuranathan T, et al. Genome editing of HBG1 and HBG2 to induce fetal hemoglobin. Blood Adv 2019;3(21):3379–92.
66. Jeong YK, Song B, Bae S. Current Status and Challenges of DNA Base Editing Tools. Mol Ther 2020;28(9):1938–52.
67. Kim YB, Komor AC, Levy JM, et al. Increasing the genome-targeting scope and precision of base editing with engineered Cas9-cytidine deaminase fusions. Nat Biotechnol 2017;35(4):371–6.
68. Komor AC, Zhao KT, Packer MS, et al. Improved base excision repair inhibition and bacteriophage Mu Gam protein yields C:G-to-T:A base editors with higher efficiency and product purity. Sci Adv 2017;3(8):eaao4774.
69. Wang J, Exline CM, DeClercq JJ, et al. Homology-driven genome editing in hematopoietic stem and progenitor cells using ZFN mRNA and AAV6 donors. Nat Biotechnol 2015;33(12):1256–63.
70. Bak RO, Dever DP, Porteus MH. CRISPR/Cas9 genome editing in human hematopoietic stem cells. Nat Protoc 2018;13(2):358–76.
71. Beerman I, Seita J, Inlay MA, et al. Quiescent hematopoietic stem cells accumulate DNA damage during aging that is repaired upon entry into cell cycle. Cell Stem Cell 2014;15(1):37–50.
72. Schiroli G, Conti A, Ferrari S, et al. Precise Gene Editing Preserves Hematopoietic Stem Cell Function following Transient p53-Mediated DNA Damage Response. Cell Stem Cell 2019;24(4):551–65.e558.
73. Charlesworth CT, Camarena J, Cromer MK, et al. Priming Human Repopulating Hematopoietic Stem and Progenitor Cells for Cas9/sgRNA Gene Targeting. Mol Ther Nucleic Acids 2018;12:89–104.
74. Ferrari S, Jacob A, Beretta S, et al. Efficient gene editing of human long-term hematopoietic stem cells validated by clonal tracking. Nat Biotechnol 2020; 38(11):1298–308.
75. Boitano AE, Wang J, Romeo R, et al. Aryl hydrocarbon receptor antagonists promote the expansion of human hematopoietic stem cells. Science 2010; 329(5997):1345–8.
76. Pavel-Dinu M, Wiebking V, Dejene BT, et al. Gene correction for SCID-X1 in long-term hematopoietic stem cells. Nat Commun 2019;10(1):1634.

77. Essers MA, Offner S, Blanco-Bose WE, et al. IFNalpha activates dormant hae-matopoietic stem cells in vivo. Nature 2009;458(7240):904–8.

78. Liu J, Guo YM, Hirokawa M, et al. A synthetic double-stranded RNA, poly I:C, induces a rapid apoptosis of human CD34(+) cells. Exp Hematol 2012;40(4): 330–41.

79. Piras F, Kajaste-Rudnitski A. Antiviral immunity and nucleic acid sensing in hae-matopoietic stem cell gene engineering. Gene Ther 2021;28(1–2):16–28.

80. Sato T, Onai N, Yoshihara H, et al. Interferon regulatory factor-2 protects quies-cent hematopoietic stem cells from type I interferon-dependent exhaustion. Nat Med 2009;15(6):696–700.

81. Hendel A, Bak RO, Clark JT, et al. Chemically modified guide RNAs enhance CRISPR-Cas genome editing in human primary cells. Nat Biotechnol 2015; 33(9):985–9.

82. Vakulskas CA, Dever DP, Rettig GR, et al. A high-fidelity Cas9 mutant delivered as a ribonucleoprotein complex enables efficient gene editing in human he-matopoietic stem and progenitor cells. Nat Med 2018;24(8):1216–24.

83. Cromer MK, Vaidyanathan S, Ryan DE, et al. Global Transcriptional Response to CRISPR/Cas9-AAV6-Based Genome Editing in CD34(+) Hematopoietic Stem and Progenitor Cells. Mol Ther 2018;26(10):2431–42.

84. De Ravin SS, Brault J, Meis RJ, et al. Enhanced homology-directed repair for highly efficient gene editing in hematopoietic stem/progenitor cells. Blood 2021;137(19):2598–608.

85. Joglekar AV, Hollis RP, Kuftinec G, et al. Integrase-defective lentiviral vectors as a delivery platform for targeted modification of adenosine deaminase locus. Mol Ther 2013;21(9):1705–17.

86. Banasik MB, McCray PB Jr. Integrase-defective lentiviral vectors: progress and applications. Gene Ther 2010;17(2):150–7.

87. Genovese P, Schiroli G, Escobar G, et al. Targeted genome editing in human re-populating haematopoietic stem cells. Nature 2014;510(7504):235–40.

88. Hoban MD, Cost GJ, Mendel MC, et al. Correction of the sickle cell disease mu-tation in human hematopoietic stem/progenitor cells. Blood 2015;125(17): 2597–604.

89. Hirsch ML. Adeno-associated virus inverted terminal repeats stimulate gene ed-iting. Gene Ther 2015;22(2):190–5.

90. Schiroli G, Ferrari S, Conway A, et al. Preclinical modeling highlights the thera-peutic potential of hematopoietic stem cell gene editing for correction of SCID-X1. Sci Transl Med 2017;9(411):eaan0820.

91. Sweeney CL, Pavel-Dinu M, Choi U, et al. Correction of X-CGD patient HSPCs by targeted CYBB cDNA insertion using CRISPR/Cas9 with 53BP1 inhibition for enhanced homology-directed repair. Gene Ther 2021;28(6):373–90.

92. Hubbard N, Hagin D, Sommer K, et al. Targeted gene editing restores regulated CD40L function in X-linked hyper-IgM syndrome. Blood 2016;127(21):2513–22.

93. Kuo CY, Long JD, Campo-Fernandez B, et al. Site-Specific Gene Editing of Hu-man Hematopoietic Stem Cells for X-Linked Hyper-IgM Syndrome. Cell Rep 2018;23(9):2606–16.

94. Vavassori V, Mercuri E, Marcovecchio GE, et al. Modeling, optimization, and comparable efficacy of T cell and hematopoietic stem cell gene editing for treat-ing hyper-IgM syndrome. EMBO Mol Med 2021;13(3):e13545.

95. Rai R, Romito M, Rivers E, et al. Targeted gene correction of human hematopoi-etic stem cells for the treatment of Wiskott - Aldrich Syndrome. Nat Commun 2020;11(1):4034.

96. Gray DH, Villegas I, Long J, et al. Optimizing Integration and Expression of Transgenic Bruton's Tyrosine Kinase for CRISPR-Cas9-Mediated Gene Editing of X-Linked Agammaglobulinemia. CRISPR J 2021;4(2):191–206.
97. Gardner CL, Pavel-Dinu M, Dobbs K, et al. Gene Editing Rescues In vitro T Cell Development of RAG2-Deficient Induced Pluripotent Stem Cells in an Artificial Thymic Organoid System. J Clin Immunol 2021;41(5):852–62.
98. Dever DP, Bak RO, Reinisch A, et al. CRISPR/Cas9 β-globin gene targeting in human haematopoietic stem cells. Nature 2016;539(7629):384–9.
99. Cromer MK, Camarena J, Martin RM, et al. Gene replacement of α-globin with β-globin restores hemoglobin balance in β-thalassemia-derived hematopoietic stem and progenitor cells. Nat Med 2021;27(4):677–87.
100. Kalhor R, Kalhor K, Mejia L, et al. Developmental barcoding of whole mouse via homing CRISPR. Science 2018;361(6405):eaat9804.
101. McKenna A, Findlay GM, Gagnon JA, et al. Whole-organism lineage tracing by combinatorial and cumulative genome editing. Science 2016;353(6298): aaf7907.
102. Román-Rodríguez FJ, Ugalde L, Álvarez L, et al. NHEJ-Mediated Repair of CRISPR-Cas9-Induced DNA Breaks Efficiently Corrects Mutations in HSPCs from Patients with Fanconi Anemia. Cell Stem Cell 2019;25(5):607–21.e607.
103. Demirci S, Zeng J, Wu Y, et al. BCL11A enhancer-edited hematopoietic stem cells persist in rhesus monkeys without toxicity. J Clin Invest 2020;130(12): 6677–87.
104. Sharma R, Dever DP, Lee CM, et al. The TRACE-Seq method tracks recombination alleles and identifies clonal reconstitution dynamics of gene targeted human hematopoietic stem cells. Nat Commun 2021;12(1):472.
105. Doulatov S, Notta F, Laurenti E, et al. Hematopoiesis: a human perspective. Cell Stem Cell 2012;10(2):120–36.
106. Brendel C, Rio P, Verhoeyen E. Humanized mice are precious tools for evaluation of hematopoietic gene therapies and preclinical modeling to move towards a clinical trial. Biochem Pharmacol 2020;174:113711.
107. Wu Y, Zeng J, Roscoe BP, et al. Highly efficient therapeutic gene editing of human hematopoietic stem cells. Nat Med 2019;25(5):776–83.
108. Xu S, Luk K, Yao Q, et al. Editing aberrant splice sites efficiently restores β-globin expression in β-thalassemia. Blood 2019;133(21):2255–62.
109. Frangoul H, Altshuler D, Cappellini MD, et al. CRISPR-Cas9 Gene Editing for Sickle Cell Disease and β-Thalassemia. N Engl J Med 2021;384(3):252–60.
110. Frangoul H, Bobruff Y, Cappellini MD, et al. Safety and Efficacy of CTX001 in Patients with Transfusion-Dependent β-Thalassemia and Sickle Cell Disease: Early Results from the Climb THAL-111 and Climb SCD-121 Studies of Autologous CRISPR-CAS9-Modified CD34+ Hematopoietic Stem and Progenitor Cells. Blood 2020;136(Supplement 1):3–4.

Adeno-Associated Virus Vector Design–Moving the Adeno-Associated Virus to a Bioengineered Therapeutic Nanoparticle

Nico Jäschke, PhD[a], Hildegard Büning, PhD[a,b,c,*]

KEYWORDS

- Adeno-associated virus (AAV) vectors • Gene therapy • Gene transfer
- Vector genome engineering • Capsid engineering

KEY POINTS

- Gene therapy is becoming an integral part of modern medicine.
- While initiated to offer a treatment of monogenic diseases, gene therapy is reaching far beyond offering now also novel treatment strategies in oncology or infectious diseases to name a few examples.
- The success of gene therapy depends on efficient and safe gene delivery tools.
- Vectors based on the adeno-associated virus (AAV) are the most frequently applied delivery tools for *in vivo* gene therapy.
- Vector engineering is applied to improve the efficacy of first-generation AAV vectors.

INTRODUCTION

Recently, the field has acknowledged the 31st anniversary of the first human gene therapy in which Michael Blaese and colleagues[1] reinfused autologous T lymphocytes modified to contain a functional copy of the adenosine deaminase (*ADA*) gene to patients suffering from ADA-severe combined immunodeficiency (ADA-SCID). This first and all subsequent human clinical trials were inspired by the idea of a gene therapy offering the possibility to treating a disease at "its genetic roots."[2] Gene therapy

[a] Institute of Experimental Hematology, Hannover Medical School, Carl-Neuberg-Str.1, Hannover 30625, Germany; [b] REBIRTH Research Center for Translational Regenerative Medicine, Hannover Medical School, Carl-Neuberg-Str.1, Hannover 30625, Germany; [c] German Center for Infection Research, Partner Site Hannover-Braunschweig
* Corresponding author. Hildegard Büning, Institute of Experimental Hematology, Hannover Medical School, Carl-Neuberg-Str. 1, Hannover 30625, Germany.
E-mail address: buening.hildegard@mh-hannover.de

Hematol Oncol Clin N Am 36 (2022) 667–685
https://doi.org/10.1016/j.hoc.2022.04.002
0889-8588/22/© 2022 Elsevier Inc. All rights reserved.
hemonc.theclinics.com

strategies were initially restricted to providing a functional copy of the malfunctioning or missing gene, or to silencing the expression of a distinct gene. As technologies have advanced, new options are becoming available. Specifically, newly developed gene-editing techniques are making it possible to repair genetic defects directly.

Gene therapy has impacted modern medicine far beyond monogenic diseases, its initial target, as through gene therapy and its accompanied technological advancements innovative treatment strategies became available for example, also in oncology, infectious disease, and vaccine development. In the Western World, gene therapy left its childhood and entered clinical reality in 2012 when the European Medicines Agency (EMA) granted the first market authorization for a gene therapy.[3] This first drug was designed as local *in vivo* gene therapy delivering a gain-of-function variant of the lipoprotein lipase (*LPL*) gene to muscle cells for the treatment of LPL deficiency, an ultra-rare monogenic disease.[4] The list of approved drugs is constantly growing, encompassing *ex vivo* gene therapies targeting autologous hematopoietic stem cells to treat monogenic disease (ADA-SCID, β-Thalassemia, metachromatic leukodystrophy, early cerebral adrenoleukodystrophy) or autologous T lymphocytes in cancer immunotherapy (Chimeric antigen receptor (CAR) T cells in CD19+ leukemias and B cell maturation antigen-positive Multiple Myeloma, respectively) as well as additional *in vivo* gene therapies (RPE65-related Leber congenital amaurosis, spinal muscular atrophy type 1 (SMA1), melanoma). All *in vivo* gene therapies for the treatment of monogenic diseases receiving market authorization by EMA (as well as the US Food & Drug Administration (FDA)) are using the same delivery vehicle, adeno-associated virus (AAV) vectors. Indeed, AAV vectors have become the most frequently used delivery system for *in vivo* gene therapy with at least 136 unique human clinical trials[5,6] for a total of so far 55 different disease indications mainly from the areas of blood, central nervous system, eye, lysosomal storage, and neuromuscular disorders.[5]

FROM VIRUS TO VECTOR

AAV vectors are derived from AAVs belonging to the genus *Dependoparvovirus* of the *Parvoviridae* family. The first member was discovered in 1965, nearly 57 years ago, as contamination of adenovirus preparations (reviewed in[7]). Since then, the size of this genus is constantly increasing as new serotypes and variants are added, discovered in tissues of various vertebrate species including humans and nonhuman primates and even in "fossils" like the germline of marsupial species to which kangaroos and wallabies belong[8].

AAVs are composed of an icosahedral capsid of approximately 25 nm in diameter protecting and transporting a single-stranded DNA viral genome (**Fig. 1**). The capsid itself is assembled in a 1:1:10 ratio from three viral protein (VP) subunits (VP1, VP2, and VP3).[9] The size of the AAV wild-type genome is approximately 4.7 kb differing slightly in length between serotypes. The left and the right-hand ends of the genome form T-shaped structures, termed inverted terminal repeats (ITRs), protecting the genome from degradation. In addition, the ITRs, which also differ in sequence between serotypes, function as the origin of replication and packaging signals, possess a weak promoter activity, and are required for second-strand synthesis, ie, to convert the single-stranded AAV genome into a DNA double-strand.[10]

So far, 2 viral genes with multiple open reading frames (ORFs) have been identified (see **Fig. 1**A). The *rep* gene is the most 5′ located gene and encodes the Rep proteins. They control viral replication and transcription, are required for viral genome packaging, and for site-specific integration of AAV viral genomes into the host genome,

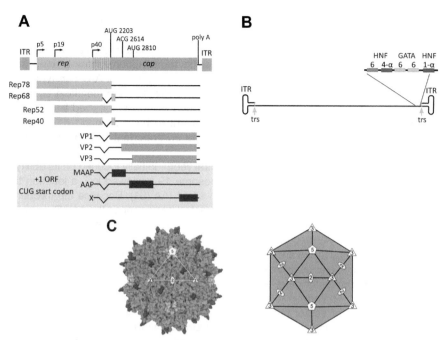

Fig. 1. The wild-type AAV2 genome. Schematic overview of the genome structure (*A*). AAV genome contains two genes with multiple open reading frames (ORFs) flanked by inverted terminal repeats (ITRs). The *rep* gene (*orange*) codes for four nonstructural, multifunctional proteins. Whereas Rep78 and Rep68 are initiated by the p5 promoter, Rep52 and Rep40 are initiated by the p19 promoter. The *cap* gene codes for the capsid proteins VP1, VP2, and VP3 (*green*). All transcripts are started from the p40 promoter and do not differ in length. Three different start codons lead to the expression of VP1 (AUG 2203), VP2 (ACG 2614), or VP3 (AUG 2810) in case of AAV2. The *cap* gene codes for three additional proteins coded by +1 frame shift using the alternative start codon CUG (*gray box*): membrane-associated accessory protein (MAAP), assembly activating protein (AAP), and the X protein (all shown as lilac filled rectangles). All six transcripts use the same poly(A) signal at the end of the *cap* gene. *Details on ITRs and adjacent regions (B).* AAV is a single-stranded DNA virus, whereas ITRs form partial double-stranded structures needed for genome packaging and second-strand synthesis. The terminal resolution sites (trs) are sequence elements necessary for the cleavage of AAV genome for DNA replication. Adjacent to the right-handed ITR, several transcription factor binding sites (TFBS) are located. One copy of TFBS for hepatocyte nuclear factor (HNF) 1-α (*pink*), 4-α (*red*), and 6 (*gray*) and two copies of GATA6 (*green*) binding site are depicted. *Structure of AAV capsid (C).* *Left*: 3D model of AAV (PDB ID 1LP3) with annotated 5-fold symmetry axis (*orange*) and 3-fold symmetry axis formed by highest (*red*) and second highest (*blue*) peak of capsid.[106] *Right*: schematic view of AAV capsid with 2-, 3-, and 5-fold axis shown.

a unique feature of AAV (reviewed in[11]). The second gene, *cap*, encodes the capsid proteins (viral protein (VP)1-VP3) and at least 3 further nonstructural proteins, namely the assembly activating protein (AAP),[12] the membrane-associated accessory protein (MAAP),[13] and the X protein.[14] While X protein is presumably involved in viral replication,[14] AAP transports newly synthesized VP proteins to the nucleus[12,15] and promotes capsid assembly of most serotypes.[16] AAP independent capsid assembly was so far reported for AAV4, AAV5 and AAV11 [16]. The function of MAAP is not fully understood. It seems to facilitate viral progeny production and egress from host cells[10,17] and is involved in viral genome packaging as well as in destabilizing VP proteins and capsids.[10]

The sequence that follows the *cap* gene downstream has attracted attention as this sequence contains multiple hepatocyte-specific transcription factor binding sites (TFBS) (see **Fig. 1**B).[18] When aligning the wild-type sequence of AAV serotypes 1 to 7, TFBS for hepatocyte nuclear factor (HNF)6 and HNF4α were identified upstream of a GATA6 sequence, which in case of AAV2 and AAV3B is followed by a second GATA6 and an HNF1α TFBS immediately adjacent to the right-hand ITR.[18] Based on these findings, liver might be considered as an important host organ for wild-type AAV.[18]

The interest for developing AAV toward a viral vector initially focused on its ability to integrate site-specifically into human chromosome 19 (reviewed in[7]), a location that has, therefore, been named AAV integration site 1 (AAVS1). Because the frequency of AAVS1 integration is lower than initially expected and because the AAV Rep protein (Rep78) required to mediate that integration would occupy half of the vector genome coding sequence, AAV vector design quickly changed to the "gut-less concept" (**Fig. 2**). Thus, all viral ORFs are replaced by the gene sequence of interest. The latter is either a transgene expression cassette including promoter/enhancer and poly(A) sequences or a template for gene editing. The gene of interest (GOI) is flanked at both ends by the ITRs. Analogous to the virus, ITRs in AAV vector genomes are required for the replication of vector genomes and as packaging signals for encapsidation, both in vector production, and for second-strand synthesis in cell transduction. Further attractive features that fostered the development of AAV vectors are that the parental virus is considered nonpathogenic and has even been associated with tumor-protective activities.[19–21] This view has been challenged by the detection of wild-type AAV genome fragments (small parts of the 3' genomic region including parts of the ITRs) in a few hepatocellular carcinomas (HCC) of unknown etiologies.[22,23]

AAVs are noninflammatory,[24] remain infectious over a broad pH and temperature range, and survive multiple rounds of thaw–freezing and even lyophilization.[25] Furthermore, AAVs depend on helper viruses such as adenovirus or members of the herpes virus family for efficient replication (reviewed in[26]). This feature adds to vector safety as

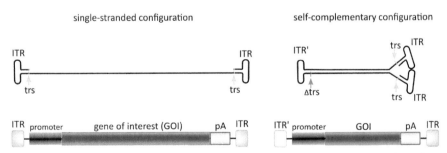

Fig. 2. AAV vector genome configurations. In the AAV vector genome *rep* and *cap* have been removed, while the ITRs are maintained to serve as the origin of replication, as primers for second-strand synthesis, and as packaging signals. The viral genes are replaced by a transgene expression cassette. A promoter sequence (*filled black rectangle*) of choice and a gene sequence of interest (*filled red rectangle*) with a strong poly(A) signal (*filled light lilac rectangle*) flanked by ITRs with a length of approximately 5 kb can be packaged by conventional single-stranded AAV vectors (*left*) or of 2.5 kb when using the self-complementary genome configuration (*right*). Self-complementary genomes can be created by destroying one of the trs motifs (Δtrs).

vector mobilization following gene therapy is likely impossible. However, it adds an additional step to the complexity of AAV vector production as either a helper virus or respectively helper virus proteins need to be present during vector production.[27]

There are also several disadvantages. The cargo capacity, ie, the length of the vector genome that can be transported by AAV vectors, is with 5 kb quite limited.[28] In addition, as humans get frequently infected by AAVs in childhood (together with an adenovirus infection)[29] seroprevalence at least for certain AAV serotypes is high with values close to 70% for AAV1 and AAV2 (reviewed in[30]). In addition, high vector doses are required to achieve therapeutic effects in patients, partly due to the broad tropism of AAV resulting in loss of vector particles to off-target cell types and partly due to the low efficacy of first-generation AAV vectors as indicated by the high particle-per-cell ratios that must be applied to achieve transduction (reviewed in[31]). The high vector doses (eg, $1.1 \times 10e14$ AAV particles per kg body weight for Zolgensma, the AAV9 vector-based gene therapy for the treatment of SMA1) pose a challenge to the patients' immune system and also for vector manufacturing (reviewed in[32]). Consequently, both vector genomes and capsids have become the targets of engineering to increase efficacy, lower the risk of off-target transduction, and tackle the issue of preexisting immunity.

ENGINEERING VECTOR GENOMES TO IMPROVE EFFICACY, CARGO CAPACITY, AND FATE

According to Au and colleagues,[5] 129 of the 136 human clinical trials use AAV vectors with the natural genome conformation, that is, a single-stranded DNA genome with 2 ITRs (see **Fig. 2**). Since AAV2 was the first serotype to be vectorized, vector genomes commonly possess AAV2-derived ITRs. If AAV2 Rep proteins are provided during vector production, AAV2-ITR flanked vector genomes can be packaged into capsids of serotypes other than AAV2 (and of engineered capsids) enabling an easy switch between serotypes.[33]

The first AAV plasmid, pSUB201, cloned by Jude Samulski, contains 2 identical ITRs, because the right-hand ITR was duplicated and substituted for the wild-type left-hand ITR.[7,18] In this process also the HNF1α TFBS adjacent to the left-hand ITR was relocated. Consequently, pSUB201 plasmid-derived AAV vector genomes in which these 49-nucleotide sequences were maintained are prone to show promoter or enhancer activity in liver tissue, explaining off-target activities with tissue-specific promoters or promoter-less constructs.[18]

Once delivered to the cell nucleus and released from the viral capsid (uncoating), single-stranded AAV vector genomes must be converted to a double-stranded DNA genome to enable transcription. *Dependoparvoviridae* (in contrast to autonomous parvoviruses) package both sense and antisense viral genomes; therefore, both orientations are delivered and might form a DNA double-strand by interstrand hybridization (reviewed in[34]). In general, though, second-strand synthesis is required, a step identified as rate-limiting and sometimes even as a barrier toward transduction. To overcome this limitation, an artificial vector genome configuration was developed (reviewed in[35]). Specifically, by inhibiting the function of one of the two ITRs in genome replication, a vector genome is produced that contains the sense and the antisense sequence separated by an additional ITR as a single molecule (see **Fig. 2**). These so-called self-complementary AAV vector genomes are packaged as single-stranded DNA into the preformed AAV capsids on vector production. Then, once released from the capsids, they form the transcriptionally active double-stranded DNA by intramolecular hybridization which is an immediate template for transcription.

Expression from self-complementary AAV vectors occurs sooner and at higher level compared with conventional AAV vectors and enabled the transduction of cell types unable to perform second-strand synthesis (reviewed in[35]). The downside of self-complementary AAV vectors is the reduction of the cargo capacity by half. The additional ITR might also result in a higher immunogenicity[36] and the impaired ITR function in replication might be responsible for the significantly higher levels of non-AAV vector genome sequences detected in self-complementary compared with conventional single-stranded AAV vector productions.[37] Nevertheless, the increase in efficacy argued for using self-complementary vector genomes in human clinical trials with their first application in 2010 as self-complementary AAV8 vectors encoding for factor IX in a liver-directed hemophilia B trial.[38] The AAV9 vectors encoding for survival motor neuron 1 (SMN1), the approved gene therapy to treat infants with SMA1, is using this vector genome design (reviewed in[34]).

The meta-analysis by Au and colleagues[5] also revealed that only 27 different promoters are in clinical use, with half of them being the cytomegalovirus (CMV), the chicken beta-actin (CBA), or the so-called CAG promoter. The latter combines a CMV enhancer and CBA promoter with a β-globin intron sequence from rabbit. These are strong ubiquitous promoters enabling high transcriptional activity in various tissues (**Fig. 3**). As virus-derived promoters are prone to being silenced, host-derived promoters such as elongation factor 1 alpha (EF1α) are used, albeit at the expense of lower transcriptional activity. In cases whereby transgene expression should be restricted, tissue-specific promoters are used. An example is the liver-specific promoter used in the above-mentioned hemophilia B trial.[38] A novel avenue that is followed to improve efficacy and selectivity of transgene expression is *in silico* design. VandenDriessche, Chuah, and colleagues pioneered this strategy which is based on identifying tissue-specific transcription *cis*-regulatory modules, which are then newly combined and added to a tissue-specific promoter. Thereby, a 10 to 100-fold increase in liver-specific promoter activity[39] and up to a 400-fold increase in muscle-specific gene transcription[40] were achieved, revealing the potency of this strategy.

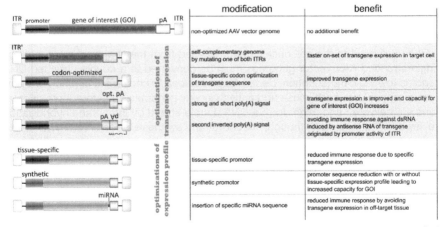

Fig. 3. Engineering AAV vector genomes. Modifications to the AAV genome and their possible benefits to vector efficacy are depicted. All modifications can be applied separately or in combination.

Besides promoter/enhancer regions, the transgene expression cassette itself can be optimized to increase transgene production (see **Fig. 3**). The most successful strategy in this regard is codon-optimization, which is based on the observation that the concentration of distinct tRNAs varies between species, tissues, and cell types (reviewed in[34]). Inclusion of WPRE or other posttranscriptional regulatory elements further impacts on efficiency,[41] while the inclusion of microRNA targeting sites has been used to avoid expression in off-target cell types.[42] Inclusion of miR-142 and miR-652 binding sites into the AAV vector genomes to avoid transgene expression in antigen-presenting cells resulted for example, in higher transgene expression levels in muscle (the target tissue of that study), inhibited antibody response against the transgene, and reduced cytotoxic T lymphocyte activation.[43] Finally, as the cargo capacity of AAV vectors is limited, choosing a small but effective poly(A) sequence is advised. Adding a second inverted poly(A) might reduce immune responses as reviewed in.[34]

The cargo capacity of single-stranded AAV vectors is limited to approximately 5 kb. Self-complementary AAV vectors transport vector genomes of the same size, but since they contain sense and antisense sequences separated by the nonfunctional ITR, the coding capacity is reduced by half. This size constraint limits the usage of AAV vectors as a number of therapeutic genes are substantially larger, with the dystrophin gene being one extreme example.[28] In addition, the use of AAV vectors in gene editing is difficult due to the size of the designer nucleases, particularly when aiming for homologous DNA repair. In response, dual or triple vector approaches are performed in which each of the vectors is delivering part of the cargo. In an excellent review, Tornabene and Tranpani describe how intracellular reconstruction of large genes delivered by separate vectors is achieved by trans-splicing, overlapping or hybrid approaches.[28] Further strategies use mRNA trans-splicing or even protein trans-splicing (reviewed in[28]).

AAV vectors are considered a nonintegrating delivery system. On vector uncoating, AAV genomes form episomes which persist in the nucleus commonly as higher order concatemers.[44] In slowly or nonproliferating cell types, stable and long-term transgene expression is achieved. However, in proliferating cells, transgene expression levels decrease quickly as the number of episomes per cell is reduced with every cell division. In an attempt to overcome this limitation without the need to integrate AAV vector genomes into the host cell, scaffold matrix attachment region (S/MAR) elements, which serve as autonomous replication units, have been included in AAV vector genomes and indeed resulted in long-term transgene expression in proliferating cells from AAV episomes.[45]

ENGINEERING THE CAPSID TO IMPROVE EFFICACY AND SELECTIVITY

As mentioned, the three capsid proteins VP1–VP3 are encoded by the *cap* gene. They are transcribed from a single mRNA and share most of their amino acids[46] (see **Fig. 1**). The minor capsid protein VP1 is the largest of the three capsid proteins with a unique sequence of 137 amino acids at its N-terminus (VP1 unique), followed by 65 amino acids shared with the second minor capsid protein VP2 (information relates to AAV2).[47] The remaining 533 amino acids are shared by all three VPs.[47] These common VP3 regions are the building blocks of the capsid, while the N-termini of VP2 and VP1 are directed toward the capsid interior on capsid assembly. During cell infection or transduction these N-termini are externalized through "channel-like structures" or pores at the 5-fold symmetry axis of the viral capsid (see **Fig. 1C**). These pores also serve as entry sites for viral/vector genomes during virus and vector production, whereby genomes are forced into the preassembled capsids by the viral Rep proteins. Other prominent structures are protrusions at the 3-fold symmetry axis which contain cell attachment and receptor binding sites and are targets of the humoral immune system (reviewed in[48]) (see **Fig. 1**C).

AAV infection, like AAV vector transduction, is initiated by the attachment of the viral capsid to cell surface proteoglycans (reviewed in[49]). This initial binding might be stabilized by interactions with coreceptors and is followed by vector entry mediated by internalization receptors (reviewed in[49]). As AAV serotypes differ in receptors used for cell attachment and/or internalization, serotypes differ in tropism, ie, in cell types they transduce preferentially (reviewed in[11]). Receptor-mediated endocytosis through clathrin-coated pits is considered the main cell entry route, although other routes are used and might be preferred depending on the target cell type.[50,51]

Once AAV vectors enter the endosomal system, vectors are transported toward the nucleus along the cytoskeleton network of the cell (reviewed in[52]). Interestingly, vector-containing endosomes have been reported to be transported faster than other vesicles.[53] On maturation, the pH of endosomal vesicles is lowered, a step that triggers a conformational change in the AAV capsid structure and results in the already mentioned externalization of the N-termini of VP2 and VP1.[54] This is an energy-consuming step as the N-termini must unfold to pass through the pores.[55] The N-termini contain domains with distinct functions, such as the phospholipase A2 domain within the unique VP1 region or basic regions in VP1 and VP2 that function as nuclear localization signals (NLS).[56–58] Additional changes to the capsid might prime the capsid for uncoating.[59] AAV vectors are released from the endosomal compartment through pores formed by the inherent phospholipase activity of VP1 and further guided to the nucleus via the NLS.[56-58]

By gene trapping, Pillay and colleagues[60] identified the adeno-associated virus receptor (AAVR), a transmembrane protein involved in retrograde transport to the trans-Golgi network, as an essential host factor for AAV1, AAV2, AAV3b, AAV5, AAV6, AAV8, and AAV9. The interaction of AAV with AAVR, which interestingly occurs in a serotype-specific manner with distinct parts of AAVR, is required for proper intracellular trafficking of the particles.[61] GPR108 is another recently described essential host factor.[62] GPR108 is present in late endosomes and the trans-Golgi network, acts downstream of AAVR and binds to the N-terminus of VP1, thus following the pH-induced conformational change in the capsid, perhaps supporting endosomal escape and nuclear delivery.[62] So far, details on the precise mechanisms of nuclear delivery are missing. Likewise, it is unclear how vector genomes are released from the capsid. Based on imaging studies using atomic force microscopy, release through pores at the 5-fold symmetry axis is one option, while complete capsid degradation represents the second option.[63] Anyway, AAVs' final destination is the cell nucleus where vector genomes form the above-mentioned episomes.

As the capsid is involved in most of the early steps in cell transduction, engineering of the capsid has emerged as a powerful strategy to improve the host–vector interaction, and thus efficacy and safety of AAV vectors (reviewed in[11,34,64,65]). In principle, two overarching strategies can be distinguished: genetic and nongenetic approaches.

Genetic Capsid Engineering Strategies

About swapping and shuffling

AAV serotypes differ in distinct features including tropism. To combine advantageous features of different serotypes, AAV hybrid vectors were developed in which whole capsid proteins from different serotypes are combined within a single hybrid capsid.[66,67] Besides combining whole capsid proteins anew, domains or surface loops may be swapped, equipping respective capsid variants with new features such as binding to heparan sulfate proteoglycan (HSPG) or improved liver transduction.[68,69] This idea was moved to a higher level by the development of shuffled AAV capsid libraries, which consist of AAV capsid variants with newly combined capsid protein fragments[70] (**Fig. 4**). The shuffling process occurs on the DNA level, whereby

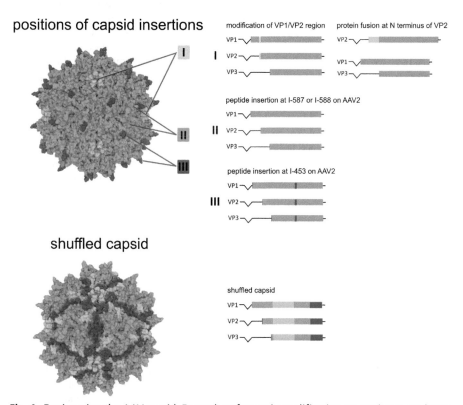

Fig. 4. Engineering the AAV capsid. Examples of genetic modification strategies to engineer AAV capsid properties are depicted, mainly to change the tropism of AAV vectors. Insertions of small sequences close to the VP1 N-terminus are accepted (not shown).[107] Also, insertion within the VP1/VP2 common region resulting in N-terminal fusion to VP2 and display of peptide within VP1 has been explored for targeting.[86,107–109] To restrict the presentation of peptides/proteins as VP2 N-terminal fusion, fusion proteins have to be cloned on a separate plasmid and combined during vector production with a plasmid providing the VP1 and VP3 coding sequence. Insertions at position I-587, I-588, or I-453 are used in AAV peptide display library approaches to select for AAV capsid variants with selective tropism for distinct target cells/tissues (see main text). Depicted structures show the predicted location of VP2 fusion proteins at 5-fold axis (orange (fusion protein not shown)), red marked structures showing I-453 position at highest peak, and the I-587 or I-588 position is shown in blue (both without insertion). Shuffled AAV capsids have shown promise in identifying variants with increased efficacy in transduction and immune escape features (see main text). Both 3D models were generated by using the RCSB structure model of AAV2 (PDB ID 1LP3).[106] Model "positions of capsid insertions" shows regions that are modified: 5-fold axis: fusion proteins to VP2 are externalized through pores (amino acids 324–331 in orange), highest peak at 3-fold axis: peptide insertions at I-453 (amino acids 451–458 in red), and second highest peak at 3-fold axis: peptide insertion at I-587 or I-588 (amino acids 583–590 in blue). Model "shuffled capsid" was colored on amino acids 217 to 439 green and 608 to 735 blue/lilac.

cap genes of different serotypes are enzymatically digested and then reassembled by a primer-less PCR.[70] The newly assembled *cap* gene sequences are cloned into an AAV production plasmid leading thereby to a plasmid library pool. This plasmid pool is used to produce the shuffled AAV capsid library, commonly in HEK293 cells. The library is then screened in multiple rounds in cell culture or *in vivo* for variants with improved transduction efficacy for the respective target cell type. This strategy was first introduced by Grimm and colleagues and has since emerged as one of the most successful strategies to develop new capsids (reviewed in[11,34,64,65]). One of these capsids, AAV-LK03, has entered human clinical trials, being thereby the second capsid-engineered AAV vector that moved from the preclinical toward the clinical trial setting. The pioneer in this regard was AAV2.5 (see later in discussion).[71]

When AAP was identified, concerns were raised that the shuffling process might negatively impact on AAP function. Studies performed by Grimm and colleagues[72] alleviated this concern, showing in a comprehensive study that AAP was not a limiting factor in shuffled AAV capsid library production. As the whole procedure is relying on the presence of related sequences, shuffled AAV capsid libraries suffered from the underrepresentation of *cap* gene fragments derived from more distantly related serotypes or variants. This limitation was overcome by codon optimization, although a new algorithm had to be developed that uses only codons already in use by natural serotypes, rather than relying on the conventional codon-optimization strategy based on tRNA representation.[73]

Minor changes can make huge differences

The first capsid-engineered AAV vector that was applied in a human clinical trial was AAV2.5. AAV2.5 is an AAV2-derived capsid variant containing five capsid amino acids from AAV1.[71] Specifically, four amino acid substitutions (Q263A, N705A, V708A, T716N, amino acid numbering according to AAV2) and one insertion (T265) were introduced into the AAV2 *cap* gene sequence.[71] AAV2.5 showed enhanced transduction of muscle and a reduced sensitivity toward anti-AAV2 and anti-AAV1 antibodies.[71] These features made AAV2.5 an attractive candidate for muscle-directed gene therapy. Thus, AAV2.5 was explored in the phase I clinical trial to transfer a mini-dystrophin gene to patients with Duchenne muscular dystrophy (DMD) via intramuscular injection.[71]

A very successful approach to improve vector efficacy by single amino acid substitutions was inspired by the observation that AAV2 capsids might become ubiquitinated when entering the cytoplasm, a modification that flags capsids for degradation by proteasomes,[74] and that the phosphorylation of capsid tyrosine residues served as a signal for ubiquitination.[74,75] On this background, capsid surface-exposed residues prone to posttranslational modifications were substituted by rational design. Initial studies focused on the AAV2 capsid and tyrosine (Y) residues revealing that changing Y444, Y500, or Y730 to phenylalanine improved transduction efficiency compared with the wild-type AAV2 capsid.[76] Efficacy was further improved by combining amino acid substitutions.[76] Interestingly, the triple-mutant AAV2 vector was shown not only to transduce hepatocytes with higher efficiency but also to reduce adaptive immune responses directed against vector-transduced cells, presumably by the reduced presentation of capsid epitopes to antigen-presenting cells.[77] Subsequently, further predicted targets of phosphorylation and ubiquitination were modified, likewise resulting in significant improvements in transduction efficacy in cell culture and *in vivo*. Specifically, serine and threonine residues were changed to valine and lysine residues to glutamic acid (reviewed in[11]). This strategy also improved the transduction efficacy of serotypes other than AAV2 including AAV3, AAV5, AAV6, and AAV8 (reviewed in[11]).

In the absence of knowledge on the function of distinct capsid amino acid residues, high-throughput selection screens of AAV capsid variants with point mutations introduced by an Error-Prone PCR mutagenesis step can be used. Initially established by Perabo and colleagues[78] and Maheshri and colleagues,[79] such libraries have mainly been used to identify epitopes recognized by neutralizing antibodies and to select for variants that transduce target cells despite the presence of neutralizing antibodies. A different approach was followed by the Vandenberghe group who performed an ancestral sequence reconstruction (ASR) to predict - based on the available *cap* gene sequence information – how an ancestral AAV capsid monomer was likely composed.[80] Thereby, Anc80 was designed, a capsid variant that is a predicted ancestor of AAV1, AAV2, AAV8 and AAV9, and which outperformed natural AAV serotypes in transducing liver, muscle, and retina.[80]

Insertion of peptides or targeting moieties to change vector tropism

Through changing the vector–receptor interaction, vector tropism is modified. In principle, the tropism can be made broader by adding an additional receptor binding motif to the capsid while leaving the natural receptor binding sites untouched, or the tropism can be made specific for a new, customer-defined receptor if the natural receptor–ligand interaction is destroyed and a new receptor-targeting moiety with the desired specificity is introduced into the capsid. As receptor-binding induces an intracellular signaling cascade, a change in the target receptor might also change the intracellular processing of the capsid-modified vector.

Genetic capsid engineering approaches to change vector tropism rely on the insertion of DNA sequences of either receptor binding ligands or structures such as Designed ankyrin repeat proteins (DARPins) or nanobodies specifically recognizing their cognate cell surface molecule into the *cap* gene (reviewed in[11]). The tips of the highest and second-highest protrusion at the 3-fold axis of symmetry (insertion (I) positions I-587, I-588, and I-453 in case of AAV2) as well as the N-terminus of VP1 and VP2 (see **Fig. 4**) can be modified with foreign sequences that enable efficient binding to the new receptor without impairing capsid assembly.

Peptide insertions at I-587 of AAV2 separate two of the main residues (arginine (R) 585, R588) of the HSPG binding motif, which serves as attachment receptor of AAV2. While this depends on the exact sequence and charge of the inserted peptide, capsid variants might obtain HSPG independence and thus rely solely on the newly inserted peptide for cell transduction.[81,82] Similarly, in case of I-588, peptide insertion might impact accessibility toward the HSPG binding motif. When I-453 or the N-termini of VP1 or VP2 are used for capsid engineering, natural receptor binding sites need to be destroyed by site-directed mutagenesis to redirect vector tropism toward the new target receptor.

I-587, I-588, and I-453 are located in the common VP3 region; insertions at those sites thus are present in each of the 60 subunits, enabling the display of 60 receptor binding ligands, providing ample possibilities for the capsid-engineered vectors to bind the cognate receptor. When larger sequences were inserted within the VP3 common region, production of hybrid capsids consisting of unmodified and insert-containing VP proteins showed success.[83-85] Alternatively, larger peptides or whole proteins can be fused to the N-terminus of VP2. This position tolerated even the insertion of proteins that adapt their own 3D structures such as eGFP or luciferase without impairing capsid assembly.[86-88] However, as VP2 is not an essential protein for capsid assembly, capsids containing the fusion protein and VP1/VP3-only capsids will be produced, necessitating a further purification step to deplete the vector preparation of fusion protein-deficient particles.[89,90] The same strategies described here for AAV2 can be applied to other serotypes using the analogous sites for genetic engineering as reviewed in.[11,34,64,65]

Suitable receptor binding ligands are frequently identified by library screens. Phage display libraries have been applied successfully for this purpose. However, such ligands did not always remain functional within the tight structure of the AAV capsid. In addition, cell binding alone is insufficient to mediate cell transduction; the newly inserted ligand needs to induce receptor-mediated endocytosis and all subsequent steps of the intracellular processing. Consequently, AAV peptide display libraries have been developed (reviewed in[11]). To produce these libraries, oligonucleotides of random sequence are inserted into the *cap* gene at sites corresponding to I-587, I-588, or I-453 when the AAV2 capsid serves as a library scaffold. As in the examples discussed above, libraries are screened by repetitive rounds of selection for those capsid variants that best meet the selection criteria. The first AAV peptide display library screenings were reported in 2003 and used AAV2 as backbone.[91,92] AAV peptide display screens have since moved from screens in cell cultures toward *in vivo* screens, using, for example, libraries that are depleted for variants that bind with equal or higher affinity toward the natural attachment receptors, as those variants likely possess broad but not selective tropism.[93] Further technical advances are the development of libraries and subsequent screens which select not only for the accumulation of capsid variants in target cells but also for those which perform best with regard to transgene expression (reviewed in[49,94]).

Nongenetic Capsid Engineering Strategies

To alter the tropism of AAV vectors in a nongenetic way, bispecific antibodies were explored in which a wild-type capsid-specific antibody was combined with an antibody recognizing a cell surface receptor.[95] An alternative strategy is based on capsid biotinylation followed by decorating the capsid with receptor-binding ligands produced as fusion protein with streptavidin.[96] A more recently applied strategy used chemical coupling to link receptor binding molecules to the AAV capsid.[97] Specifically, N-acetylgalactosamine molecules were linked to the capsid of AAV2 vectors to improve the transduction of hepatocytes by targeting the asialoglycoprotein receptor.[97]

Combining Genetic and Nongenetic Capsid Engineering Strategies

One flexible receptor targeting platform used a combined genetic and nongenetic targeting approach to introduce a biotin acceptor site into the *cap* gene and produce viral vector particles in the presence of a biotin ligase.[98] Targeting ligands can then be added – like in the example of Ponnazhagan and colleagues - as fusion protein to streptavidin or avidin. Kelemen and colleagues[99] established an alternative platform that is based on the incorporation of nonnatural amino acids into the AAV capsid, which then serves as acceptor sites for chemical conjugation of targeting ligands.

Adeno-associated Virus Exosomes–an Alternative Mode of Cell Transduction

Ten years ago, Maguire and colleagues[100] isolated AAV vectors that were contained within an envelope from the supernatant of AAV producer cells. These exosome-embedded AAVs or so-called vexosomes showed several beneficial effects such as transduction in the presence of neutralizing antibodies and an increased tropism to target cells in *in vitro* and *in vivo* studies.[100-103] Hull and colleagues[104] recently proposed a role of MAAP in the production of these enveloped AAVs. Production and purification of enveloped AAVs are still in their infancy, but nevertheless of importance, as the purity of exosome-embedded AAVs impacts their antibody escape feature.[105] Besides the possible therapeutic use of exosome-embedded AAVs, the natural egress of AAV by the exosomal pathway has revealed new insights in the infection biology of AAV.

SUMMARY AND PERSPECTIVES

Sergei Zolotukhin and Luk Vandenberghe closed their recent review with the words "AAV is now a medicine: we had better get this right."[65] Indeed, it has been a long journey from a virus identified in 1965 to a vector approved for *in vivo* gene therapy. Despite the success of vectors using natural serotypes, barriers toward using AAVs' full potential as a delivery tool in gene therapy became obvious. These challenges fostered impressive technological progress resulting in an AAV toolbox filled with second-generation vectors that outcompete natural serotypes. This promising new generation of AAV vectors is entering human clinical trials, while the developing pipeline continues to focus on further improving the efficacy of these bioengineered nanoparticles.

ACKNOWLEDGMENTS

We thank the French Muscular Dystrophy Association (AFM Telethon), BMBF, and German Research Foundation (DFG) for their support. The authors apologize to investigators whose work was not cited owing to limited space.

DISCLOSURES

The authors declare no relevant conflicts of interest.

REFERENCES

1. Blaese RM, Culver KW, Miller AD, et al. T lymphocyte-directed gene therapy for ADA- SCID: initial trial results after 4 years. Science 1995;270(5235):475–80.
2. Naldini L. Gene therapy returns to centre stage. Nature 2015;526(7573):351–60.
3. Buning H. Gene therapy enters the pharma market: the short story of a long journey. EMBO Mol Med 2013;5(1):1–3.
4. Gaudet D, Methot J, Dery S, et al. Efficacy and long-term safety of alipogene tiparvovec (AAV1-LPLS447X) gene therapy for lipoprotein lipase deficiency: an open-label trial. Gene Ther 2013;20(4):361–9.
5. Au HKE, Isalan M, Mielcarek M. Gene therapy advances: a meta-analysis of AAV Usage in clinical settings. Front Med (Lausanne) 2021;8:809118.
6. Kuzmin DA, Shutova MV, Johnston NR, et al. The clinical landscape for AAV gene therapies. Nat Rev Drug Discov 2021;20(3):173–4.
7. Hastie E, Samulski RJ. Adeno-associated virus at 50: a golden anniversary of discovery, research, and gene therapy success–a personal perspective. Hum Gene Ther 2015;26(5):257–65.
8. Smith RH, Hallwirth CV, Westerman M, et al. Germline viral "fossils" guide in silico reconstruction of a mid-Cenozoic era marsupial adeno-associated virus. Sci Rep 2016;6:28965.
9. Havlik LP, Simon KE, Smith JK, et al. Coevolution of Adeno-associated Virus Capsid Antigenicity and Tropism through a Structure-Guided Approach. J Virol 2020;94(19). https://doi.org/10.1128/JVI.00976-20.

10. Galibert L, Hyvonen A, Eriksson RAE, et al. Functional roles of the membrane-associated AAV protein MAAP. Sci Rep 2021;11(1):21698.
11. Buning H, Srivastava A. Capsid modifications for targeting and improving the efficacy of AAV vectors. Mol Ther Methods Clin Dev 2019;12:248–65.
12. Sonntag F, Schmidt K, Kleinschmidt JA. A viral assembly factor promotes AAV2 capsid formation in the nucleolus. Proc Natl Acad Sci U S A 2010;107(22):10220–5.
13. Ogden PJ, Kelsic ED, Sinai S, et al. Comprehensive AAV capsid fitness landscape reveals a viral gene and enables machine-guided design. Science 2019;366(6469):1139–43.
14. Cao M, You H, Hermonat PL. The X gene of adeno-associated virus 2 (AAV2) is involved in viral DNA replication. PLoS One 2014;9(8):e104596.
15. Sonntag F, Kother K, Schmidt K, et al. The assembly-activating protein promotes capsid assembly of different adeno-associated virus serotypes. J Virol 2011;85(23):12686–97.
16. Earley LF, Powers JM, Adachi K, et al. Adeno-associated Virus (AAV) Assembly-Activating Protein Is Not an Essential Requirement for Capsid Assembly of AAV Serotypes 4, 5, and 11. J Virol 2017;91(3). https://doi.org/10.1128/JVI.01980-16.
17. Elmore ZC, Patrick Havlik L, Oh DK, et al. The membrane associated accessory protein is an adeno-associated viral egress factor. Nat Commun 2021;12(1):6239.
18. Logan GJ, Dane AP, Hallwirth CV, et al. Identification of liver-specific enhancer-promoter activity in the 3' untranslated region of the wild-type AAV2 genome. Nat Genet 2017;49(8):1267–73.
19. Buning H, Schmidt M. Adeno-associated vector toxicity-to be or not to be? Mol Ther 2015;23(11):1673–5.
20. Berns KI, Byrne BJ, Flotte TR, et al. Adeno-Associated Virus Type 2 and Hepatocellular Carcinoma? Hum Gene Ther 2015;26(12):779–81.
21. Alam S, Bowser BS, Israr M, et al. Adeno-associated virus type 2 infection of nude mouse human breast cancer xenograft induces necrotic death and inhibits tumor growth. Cancer Biol Ther 2014;15(8):1013–28.
22. La Bella T, Imbeaud S, Peneau C, et al. Adeno-associated virus in the liver: natural history and consequences in tumour development. Gut 2020;69(4):737–47.
23. Nault JC, Datta S, Imbeaud S, et al. Recurrent AAV2-related insertional mutagenesis in human hepatocellular carcinomas. Nat Genet 2015;47(10):1187–93.
24. Sudres M, Cire S, Vasseur V, et al. MyD88 signaling in B cells regulates the production of Th1-dependent antibodies to AAV. Mol Ther 2012;20(8):1571–81.
25. Gruntman AM, Su L, Su Q, et al. Stability and compatibility of recombinant adeno-associated virus under conditions commonly encountered in human gene therapy trials. Hum Gene Ther Methods 2015;26(2):71–6.
26. Rodrigues GA, Shalaev E, Karami TK, et al. Pharmaceutical Development of AAV-Based Gene Therapy Products for the Eye. Pharm Res 2018;36(2):29.
27. Penaud-Budloo M, Francois A, Clement N, et al. Pharmacology of Recombinant Adeno-associated Virus Production. Mol Ther Methods Clin Dev 2018;8:166–80.
28. Tornabene P, Trapani I. Can adeno-associated viral vectors deliver effectively large genes? Hum Gene Ther 2020;31(1–2):47–56.
29. Calcedo R, Morizono H, Wang L, et al. Adeno-associated virus antibody profiles in newborns, children, and adolescents. Clin Vaccin Immunol 2011;18(9):1586–8.
30. Vandamme C, Adjali O, Mingozzi F. Unraveling the complex story of immune responses to AAV vectors trial after trial. Hum Gene Ther 2017;28(11):1061–74.

31. Rodriguez-Marquez E, Meumann N, Buning H. Adeno-associated virus (AAV) capsid engineering in liver-directed gene therapy. Expert Opin Biol Ther 2020;1–18. https://doi.org/10.1080/14712598.2021.1865303.

32. Muhuri M, Maeda Y, Ma H, et al. Overcoming innate immune barriers that impede AAV gene therapy vectors. J Clin Invest 2021;131(1).

33. Rabinowitz J, Rolling F, Li C, et al. Cross-Packaging of a Single Adeno-Associated Virus (AAV) Type 2 Vector Genome into Multiple AAV Serotypes Enables Transduction with Broad Specificity. J Virol 2002;76(2):791–801.

34. Li C, Samulski RJ. Engineering adeno-associated virus vectors for gene therapy. Nat Rev Genet 2020;21(4):255–72.

35. McCarty DM. Self-complementary AAV vectors; advances and applications. Mol Ther 2008;16(10):1648–56.

36. Martino AT, Suzuki M, Markusic DM, et al. The genome of self-complementary adeno-associated viral vectors increases Toll-like receptor 9-dependent innate immune responses in the liver. Blood 2011;117(24):6459–68.

37. Schnodt M, Schmeer M, Kracher B, et al. DNA Minicircle Technology Improves Purity of Adeno-associated Viral Vector Preparations. Mol Ther Nucleic Acids 2016;5:e355.

38. Nathwani AC, Tuddenham EG, Rangarajan S, et al. Adenovirus-associated virus vector-mediated gene transfer in hemophilia B. N Engl J Med 2011;365(25):2357–65.

39. Chuah MK, Petrus I, De Bleser P, et al. Liver-specific transcriptional modules identified by genome-wide in silico analysis enable efficient gene therapy in mice and non-human primates. Mol Ther 2014;22(9):1605–13.

40. Sarcar S, Tulalamba W, Rincon MY, et al. Next-generation muscle-directed gene therapy by in silico vector design. Nat Commun 2019;10(1):492.

41. Higashimoto T, Urbinati F, Perumbeti A, et al. The woodchuck hepatitis virus post-transcriptional regulatory element reduces readthrough transcription from retroviral vectors. Gene Ther 2007;14(17):1298–304.

42. Brown BD, Naldini L. Exploiting and antagonizing microRNA regulation for therapeutic and experimental applications. Nat Rev Genet 2009;10(8):578–85.

43. Muhuri M, Zhan W, Maeda Y, et al. Novel combinatorial MicroRNA-binding sites in AAV vectors synergistically diminish antigen presentation and transgene immunity for efficient and stable transduction. Front Immunol 2021;12:674242.

44. Manini A, Abati E, Nuredini A, et al. Adeno-Associated Virus (AAV)-mediated gene therapy for duchenne muscular dystrophy: the issue of transgene persistence. Front Neurol 2021;12:814174.

45. Hagedorn C, Schnodt-Fuchs M, Boehme P, et al. Buning H. S/MAR element facilitates episomal long-term persistence of adeno-associated virus vector genomes in proliferating cells. Hum Gene Ther 2017;28(12):1169–79.

46. Van Vliet K, Blouin V, Brument N, et al. The Role of Adeno-Associated Virus Capsid in Gene Transfer. Method Mol Biol 2008;437:51–91. https://doi.org/10.1007/978-1-59745-210-6_2. Drug Delivery Systems).

47. Xie Q, Bu W, Bhatia S, et al. The atomic structure of adeno-associated virus (AAV-2), a vector for human gene therapy. Proc Natl Acad Sci U S A 2002;99(16):10405–10.

48. Tseng YS, Agbandje-McKenna M. Mapping the AAV capsid host antibody response toward the development of second generation gene delivery vectors. Front Immunol 2014;5:9.

49. Macdonald J, Marx J, Buning H. Capsid-Engineering for Central Nervous System-Directed Gene Therapy with Adeno-Associated Virus Vectors. Hum Gene Ther 2021;32(19–20):1096–119.

50. Sanlioglu S, Benson PK, Yang J, et al. Endocytosis and nuclear trafficking of adeno-associated virus type 2 are controlled by rac1 and phosphatidylinositol-3 kinase activation. J Virol 2000;74(19):9184–96.

51. Nonnenmacher M, Weber T. Intracellular transport of recombinant adeno-associated virus vectors. Gene Ther 2012;1–10. https://doi.org/10.1038/gt.2012.6.

52. Xiao PJ, Samulski RJ. Cytoplasmic trafficking, endosomal escape, and perinuclear accumulation of adeno-associated virus type 2 particles are facilitated by microtubule network. J Virol 2012;86(19):10462–73.

53. Castle MJ, Perlson E, Holzbaur EL, et al. Long-distance axonal transport of AAV9 is driven by dynein and kinesin-2 and is trafficked in a highly motile Rab7-positive compartment. Mol Ther 2014;22(3):554–66.

54. Sonntag F, Bleker S, Leuchs B, et al. Adeno-associated virus type 2 capsids with externalized VP1/VP2 trafficking domains are generated prior to passage through the cytoplasm and are maintained until uncoating occurs in the nucleus. J Virol 2006;80(22):11040–54.

55. Venkatakrishnan B, Yarbrough J, Domsic J, et al. Structure and dynamics of adeno-associated virus serotype 1 VP1-unique N-terminal domain and its role in capsid trafficking. J Virol 2013;87(9):4974–84.

56. Popa-Wagner R, Porwal M, Kann M, et al. Impact of VP1-specific protein sequence motifs on adeno-associated virus type 2 intracellular trafficking and nuclear entry. J Virol 2012;86(17):9163–74.

57. Girod A, Wobus CE, Zadori Z, et al. The VP1 capsid protein of adeno-associated virus type 2 is carrying a phospholipase A2 domain required for virus infectivity. J Gen Virol 2002;83(Pt 5):973–8.

58. Stahnke S, Lux K, Uhrig S, et al. Intrinsic phospholipase A2 activity of adeno-associated virus is involved in endosomal escape of incoming particles. Virology 2011;409(1):77–83.

59. Rossi A, Dupaty L, Aillot L, et al. Vector uncoating limits adeno-associated viral vector-mediated transduction of human dendritic cells and vector immunogenicity. Sci Rep 2019;9(1):3631.

60. Pillay S, Carette JE. Host determinants of adeno-associated viral vector entry. Curr Opin Virol 2017;24:124–31.

61. Pillay S, Zou W, Cheng F, et al. AAV serotypes have distinctive interactions with domains of the cellular receptor AAVR. J Virol 2017. https://doi.org/10.1128/JVI.00391-17.

62. Dudek AM, Zabaleta N, Zinn E, et al. GPR108 Is a Highly Conserved AAV Entry Factor. Mol Ther 2020;28(2):367–81.

63. Bernaud J, Rossi A, Fis A, et al. Characterization of AAV vector particle stability at the single-capsid level. J Biol Phys 2018;44(2):181–94.

64. Wang D, Tai PWL, Gao G. Adeno-associated virus vector as a platform for gene therapy delivery. Nat Rev Drug Discov 2019;18(5):358–78.

65. Zolotukhin S, Vandenberghe LH. AAV capsid design: a Goldilocks challenge. Trends Mol Med 2022;28(3):183–93.

66. Hauck B, Chen L, Xiao W. Generation and characterization of chimeric recombinant AAV vectors. Mol Ther 2003;7(3):419–25.

67. Rabinowitz JE, Bowles DE, Faust SM, et al. Cross-dressing the virion: the transcapsidation of adeno-associated virus serotypes functionally defines subgroups. J Virol 2004;78(9):4421–32.

68. Shen X, Storm T, Kay MA. Characterization of the relationship of AAV capsid domain swapping to liver transduction efficiency. Mol Ther 2007. https://doi.org/10.1038/sj.mt.6300293.

69. Asokan A, Conway JC, Phillips JL, et al. Reengineering a receptor footprint of adeno-associated virus enables selective and systemic gene transfer to muscle. Nat Biotechnol 2010;28(1):79–82.

70. Grimm D, Lee JS, Wang L, et al. In vitro and in vivo gene therapy vector evolution via multispecies interbreeding and retargeting of adeno-associated viruses. Journal of Virology 2008;82(12):5887–911.

71. Bowles DE, McPhee SW, Li C, et al. Phase 1 gene therapy for Duchenne muscular dystrophy using a translational optimized AAV vector. Mol Ther 2012;20(2):443–55.

72. Herrmann AK, Grosse S, Borner K, et al. Impact of the assembly-activating protein (AAP) on molecular evolution of synthetic Adeno-associated virus (AAV) capsids. Hum Gene Ther 2018. https://doi.org/10.1089/hum.2018.085.

73. Cabanes-Creus M, Ginn SL, Amaya AK, et al. Codon-optimization of wild-type adeno-associated virus capsid sequences enhances dna family shuffling while conserving functionality. Mol Ther Methods Clin Dev 2019;12:71–84.

74. Duan D, Yue Y, Yan Z, et al. Endosomal processing limits gene transfer to polarized airway epithelia by adeno-associated virus. J Clin Invest 2000;105(11):1573–87.

75. Zhong L, Li B, Jayandharan G, et al. Tyrosine-phosphorylation of AAV2 vectors and its consequences on viral intracellular trafficking and transgene expression. Virology 2008;381(2):194–202.

76. Markusic DM, Herzog RW, Aslanidi GV, et al. High-efficiency transduction and correction of murine hemophilia B using AAV2 vectors devoid of multiple surface-exposed tyrosines. Mol Ther 2010;18(12):2048–56.

77. Martino AT, Basner-Tschakarjan E, Markusic DM, et al. Engineered AAV vector minimizes in vivo targeting of transduced hepatocytes by capsid-specific CD8+ T cells. Blood 2013;121(12):2224–33.

78. Perabo L, Endell J, King S, et al. Combinatorial engineering of a gene therapy vector: directed evolution of adeno-associated virus. J Gene Med 2006;8(2):155–62.

79. Maheshri N, Koerber JT, Kaspar BK, et al. Directed evolution of adeno-associated virus yields enhanced gene delivery vectors.pdf. Nat Biotechnol 2006;24(2):198–204.

80. Zinn E, Pacouret S, Khaychuk V, et al. In Silico reconstruction of the viral evolutionary lineage yields a potent gene therapy vector. Cell Rep 2015;12(6):1056–68.

81. Perabo L, Goldnau D, White K, et al. Heparan sulfate proteoglycan binding properties of adeno-associated virus retargeting mutants and consequences for their in vivo tropism. J Virol 2006;80(14):7265–9.

82. Uhrig S, Coutelle O, Wiehe T, et al. Successful target cell transduction of capsid-engineered rAAV vectors requires clathrin-dependent endocytosis. Gene Ther 2012;19(2):210–8.

83. Gigout L, Rebollo P, Clement N, et al. Altering AAV tropism with mosaic viral capsids. Mol Ther 2005;11(6):856–65.

84. Eichhoff AM, Borner K, Albrecht B, et al. Nanobody-Enhanced Targeting of AAV Gene Therapy Vectors. Mol Ther Methods Clin Dev 2019;15:211–20.

85. Hamann MV, Beschorner N, Vu XK, et al. Improved targeting of human CD4+ T cells by nanobody-modified AAV2 gene therapy vectors. PLoS One 2021; 16(12):e0261269.

86. Warrington KH Jr, Gorbatyuk OS, Harrison JK, et al. Adeno-associated virus type 2 VP2 capsid protein is nonessential and can tolerate large peptide insertions at its N terminus. J Virol 2004;78(12):6595–609.

87. Lux K, Goerlitz N, Schlemminger S, et al. Green fluorescent protein-tagged adeno-associated virus particles allow the study of cytosolic and nuclear trafficking. J Virol 2005;79(18):11776–87.

88. Asokan A, Johnson JS, Li C, et al. Bioluminescent virion shells: new tools for quantitation of AAV vector dynamics in cells and live animals. Gene Ther 2008;15(24):1618–22.

89. Munch RC, Muth A, Muik A, et al. Off-target-free gene delivery by affinity-purified receptor-targeted viral vectors. Nat Commun 2015;6:6246.

90. Munch RC, Janicki H, Volker I, et al. Displaying high-affinity ligands on adeno-associated viral vectors enables tumor cell-specific and safe gene transfer. Mol Ther 2013;21(1):109–18.

91. Perabo L, Buning H, Kofler DM, et al. In vitro selection of viral vectors with modified tropism: the adeno-associated virus display. Mol Ther 2003;8(1):151–7.

92. Muller OJ, Kaul F, Weitzman MD, et al. Random peptide libraries displayed on adeno-associated virus to select for targeted gene therapy vectors. Nat Biotechnol 2003;21(9):1040–6.

93. Pavlou M, Schon C, Occelli LM, et al. Novel AAV capsids for intravitreal gene therapy of photoreceptor disorders. EMBO Mol Med 2021;e13392. https://doi.org/10.15252/emmm.202013392.

94. Grimm D, Buning H. Small But Increasingly Mighty: Latest Advances in AAV Vector Research, Design, and Evolution. Hum Gene Ther 2017;28(11):1075–86.

95. Bartlett JS, Kleinschmidt J, Boucher RC, et al. Targeted adeno-associated virus vector transduction of nonpermissive cells mediated by a bispecific F(ab'-gamma)2 antibody. Nat Biotechnol 1999;17(2):181–6.

96. Ponnazhagan S, Mahendra G, Kumar S, et al. Conjugate-based targeting of recombinant adeno-associated virus type 2 vectors by using avidin-linked ligands. J Virol 2002;76(24):12900–7.

97. Mével M, Bouzelha M, Leray A, et al. Chemical modification of the adeno-associated virus capsid to improve gene delivery. Chem Sci 2020;11(4): 1122–31.

98. Arnold GS, Sasser AK, Stachler MD, et al. Metabolic biotinylation provides a unique platform for the purification and targeting of multiple AAV vector serotypes. Mol Ther 2006;14(1):97–106.

99. Kelemen RE, Mukherjee R, Cao X, et al. A Precise chemical strategy to alter the receptor specificity of the adeno-associated virus. Angew Chem Int Ed Engl 2016;55(36):10645–9.

100. Maguire CA, Balaj L, Sivaraman S, et al. Microvesicle-associated AAV vector as a novel gene delivery system. Mol Ther 2012;20(5):960–71.

101. Meliani A, Boisgerault F, Fitzpatrick Z, et al. Enhanced liver gene transfer and evasion of preexisting humoral immunity with exosome-enveloped AAV vectors. Blood Adv 2017;1(23):2019–31.

102. Gyorgy B, Sage C, Indzhykulian AA, et al. Rescue of Hearing by Gene Delivery to Inner-Ear Hair Cells Using Exosome-Associated AAV. Mol Ther 2017;25(2): 379–91.
103. Gyorgy B, Fitzpatrick Z, Crommentuijn MH, et al. Naturally enveloped AAV vectors for shielding neutralizing antibodies and robust gene delivery in vivo. Biomaterials 2014;35(26):7598–609.
104. Hull JA, Mietzsch M, Chipman P, et al. Structural characterization of an envelope-associated adeno-associated virus type 2 capsid. Virology 2022; 565:22–8.
105. Cheng M, Dietz L, Gong Y, et al. Neutralizing antibody evasion and transduction with purified extracellular vesicle-enveloped adeno-associated virus vectors. Hum Gene Ther 2021;32(23–24):1457–70.
106. Sehnal D, Bittrich S, Deshpande M, et al. Mol* Viewer: modern web app for 3D visualization and analysis of large biomolecular structures. Nucleic Acids Res 2021;49(W1):W431–7.
107. Wu P, Xiao W, Conlon T, et al. Mutational Analysis of the Adeno-Associated Virus Type 2 (AAV2) Capsid Gene and Construction of AAV2 Vectors with Altered Tropism. J Virol 2000;74:8635–47.
108. Loiler SA, Conlon TJ, Song S, et al. Targeting recombinant adeno-associated virus vectors to enhance gene transfer to pancreatic islets and liver. Gene Ther 2003;10:1551–8.
109. Yang Q, Mamounas M, Yu G, et al. Development of novel cell surface CD34-targeted recombinant adenoassociated virus vectors for gene therapy. Hum Gene Ther 1998;9(13):1929–37.

Regulatory Aspects of Gene Therapy: The Regulatory Life Cycle

Najat Bouchkouj, MD*, Megha Kaushal, MD,
Poornima Sharma, MD, Kristin Baird, MD

KEYWORDS

- Pediatric • Gene therapy • Cell therapy • Food and drug administration (FDA)
- Regulations

KEY POINTS

- Food and drug administration (FDA) has vast guidance documents that can help investigators/sponsors.
- Programmatic support can be found through various meetings and incentive programs.
- Expedited Programs exist to facilitate rapid development of products that show early promise.

INTRODUCTION

In recent years, gene and gene-modified cellular therapies have shown great promise for numerous pediatric diseases. Despite this promise, the field is still relatively young, and the number of Food and Drug Administration (FDA) approved gene therapy (GT) products is limited.[1] The development of these products is inherently complicated, products are moving rapidly from the laboratory to the clinic, product manufacturing is intricate, and the regulatory requirements are rigorous. Due to additional ethical and regulatory considerations for the protection of human subjects, particularly vulnerable subjects, the development of these products in the pediatric population adds an additional layer of complexity. Although there are obstacles, there are many resources available to help guide investigators through these challenges and FDA has the ability to use regulatory flexibility for rare diseases and conditions with unmet medical needs. This article will focus on the regulatory fundamentals from early to late-phase product development and highlight not only the challenges but also the opportunities for expedited product development and provide guidance on navigating the multifaceted regulatory landscape in pediatric GT.

Office of Tissue and Advanced Therapies, Center for Biologics Evaluation and Research, U.S. Food and Drug Administration, 10903 New Hampshire Avenue, WO71, Silver Spring, MD 20993, USA
* Corresponding author.
E-mail address: Najat.Bouchkouj@fda.hhs.gov

Hematol Oncol Clin N Am 36 (2022) 687–699
https://doi.org/10.1016/j.hoc.2022.03.004
0889-8588/22/© 2022 Elsevier Inc. All rights reserved.

EARLY PHASE INTERACTIONS WITH THE FOOD AND DRUG ADMINISTRATION

The development of innovative, investigational products is inherently complicated given the unique issues related to unknown safety profiles, complex manufacturing processes, and the use of cutting-edge technologies and testing methodologies. Therefore, it is important to optimize interactions with the FDA throughout all stages of product development. At FDA, the regulation of gene therapies occurs in the Center for Biologics Evaluation and Research (CBER) **Fig. 1**. Before submission of an initial Investigational new drug (IND) application to FDA, typically years of preclinical development have ensued resulting in data that will inform subsequent drug development. It is during this time, even before formal interactions with the regulatory authorities that regulatory issues should be considered. Data should be collected and collated in a manner that meets regulatory standards and requirements. It is also at this time when informal interactions with the Agency can begin (**Fig. 2**).

The first interaction with CBER can be initiated through INitial Targeted Engagement for Regulatory Advice on CBER ProducTs (INTERACT) meetings between CBER representatives and regulated industry and/or individual sponsor-investigators.[2] Through an INTERACT meeting, sponsors can obtain initial, nonbinding advice from FDA regarding chemistry, manufacturing and controls (CMC), pharmacology/toxicology, and/or clinical aspects of the development program. The purpose of this informal meeting is to assist sponsors in conducting early product characterization and preclinical proof-of-concept studies, inform sponsors about early-phase clinical trial design elements, and identify any other critical issues or deficiencies for sponsors to address early in the development of unique and novel products. INTERACT meetings are intended for earlier stages of development when a sponsor is not yet at the pre-IND stage. Of note, INTERACT meetings are not required before requesting a pre-IND meeting.[3]

Before submission of an IND, FDA encourages sponsors to request a pre-IND meeting to seek guidance on efficient product development and readiness for submission of a complete IND. The pre-IND meeting should focus on the specific questions from all disciplines related to the planned clinical trials. This includes starting doses, patient population, and also should include a discussion of various scientific and regulatory aspects of the product as they relate to safety and/or potential clinical hold

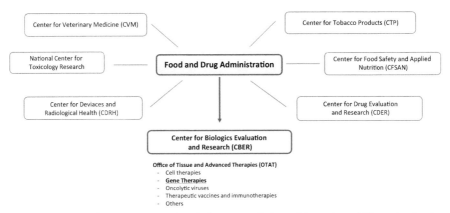

Fig. 1. Abbreviated FDA Organizational Chart: Regulation of Gene-Based Therapies for Pediatric Blood Diseases. The regulation of gene-based therapies for pediatric blood diseases occurs in the Center for Biologics Evaluation and Research (CBER), Office of Tissue and Advanced Therapies (OTAT).

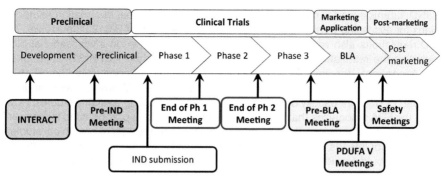

Fig. 2. Opportunities for Formal and Informal Interaction with FDA. There are multiple opportunities for formal and informal interactions with FDA throughout the course of product development. The most common meeting types and their timing are illustrated here. Additional meetings can be requested for stalled development or other unique situations.[5] Additional required meetings can occur with the Expedited Development Programs (see **Table 1**). BLA, biologics license applications; IND, investigational new drug; INTERACT, INitial Targeted Engagement for Regulatory Advice on CBER products; PDUFA, prescription drug user fee amendments; Ph, Phase.

issues before initiating a first-in-human trial. The pre-IND meeting is an opportunity for sponsors to gain valuable feedback from the Agency to help ensure that the product development plan and proposed clinical trial are going to be acceptable to the FDA.[4,5]

EARLY PHASE CONSIDERATIONS FOR THE DEVELOPMENT OF GENE THERAPY PRODUCTS IN PEDIATRIC SUBJECTS

Some GT products are developed specifically for pediatric conditions. Sponsors who are developing GT products to treat pediatric diseases should consider how they will incorporate the additional safeguards for pediatric subjects in clinical investigations into the overall development program.[6] Before conducting clinical trials in pediatric subjects, initial safety and tolerability data are typically obtained in adults to meet requirements of Title 21 CFR Part 50 Subpart D (Subpart D),[7] which provides additional safeguards for children in clinical investigations. A detailed discussion of the individual provisions of Subpart D is beyond the scope of this article, and the FDA has published other documents for that purpose.[8] However, it is important to remain mindful that the special features associated with GT products usually present more than a minor increase over minimal risk, and therefore would need to meet the requirements of 21 CFR 50.52.

Clinical trials presenting greater than minimal risk may proceed only after the Institutional Review Board (IRB) finds either that the intervention or procedure presenting that risk holds out the prospect of direct benefit for the individual pediatric subjects, or that the monitoring procedure presenting that risk is likely to contribute to the subject's well-being. In addition, the IRB must find that:

- the risk is justified by the anticipated benefit to the subjects;
- the relation of the anticipated benefits to the risk is at least as favorable to the subjects as that presented by available alternative approaches; and
- adequate provisions are made for soliciting the assent of the children and the permission of their parents or guardians (21 CFR 50.52 and 50.55).
- When an IRB determines that existing data are inadequate to support the findings required under these regulations, it may not permit the study to proceed.

IND submissions for pediatric trials must provide additional information related to plans for assessing pediatric safety and effectiveness (21 CFR 312.23(a) (10(iii)). The IND regulations also require the sponsor to submit to FDA an investigational plan, including the rationale for the drug or the research study (21 CFR 312.23(a) (3) (iv) (a)). Accordingly, the sponsor should provide a rationale for conducting the GT study on children. To obtain the information necessary for a benefit-risk assessment under Subpart D, data are usually obtained in adults before initiating pediatric studies. However, the FDA recognizes that in some situations, it may be appropriate to initiate clinical studies of GT products in children based only on the results of preclinical studies. If the sponsor intends to conduct a pediatric trial without prior evaluation in adults, the sponsor should provide a rationale as to why adult studies are unethical or infeasible.

AVAILABLE INCENTIVE PROGRAMS

The Rare Pediatric Disease (RPD) Designation and voucher programs[9] under the implementation of section 908 of the Food and Drug Administration Safety and Innovation Act (FDASIA), section 529,[10] state that the FDA will award priority review (PR) vouchers to sponsors of certain rare pediatric disease product applications that meet the criteria specified in that section. Section 529 of the FD&C Act is intended to encourage the development of new drug and biological products for the prevention and treatment of certain rare pediatric diseases. Although there are existing incentive programs to encourage the development and study of drugs for rare diseases, pediatric populations, and unmet medical needs, section 529 provides an additional incentive for rare pediatric diseases, which may be used alone or in combination with other incentive programs.[11] These other incentive programs include: orphan-drug designation (ODD)[12] and the associated benefits under the Orphan Drug Act[13] for rare disease therapies; programs that encourage or require the study of drugs used in pediatric populations under the Best Pharmaceuticals for Children Act (BPCA) and the Pediatric Research Equity Act (PREA); and various programs to facilitate and expedite development and review of new drugs to address the unmet medical needs in the treatment of serious or life-threatening conditions (see Expedited Programs later in discussion). Even so, Congress has recognized that there remain unmet medical needs among patients with rare diseases that occur primarily in pediatric populations. By enacting section 529, Congress intended to stimulate new drug development for rare pediatric diseases by offering additional incentives for obtaining FDA approval of these products.

As with other drugs, a human GT product may qualify for ODD if it is intended for the treatment of a rare disease or condition and the sponsor provides sufficient scientific rationale to establish a medically plausible basis for expecting the drug to be effective in a rare disease. ODD may provide the sponsor of a GT product with financial incentives, including tax credits for qualified clinical testing and waiver of the human drug application fee for a marketing application, and consideration for 7 years of orphan-drug exclusivity, as long as the eligibility criteria are met. To be considered for ODD, a sponsor must submit a request for designation for its investigational drug to the Office of Orphan Products Development (OOPD) following the procedures described in 21 CFR 316.20. Sponsors can apply for ODD at any point before the submission of a marketing application. In addition, under Section 505(A) of the Modernization Act, FDA is required to develop, prioritize, and publish a list of approved drugs for which additional pediatric information may produce health benefits in the pediatric populations and update it annually. As an incentive to the industry to conduct studies requested by the Agency, Section 505(A) provides for a 6-month period of marketing exclusivity (pediatric exclusivity).[14]

Finally, FDA may use regulatory discretion and flexibility for the development of GT products for rare and ultrarare diseases. Although the same statutory rigor is required for marketing approval, some latitude is permissible for clinical trial development in rare diseases. This latitude allows for creative trial design, nontraditional efficacy endpoints, biomarker evidence, and more tolerance toward the use of external comparators and historic controls, when applicable.[15]

Mid and Late Phase Considerations

Phase 2 of drug development typically provides data on the relationship of dosing and response for the intended use including "proof of concept" trials evaluating the impact of dose ranges on safety, and preliminary efficacy. An end of phase 2 meeting facilitates interaction between the FDA and sponsors who seek guidance before the initiation of phase 3 clinical efficacy-safety trials intended to support a licensing application. Discussion includes but is not limited to options for trial designs, dose selection, key clinical efficacy endpoints, and safety monitoring. Common endpoints for single-arm oncology trials include overall response rate (ORR), and duration of response (DOR). In a single-arm trial, time-to-event endpoints such as overall survival (OS) and progression-free survival (PFS) are uninterpretable as there is no randomization or comparator arm.

Late phase trials (including phase 2 trials in GT) evaluate the overall benefit and risk profile of the investigational product and are intended to gather data to provide substantial evidence of effectiveness to support marketing approval. Generally, larger number of subjects is included to provide the basis for extrapolation to the general population. For GT, FDA may rely on a single adequate well-controlled efficacy trial with confirmatory evidence in this unmet need population when a clinically meaningful effect is shown, results are statistically significant and robust, and treatment effects are internally consistent.

To support a licensing application, FDA requires substantial evidence of effectiveness derived from these adequate and well-controlled investigations (1962 amendment to Food, Drug and Cosmetic Act). Clinical benefit is demonstrated by showing a benefit in how patients feel, function, or survive or in a validated surrogate endpoint, which can form the basis for a traditional approval. An effect on a surrogate endpoint that is reasonably likely to predict clinical benefit or an intermediate clinical endpoint (a measurement of a therapeutic effect that can be measured earlier than an effect on irreversible morbidity or mortality (IMM)) can support accelerated approval (AA) (see later in discussion for information on expedited programs).

Pediatric Study Plans

The FDA has worked to address the problem of inadequate testing of drugs in pediatric populations and in drug labeling [labeling regulations for prescription drugs: 0–16 years old [21 CFR 201.57(c) (9) (iv)]. A sponsor who is planning to submit a marketing application (or supplement to an application) for a new active ingredient, new indication, new dosage form, new dosing regimen, or new route of administration is required to submit an initial pediatric study plan (iPSP)[16] unless the drug is for an indication for which orphan designation has been granted.[13] The FDA Reauthorization Act of 2017 (FDARA) further updated Pediatric Research Equity Act (PREA) with respect to certain drugs intended for the treatment of adult cancer and directed at a molecular target determined to be substantially relevant to the growth or progression of pediatric cancer, and for which an original marketing application is submitted on or after August 18, 2020.[16] This removes the orphan designation exception for oncology products with potential to treat pediatric oncologic indications.

A sponsor must submit an iPSP, if required under PREA, before the date on which the sponsor submits the required assessments or investigation and no later than either 60 calendar days after the date of the end-of-phase 2 meeting, 210 days before a BLA submission, or such other time as agreed on between FDA and the sponsor.[16]

Licensing/postmarketing Considerations

The Biologics License Application (BLA) is a request for permission to obtain marketing approval for a biological product. Applicants should demonstrate substantial evidence of the effectiveness of their products through the conduct of adequate and well-controlled studies. Although FDA's evidentiary standard for effectiveness has not changed over the years, the evolution of drug development and science has led to changes in the types of drug development programs submitted to the FDA (eg, programs studying serious diseases lacking effective treatment, more programs in rare diseases, and more programs for therapies targeted at disease subsets). Therefore, FDA has been flexible in the amount and type of evidence needed to meet the substantial evidence standard to reflect the evolving landscape of drug development.[17] Notably, the effectiveness of a drug for pediatric use may sometimes be based on FDA's previous findings of the effectiveness of the drug in adults, together with scientific evidence that justifies such reliance. The scientific evidence may include, for example, evidence supporting a conclusion of similar disease course and pathophysiologic basis in adult and pediatric populations, and similar pharmacologic activity of the drug in adults and children. However, because the GT products are "living drugs" extrapolation of clinical pharmacology data from adults to the pediatric population may not be feasible.

Risk Evaluation and Mitigation Strategy

The statutory standard for FDA approval of a drug is that the drug is safe and effective for its labeled indications under its labeled conditions of use. Risk management is a key factor in FDA's risk-benefit assessment and the goal of risk mitigation is to preserve a drug's benefits while reducing its risks to the extent possible. The Food and Drug Administration Amendments Act of 2007 (FDAAA) created section 505-1 of the FD&C Act, which establishes FDA's REMS authority. A REMS is a risk management program that may be required to ensure that the benefits of a drug outweigh the risks. If FDA determines that a REMS is necessary, the Agency may require one or more REMS elements, which could include a Medication Guide, a patient package insert, and/or a communication plan. FDA may also require elements to assure safe use (ETASU) as part of a REMS. FDA can require a REMS before the initial approval of a new drug application or after the drug/biologic has been approved. If FDA becomes aware of new safety information about a drug postapproval, the Agency may determine that a REMS is necessary to ensure that the benefits of the drug outweigh its risks.[18]

Postmarketing Requirements and Postmarketing Commitments

Postmarketing requirement (PMR) studies and clinical trials (that sponsors are *required* to conduct under one or more statutes or regulations) and postmarketing commitment (PMC) studies (that a sponsor has agreed to conduct, but that are *not required* by a statute or regulation), are conducted after a drug or biological product has been approved by FDA.[19]

Under various statutory and regulatory authorities, FDA can require manufacturers of certain drug products to conduct postmarketing studies or clinical trials, if FDA becomes aware of new safety information which may include data about a serious risk or an unexpected serious risk associated with the use of the drug. The sponsor is required to provide information to FDA in periodic reports (eg, annually).

If pediatric studies were deferred at the time of BLA approval, FDA will require PMR studies to fulfill the PREA requirement.[20]

Special Consideration for GT products, Long-Term Follow-Up

GT products have unique characteristics that may be associated with delayed adverse events which include the integration of retroviral vectors (eg, vectors derived from gammaretrovirus, lentivirus, foamy virus, and so forth) and transposon elements. Such integration is not directed to specific sites in the human genome, and this raises the potential for the disruption of critical genes at the site of integration, or the activation of proto-oncogenes near the integration site(s) and, thereby, the potential risk for malignancies. Genome editing-based GT products impart their biological activity through site-specific changes in the human genome but may also have off-target effects and may produce undesirable changes in the genome. In addition, GT products that are replication-competent viruses have the potential to establish persistent infections in immunocompromised patients leading to the risk of developing a delayed but serious infection. In addition to product-related factors, the long-term risk profile of a GT product should also take into consideration the target cell/tissues/organ, and the patient population (age, immune status, risk of mortality, and so forth), and the relevant disease characteristics.

Given these unique issues with GT products, long-term follow-up (LTFU) of patients administered GT products is critically important. The objective of LTFU observations in the clinical development of a GT product is to identify and mitigate the long-term risks to patients receiving the GT product. The LTFU protocol for GT trials is primarily designed to capture delayed adverse events in study subjects as well as to understand the persistence of the GT product.

In general, FDA recommends the following for the duration of an LTFU protocol based on the product type[21]:

- Fifteen years for integrating vectors such as gammaretroviral and lentiviral vectors and transposon elements.
- Up to 15 years for herpes virus vectors (or oncolytics) that can establish latency.
- Up to 15 years for microbial vectors that are known to establish persistent infection.
- Up to 15 years for genome editing products.
- Up to 5 years for AAV vectors (can be longer depending on additional modifications).

An investigator or a sponsor may cease to operate or may decide to inactivate, transfer, or withdraw an IND before the completion of LTFU observations for all subjects exposed to the GT product under its IND. Under such circumstances, before inactivating, transferring, or withdrawing an IND, or ceasing to operate, FDA recommends that the sponsor consults with FDA on the plans for the completion of LTFU observation.

Additional Considerations, Expedited Programs

In 1988, FDA issued regulations in 21 CFR Part 312 (Subpart E) to expedite the development of therapies for patients with serious conditions.[22,23] In subsequent years, the Federal Food, Drug, and Cosmetic (FD&C) Act has been amended to include several new programs for expedited product development and review, including fast track designation (FTD), AA, and breakthrough therapy designation (BTD).[24]

In December 2016, Congress amended section 506 of the FD&C Act by the 21st Century Cures Act adding a new section 506(g), which specifically addresses the expedited development and review of certain regenerative medicine therapies designated as regenerative medicine advanced therapies (RMATs).[25]

The FDA has 5 programs that are intended to facilitate and expedite the development of new therapies to address unmet medical needs in the treatment of serious or life-threatening conditions: FTD, BTD, RMAT designation, AA, and PR designation[26] (**Table 1**). The purpose of these expedited programs is to speed up the availability of therapies to patients while maintaining the evidentiary standards for safety and effectiveness. Except the RMAT program, which is limited to regenerative medicine therapies, the remaining 4 programs are applicable to both biologics and drugs that have a direct impact on serious conditions including mitigating serious treatment-related side effects. Diagnostic products intended to improve the detection of a serious condition resulting in improved outcomes can also be considered for expedited programs. For the purpose of the expedited programs, FDA considers available therapy to be agents that are licensed in the US for the same indication being considered for the new therapy. In addition, therapies that are considered standard of care based on recommendations of scientific bodies, such as the National Comprehensive Cancer Network (NCCN), American Society of Pediatric Hematology/Oncology (ASPHO), and American Society of Clinical Oncology (ASCO), and so forth may also be considered available therapies. Therapies that are granted AA based on a surrogate or intermediate clinical endpoint are not considered available therapies unless the reason for AA is due to restricted distribution and the study population for the new therapy under development is eligible to receive the approved drug under the restricted distribution program. In diseases with a rapidly evolving treatment landscape, available therapies may change over the span of a product's clinical development. The Agency addresses this by having an ongoing discussion with the sponsor about what is considered available therapy through different phases of product development. FDA may also advise that a sponsor consider a randomized controlled trial with a contemporaneous control arm that incorporates changing standards of care to address this issue.

These expedited programs are briefly summarized later in discussion including the qualifying criteria for each and the benefit that is received.[24,26]

- FTD applies to therapies that are intended to treat a serious condition or serious aspect of a condition AND if preclinical or clinical data demonstrate the potential to address unmet medical needs depending on the stage of drug development (506 (b) of the FD&C Act). The fast-track submission should include a product development plan that is adequately designed to determine whether the therapy addresses the same unmet need which is the basis for FT designation. Benefits of fast-track designation include actions to expedite development and review including the possibility of PR if clinical data meet requirements for PR.
- BTD applies to therapies that are intended to treat a serious or life-threatening condition AND preliminary clinical evidence indicates that the therapy may demonstrate substantial improvement over existing therapies on a clinically significant endpoint (Section 506 (a) of the FD&C Act). It should be noted that the level of evidence required for BTD is higher than for fast-track designation. FDA has granted BTD based on substantial efficacy observed in early phase single-arm trials of CAR T therapies in relapsed refractory malignancies with limited available therapies. The decision to grant BTD was based on ORR, complete response rate, and DOR with follow-up of at least 6 to 9 months from the onset of response. The efficacy was based on investigators' assessment in these

Table 1
Expedited programs: Criteria & features[24,26]

	Fast Track (FT)	Breakthrough Therapy Designation (BTD)	Regenerative Medicine Advanced Therapy (RMAT)	Accelerated Approval (AA)	Priority Review (PR)
Criteria	• Serious condition AND • Nonclinical or clinical data demonstrate the *potential* to address unmet medical need Note: Information to demonstrate *potential* depends on the stage of development at which FT is requested	• Serious condition AND • Preliminary clinical evidence indicates that the drug may demonstrate substantial improvement over available therapy on one or more clinically significant endpoints	• Serious condition AND • It is a regenerative medicine therapy • Preliminary clinical evidence indicates that the drug has the potential to address unmet medical needs for such disease or condition	• Serious condition AND • Meaningful advantage over available therapies • Demonstrates an effect on either: a surrogate endpoint or an intermediate clinical endpoint	• Serious condition AND • Demonstrates potential to be a significant improvement in safety or effectiveness
Features	Frequent meetings Frequent interactions with the review team Eligibility for [a]: • Priority Review • Rolling Review	All of FT Features Plus: • Intensive guidance on an efficient drug development program, beginning as early as Phase 1 • Organizational commitment involving senior managers	All of BT Features	Approval based on surrogate or intermediate clinical endpoints	• Shorter Review Clock • FDA will Take action on an application within 6 mo (compared with 10 mo under standard review).

[a] if relevant criteria are met.

early phase trials. The review team examined the study population characteristics to ensure that they reflected unmet medical needs. Efficacy in the leukaphersed or the enrolled population was analyzed in addition to the treated population to ensure the robustness of the efficacy data.

Advantages of BTD designation incorporate all the benefits of fast-track designation and also include intensive FDA guidance on efficient drug development in form of meetings with the review division, and an organizational commitment to involve senior management in facilitating the product's development program.

- RMAT designation applies to cell therapies (allogeneic and autologous), therapeutic tissue engineering products, human cell and tissue products, and combination products when the biological product constituent part is a regenerative medicine therapy and provides the greatest contribution to the overall intended therapeutic effects of the combination product. Human gene therapies, including genetically modified cells that lead to a sustained effect on cells or tissues, are also interpreted to meet the definition of a regenerative medicine therapy (Section 506 (g) FD& C Act).[25,26] Additionally xenogeneic cell products may also meet the definition of a regenerative medicine therapy.

RMAT designation applies to regenerative medicine therapies that are intended to treat a serious condition AND preliminary clinical evidence indicates that the therapy has the potential to address unmet medical needs for such condition. Given that the manufacturing process for cell and gene therapies can change during clinical development resulting in significant changes in product attributes, it is essential that the preliminary clinical evidence be generated using the product that the sponsor intends to use for clinical development. As opposed to BTD, RMAT designation is based on preliminary clinical data and does not require evidence that a product may demonstrate substantial improvement over available therapies. Advantages of an RMAT designation include all BTD features including early interactions to discuss any potential surrogate or intermediate endpoints that may support AA and advice regarding postapproval requirements. Additionally, for RMAT-designated products, the statue discusses potential ways to address postapproval requirements for AA.

FT, RMAT, and BTD designations may be rescinded if the product no longer meets the designation -specifying qualifying criteria later in product development.

- AA is considered for therapies that provide a meaningful advantage over available therapies in the treatment of a serious condition AND demonstrate an effect on a surrogate endpoint that is reasonably likely to predict clinical benefit or on a clinical endpoint that can be measured earlier than IMM that is reasonably likely to predict an effect on IMM or other clinical benefits. Clinical development plans that use a novel surrogate endpoint require early and close collaboration with the review division.[27] This pathway has been used primarily in settings for which the disease course is long, and an extended period of time would be required to measure the intended clinical benefit. Therapies granted AA must meet the same statutory standards for safety and effectiveness as those granted traditional approval.[28] For drugs granted AA, postmarketing confirmatory trials are required to verify and describe the anticipated effect on IMM or other clinical benefits. These trials must be completed with due diligence. The protocol for a postmarketing trial should be developed as early as possible, and timelines for the trial such as timelines for enrollment and trial completion should be stipulated. There should be an agreement between FDA and the sponsor on the design and conduct of the confirmatory trial at the time of approval. FDA may withdraw a therapy or indication approved under AA if a confirmatory trial required to verify the predicted clinical benefit of the product fails to verify such benefit, if other evidence demonstrates that the product is not shown to be safe or effective under the conditions of use or if the applicant fails to conduct the required postapproval trial with due diligence.[29]

- Priority review (PR): at the time of a marketing application submission, a product that has received fast track, breakthrough therapy, or RMAT designation, may be eligible for PR, if when approved, it would provide a significant improvement in safety or effectiveness over available therapies. A PR designation means a shorter review clock for the review of marketing application (6 months compared with the 10-month standard review timeline following the filing of the application).[30]

SUMMARY

The development of GT products in the pediatric population is fundamentally complex and challenging. The FDA has many resources dedicated to aiding sponsors from the early stages of product development through licensing and beyond to promote progress in the field of pediatric drug development. This includes numerous guidance documents, informal and formal interactions/meetings, pediatric drug, and biologic incentive programs and expedited development programs. The FDA encourages sponsors to engage early and often with the FDA throughout their product development, taking advantage of the available stage-appropriate meetings and programs.

DISCLOSURE

The authors have nothing to disclose.

REFERENCES

1. Approved Cellular and Gene Therapy Products. Available at: https://www.fda.gov/vaccines-blood-biologics/cellular-gene-therapy-products/approved-cellular-and-gene-therapy-products. Accessed May 18, 2022.
2. INTERACT Meetings. Available at: https://www.fda.gov/vaccines-blood-biologics/industry-biologics/interact-meetings. Accessed May 18, 2022.
3. SOPP 8214: INTERACT Meetings with Sponsors for Drugs and Biological Products. Available at: https://www.fda.gov/media/124044/download. Accessed May 18, 2022.
4. Small Business and Industry Assistance: Frequently Asked Questions on the Pre-Investigational New Drug (IND) Meeting. Available at: https://www.fda.gov/drugs/cder-small-business-industry-assistance-sbia/small-business-and-industry-assistance-frequently-asked-questions-pre-investigational-new-drug-ind. Accessed May 18, 2022.
5. Formal Meetings Between the FDA and Sponsors or Applicants of PDUFA Products Guidance for Industry. Available at: https://www.fda.gov/media/109951/download. Accessed May 18, 2022.
6. Guidance for Industry: E11 Clinical Investigation of Medicinal Products in the Pediatric Population. Available at: https://www.fda.gov/media/71355/download. Accessed May 18, 2022.
7. CFR - Code of Federal Regulations Title 21 Part 50, Subpart D. Available at: https://www.accessdata.fda.gov/scripts/cdrh/cfdocs/cfcfr/CFRSearch.cfm?

CFRPart=50&showFR=1&subpartNode=21:1.0.1.1.21.4. Accessed May 18, 2022.

8. Division of Pediatric and Maternal Health - Pediatric Guidances. Available at: https://www.fda.gov/drugs/development-resources/division-pediatric-and-maternal-health-pediatric-guidances. Accessed May 18, 2022.

9. FDA Rare Diseases Program. Available at: https://www.fda.gov/about-fda/center-drug-evaluation-and-research-cder/rare-diseases-program. Accessed May 18, 2022.

10. Amendment to the Federal Food, Drug, and Cosmetic Act: 126 STAT. 993. Available at: https://www.govinfo.gov/content/pkg/PLAW-112publ144/pdf/PLAW-112publ144.pdf. Accessed May 18, 2022.

11. Developing Products for Rare Diseases & Conditions. Available at: https://www.fda.gov/industry/developing-products-rare-diseases-conditions. Accessed May 18, 2022.

12. Designating an Orphan Product: Drugs and Biological Products. Available at: https://www.fda.gov/industry/developing-products-rare-diseases-conditions/designating-orphan-product-drugs-and-biological-products. Accessed May 18, 2022.

13. Orphan Drug Act - Relevant Excerpts. Available at: https://www.fda.gov/industry/designating-orphan-product-drugs-and-biological-products/orphan-drug-act-relevant-excerpts. Accessed May 18, 2022.

14. Qualifying for Pediatric Exclusivity Under Section 505A of the Federal Food, Drug, and Cosmetic Act: Frequently Asked Questions on Pediatric Exclusivity (505A). Available at: https://www.fda.gov/drugs/development-resources/qualifying-pediatric-exclusivity-under-section-505a-federal-food-drug-and-cosmetic-act-frequently. Accessed May 18, 2022.

15. Human Gene Therapy for Rare Diseases: Guidance for Industry. Available at: https://www.fda.gov/media/113807/download. Accessed May 18, 2022.

16. Pediatric Study Plans: Content of and Process for Submitting Initial Pediatric Study Plans and Amended Initial Pediatric Study Plans: Guidance for Industry. Available at: https://www.fda.gov/media/86340/download, https://www.fda.gov/regulatory-information/fda-reauthorization-act-2017-fdara/reports-and-plans-mandated-fdara. Accessed May 18, 2022.

17. Draft Guidance for Industry: Demonstrating Substantial Evidence of Effectiveness for Human Drug and Biological Products. Available at: https://www.fda.gov/media/133660/download. Accessed May 18, 2022.

18. Guidance for Industry REMS: FDA's Application of Statutory Factors in Determining When a REMS Is Necessary. Available at: https://www.fda.gov/media/100307/download. Accessed May 18, 2022.

19. Guidance for Industry Postmarketing Studies and Clinical Trials — Implementation of Section 505(o)(3) of the Federal Food, Drug, and Cosmetic Act. Available at: https://www.fda.gov/media/131980/download.2. Accessed May 18, 2022.

20. Draft Guidance for Industry: How to Comply with the Pediatric Research Equity Act. Available at: https://www.fda.gov/media/72274/download. Accessed May 18, 2022.

21. Guidance for Industry: Long Term Follow-Up After Administration of Human Gene Therapy Products. Available at: https://www.fda.gov/media/113768/download. Accessed May 18, 2022.

22. Food and Drug Administration, Interim Rule, Investigational New Drug, Antibiotic, and Biological Drug Product Regulations; Procedures for Drugs Intended to Treat

Life-Threatening and Severely Debilitating Illnesses (53 FR 41516, October 21, 1988).

23. Whether a disease is serious is a matter of clinical judgement, based on its impact on survival, day to day functioning or the likelihood that the disease, if untreated will progress from a less severe to a more severe one. All life-threatening conditions are considered serious. Refer to 21 CFR 312.81 (a).

24. Guidance for Industry: Expedited Programs for Serious Conditions-Drugs and Biologics. Available at: https://www.fda.gov/media/86377/download. Accessed May 18, 2022.

25. Human cells, tissues and cellular and tissue-based products that are regulated solely under section 361 of the Public Health Service Act (PHS Act) (42 U.S.C. 264) and Title 21 of the Code of Federal Regulations Part 1271 (21 CFR Part 1271) are excluded from definition of regenerative medicine therapy.

26. Guidance for Industry: Expedited Programs for Regenerative Medicine Therapies for Serious Conditions. Available at: https://www.fda.gov/media/120267/download. Accessed May 18, 2022.

27. Surrogate Endpoint Resources for Drug and Biologic Development. Available at: https://www.fda.gov/drugs/development-resources/surrogate-endpoint-resources-drug-and-biologic-development. Accessed May 18, 2022.

28. Section 505(d) of the Food Drug and Cosmetic Act.

29. 21 CFR 314.510 and 21 CFR 601.41.

30. PDUFA Reauthorization Performance Goals and Procedures Fiscal Years 2018 through 2022. Available at: https://www.fda.gov/downloads/forindustry/userfees/prescriptiondruguserfee/ucm511438.pdf. Accessed May 18, 2022.

Chimeric Antigen Receptor T-cell Therapy

Current Status and Clinical Outcomes in Pediatric Hematologic Malignancies

Aimee C. Talleur, MD[a], Regina Myers, MD[b],
Colleen Annesley, MD[c], Haneen Shalabi, DO[d],*

KEYWORDS

- Chimeric antigen receptor T-cell therapy
- Relapsed/refractory B-cell acute lymphoblastic leukemia
- Cytokine release syndrome • Neurotoxicity • Pediatric • Immunotherapy

KEY POINTS

- CD19-CART therapy has demonstrated remarkable success as a salvage therapy for pediatric patients with B-cell ALL; however, 30% to 60% of patients who achieve remission ultimately relapse.
- Alternative targets and dual-targeting strategies in B-ALL are emerging as efficacious treatment options to provide additional therapeutic strategies for patients to prevent and/or treat post-CD19 CART relapse.
- Use of CART therapy in other pediatric hematologic malignancies (lymphoma, T-cell ALL, AML) remains an active area of clinical investigation with several clinical trials ongoing.
- Several treatment-related toxicities (eg, cytokine release syndrome, immune effector cell-associated neurotoxicity syndrome, cytopenias, infection) have emerged in the acute and subacute time period post-CART that warrant further systematic investigations.

Disclaimer: The content of this publication does not necessarily reflect the views of policies of the Department of Health and Human Services, nor does mention of trade names, commercial products, or organizations imply endorsement by the U.S. Government.

[a] Department of Bone Marrow Transplantation and Cellular Therapy, St. Jude Children's Research Hospital, 262 Danny Thomas Place, MS1130, Memphis, TN 38105, USA; [b] Division of Oncology, Children's Hospital of Philadelphia, Office 2568A, 3500 Civic Center Blvd, Philadelphia, PA 19104, USA; [c] Seattle Children's Research Institute, 4800 Sand Point Way NE, M/S MB8. 501, Seattle, WA 98145-5005, USA; [d] Pediatric Oncology Branch, Center for Cancer Research, National Cancer Institute, National Institutes of Health, Building 10, Room 1W-5750, 9000 Rockville Pike, Bethesda, MD 20892-1104, USA
* Corresponding author.
E-mail address: haneen.shalabi@nih.gov

INTRODUCTION

Chimeric antigen receptor T-cell (CART) therapy constitutes a new treatment platform for pediatric patients with relapsed/refractory malignancies. CARs are synthetic receptors engineered to combine the antibody-binding domains that target a specific antigen with T-cell signaling domains, to establish a T-cell with tumor-specific cytotoxic activity.[1,2] The CART manufacturing and infusion process includes leukapheresis, activation of T-cells, transduction with the viral vector encoding the CAR, expansion of genetically modified CART, lymphodepletion, and finally, CART infusion (**Fig. 1**).

Most CART therapies evaluated in pediatrics have targeted B-cell antigens for the treatment of patients with multiply relapsed and/or refractory B-cell acute lymphoblastic leukemia (B-ALL). Multiple clinical trials have tested different CART constructs in varied patient populations, and all have demonstrated impressive rates of remission induction. Additional data are emerging on other T- and B-cell malignancies and acute myeloid leukemia (AML). Despite high efficacy, CART therapy continues to be used as salvage therapy in high-risk patients with refractory or multiply relapsed disease. Clinical trials are ongoing to evaluate the optimal timing for CART administration in the current treatment paradigm. This review will summarize clinical outcomes post-CART

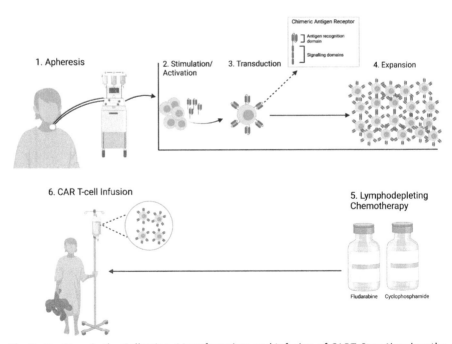

Fig. 1. Key Steps in the Collection, Manufacturing, and Infusion of CART. Step 1 involves the collection of lymphocytes (apheresis) from patient or donor; Step 2 includes the stimulation/ activation of T-cells most commonly with anti-CD3 and anti-CD28 coated paramagnetic beads in the presence of cytokines; Step 3 involves the transduction of activated T-cells with the CAR using either retroviral or lentiviral (more common) vector; Step 4 is the expansion in vitro of CART for a prescribed period of time; Step 5 describes patient receipt of lymphodepleting chemotherapy, typically fludarabine and cyclophosphamide; Step 6 depicts infusion of the CART product to the patient. (*Created with* BioRender.com.)

treatment in patients with pediatric hematologic malignancies, highlight common tox-icities and select limitations of CART seen to date, and discuss potential strategies to optimize outcomes.

CD19-CART CLINICAL TRIALS AND OUTCOMES

CD19-CART has transformed the treatment landscape for pediatric relapsed/refrac-tory B-ALL. Several clinical programs have tested different CAR constructs which have informed the safety, efficacy, and clinical utility of this therapy. The constructs varied in their single-chain variable fragment (scFv) composition (murine or human-ized), costimulatory domain (4-1BB or CD28z), type of vector used to transduce the T-cells (lentiviral or retroviral), and selection of CART cells for infusion. Direct compar-isons between products have not been feasible, however, due to fundamental differ-ences in clinical trial designs, including patient populations, lymphodepletion regimens, toxicity grading systems, and decisions about consolidative hematopoietic cell transplantation (HCT). Yet, the different products and trials have demonstrated consistently high complete remission (CR) rates, with a subset of patients achieving durable responses. A summary of key CD19-CART clinical trials is presented in **Table 1**.

Murine-based/4-1BB CD19-chimeric Antigen Receptor T-cell

Tisagenlecleucel
Tisagenlecleucel was initially developed as CTL019 by Novartis Pharmaceuticals in collaboration with Children's Hospital of Philadelphia (CHOP) and the University of Pennsylvania (Penn). The seminal trial was a phase 1-2a, single-arm, open-label study in children and adults (NCT01626495, NCT01029366). In the initial manuscript of the first 30 patients infused, the CR rate was 90% and 6-month event-free survival (EFS) was 67% (95% CI, 51–88).[3] The majority maintained B-cell aplasia (BCA), an indication of functional CART persistence, for $\geq$6 months. Updated results reported a 93% CR rate among 59 infused patients; 12-month relapse-free survival (RFS) was 76% (95% CI, 65–89).[4] Notably, 13/20 relapses had antigen escape with CD19-negative leukemic blasts.

The phase 2 study, ELIANA, was a 25-center, global registration trial (NCT02435849) which demonstrated similar efficacy to the single-center trial.[5] Among 75 patients infused, the CR rate was 81% and 12-month RFS was 59% (95% CI, 41–73). Most patients had $\geq$6 months of BCA and only 13% proceeded to consolidative HCT. Of 22 relapses, 15 were CD19-negative. These results were pivotal to tisagenle-cleucel becoming the first CART product to receive approval by the United States Food and Drug Administration (FDA), and the only such product with a pediatric indication.

Seattle Children's Hospital
Seattle children's hospital (SCH) conducted PLAT-02, a phase 1/2 trial using a CD19/4-1BB-CART product that was engineered with a defined ratio of CD4+/CD8+ cells (NCT02028455).[6] Among 43 infused patients, the CR rate was 93% and 12-month EFS was 51% (95% CI, 37–70). A greater proportion of patients (28%) proceeded to consolidative HCT compared with the tisagenlecleucel trials (10%–15%).[3,5] Impor-tantly, PLAT-02 demonstrated that loss of CART persistence was associated with increased relapse risk (hazard ratio [HR] 3.5 [95% CI, 1.01–11.88]; P = .04), and that low CD19-antigen burden and non-fludarabine/cyclophosphamide based lym-phodepletion were associated with poor persistence.

Table 1
Summary of select CD19-targeted CART clinical trials for pediatric B-cell acute lymphoblastic leukemia

Author NCT #	Programs	Phase	Construct	Vector	No. of patients Treated	Lympho-depletion	Grade ≥3 CRS	CR Rate	EFS/PFS	CART Persistence
Maude NCT01626495 NCT01029366	CHOP/Penn	I/IIa	Murine, 4-1BB (Tisagenlecleucel)	Lentiviral	30 (child, n = 25; adult, n = 5)	Flu/Cy (n = 15) or other	27%[a]	90%	6-mo EFS: 67%	68% at 6 mo[b]
Lee Shah NCT01593696	NCI	I	Murine, CD28	Retroviral	50	Flu/Cy (n = 42) or other	18%	62%	6-mo EFS: 38%	Longest persistence = 68 d[b]
Gardner NCT02028455	SCH	I/II	Murine, 4-1BB	Lentiviral	43	Flu/Cy (n = 14) or other	23%[a]	93%	12-mo EFS: 51%	Median duration, 6.4 mo (for CD19+ antigen load >15%, n = 26)[c]
Maude NCT02435849	Multicenter	II	Murine, 4-1BB (Tisagenlecleucel)	Lentiviral	75	Flu/Cy	47%	81%	12-mo EFS: 50%	83% at 6 mo[c]
Ghorashian NCT02443831	Multicenter in the UK	I	New CD19 scFv, 4-1BB (CAT CAR)	Lentiviral	14	Flu/Cy	0%	86%	12-mo EFS: 46%	Median duration, 7.6 mo; 12/14 with persistence at last follow-up[c]

Curran NCT01860937	MSKCC	I	Murine, CD28	Retroviral	25	Cy (n = 19) or Flu/Cy (n = 6)	16%	75%	EFS not reported. Median OS varied by cohort (disease burden and Cy dose)	Median duration, 7 d,[d] but 15/18 patients with response went to HCT
Benjamin NCT02808442 NCT02746952	Multicenter	I	Allogeneic, genome edited (UCART19)	Lentiviral	21 (child, n = 7; adult, n = 14)	Flu/Cy + alemtuzumab	15%	67%	6-mo PFS: 27%	3/21 patients with persistence >42 d[b,d]
Myers NCT02374333	CHOP	I	Humanized, 4-1BB (huCART19)	Lentiviral	CAR-naïve, n = 41; retreatment, n = 33	CAR-naïve, Flu/Cy	15%	CAR-naïve, 98%; retreatment, 64%	12-mo EFS: CAR-naïve, 82%; retreatment, 47%	85% (CAR-naïve) and 42% (retreatment) at 6 mo[c]

Abbreviations: NCT, national clinical trial; CRS, cytokine release syndrome; CR, complete response; EFS, event-free survival; PFS, progression-free survival; CHOP, Children's Hospital of Philadelphia; Penn, University of Pennsylvania; NCI, National Cancer Institute; SCH, Seattle Children's Hospital; UK, united kingdom; MSKCC, Memorial Sloan Kettering Cancer Center; Flu, Fludarabine; Cy, Cyclophosphamide; OS, overall survival; HCT, hematopoietic cell transplant; mo, months

[a] Classified as severe CRS, based on the requirement of intensive care unit-level support.
[b] Measured by flow cytometry for CART.
[c] Measured by the duration of B-cell aplasia.
[d] Measured by PCR.

Murine-based/CD28z CD19-chimeric Antigen Receptor T-cell

National Cancer Institute
The National Cancer Institute (NCI) conducted a phase 1 dose-escalation trial using CD19/CD28z-CART (NCT01593696). The initial manuscript reported a 70% CR rate among the first 20 infused patients with B-ALL.[7] The longest detectable CART persistence was 68 days. A subsequent long-term follow-up manuscript (median, 4.8 years) reported a 62% CR rate among 50 infused patients.[8] Fludarabine/cyclophosphamide-based lymphodepletion was associated with improved CR, EFS, and overall survival (OS). Of 28 patients who achieved CR, 21 (75%) proceeded to HCT. This subset had a 5-year EFS of 61.9% (95% CI: 38.1–78.8) compared with dismal EFS without HCT, highlighting the role of consolidative HCT in mediating durable remissions with this product. Notably, only 3/7 relapses among patients who did not undergo HCT were CD19-negative/dim.

Memorial Sloan Kettering Cancer Center
Memorial sloan kettering cancer center (MSKCC) and the Dana Farber Cancer Institute conducted a phase 1 trial with the MSKCC CD19/CD28z-CART (NCT01860937).[9] Among 24 evaluable patients, the CR rate was 75%; 83% of responders proceeded to HCT. With a median follow-up of 29 months, 6 patients experienced relapse, all CD19-positive. This highlights that CD19-antigen escape may be less common with CD28z-CART constructs due to shorter persistence.

Humanized/4-1BB CD19-chimeric Antigen Receptor T-cell

Children's Hospital of Philadelphia/University of Pennsylvania
CHOP/Penn, in conjunction with Novartis Pharmaceuticals, developed a CAR containing a humanized CD19 scFv domain (huCART19) in an effort to overcome immune-mediated rejection of murine-based CART and improve persistence. HuCART19 was tested in a phase 1 trial of patients with (retreatment) or without (CAR-naïve) prior CART exposure (NCT02374333).[10] The overall response rate, defined as CR with the establishment of BCA, was 98% among 41 CAR-naïve and 64% among 33 retreatment patients. With a median follow-up of 34.6 months, 24-month RFS was 74% (95% CI, 60–90) and 58% (95% CI, 37–90) in CAR-naïve and retreatment patients, respectively. Only 5 patients proceeded to HCT. The cumulative incidence of B-cell recovery by 6 months was 15% (95% CI, 6–28) in CAR-naïve and 58% (95% CI, 33–77) in retreatment patients. Six of 12 relapses among CAR-naïve patients had CD19-negative leukemic blasts compared to 1/8 among patients with CAR-retreatment.

Donor-derived allogeneic/4-1BB CD19-chimeric Antigen Receptor T-cell

Multi-center international study
Servier developed UCART19 to provide an immediately available CART product for patients unable to manufacture or wait for an autologous product. UCART19 lacks expression of a native TCR, minimizing the risk of developing graft versus host disease (GVHD), and has a knockout of CD52, allowing for host lymphodepletion with alemtuzumab to minimize the rejection of the allogeneic T-cells. Pooled data from multi-center, phase 1 trials of UCART19 in adults and children (NCT02808442, NCT02746952) demonstrated the feasibility of administration, CART expansion, and antileukemic activity, with 14/21 (67%) of patients achieving a CR.[11] Progression-free survival (PFS) at 6 months was 27% (95% CI, 10–47). Though rates of severe cytokine release syndrome (CRS) or neurotoxicity were low, 2 patients died of treatment-related toxicities.

BEYOND CD19-TARGETING IN B-CELL MALIGNANCIES

Although CD19-CART is now established as an effective treatment of B-ALL, relapse presents a significant clinical challenge with rates of 30% to 60%.[3,5,6,12,13] Thus, there is a critical need for alternative targeting and mechanisms to optimize CART efficacy. CD22, a pan B-cell marker, represents an alternative target. Indeed, in clinical trials, CD22-CART products have demonstrated tolerable safety profiles and antileukemia efficacy. However, antigen loss/downregulation remains a clinical conundrum after single antigen targeting. One proposed therapeutic strategy to overcome this mode of relapse is the simultaneous targeting of multiple antigens. Several clinical trials evaluating dual-antigen targeting with bivalent or bicistronic CART constructs are underway, with resultant pediatric data emerging.

CD22-chimeric Antigen Receptor T-cell

National Cancer Institute
NCI's CD22-CART trial (NCT02315612) used a fully humanized m971 scFv linked to a 4-1BB costimulatory domain in phase 1 dose-escalation trial in heavily pre-treated children and young adults (CAYA) with relapsed/refractory CD22-positive hematologic malignancies.[14–16] In the expanded experience, 58 patients were treated, a majority of whom relapsed after prior CD19-targeted therapy. Of 57 evaluable patients, the CR rate was 70.4%. With a median potential follow-up of 24 months, median OS and RFS were 13.4 months (95% CI, 7.7–20.3 months) and 6 months (95% CI, 4.1–6.5 months), respectively.[16] Response was unaffected by prior CD19-targeted therapy; however, prior CD22-targeted therapy was associated with decreased MRD-negative CR rates and shorter duration of remission. Additionally, consolidative HCT was associated with favorable outcomes. Relapses with antigen downregulation were seen post-CD22-CART, especially in those who received prior CD22-targeted therapy.

Beijing Boren Hospital
The outcomes using a different CD22/4-1BB-CART construct (ChiCTR-OIC-17013523) were reported on 34 CAYA with B-ALL, 91% of whom received prior CD19-CART. Of 30 evaluable patients, 80% achieved a CR.[17] Prior CD19-CART did not affect response rate. The 12-month RFS rate was 58% (95% CI, 35.2–81.0). Eleven of 24 patients in CR received a consolidative HCT and had a 1-year RFS of 71.6% (95% CI, 44.2–99.0). B-cell recovery occurred in all relapsed patients, suggesting that limited CART persistence contributed to relapse.

Children's Hospital of Philadelphia
This trial used the CD22 NCI construct with a longer scFv linker in 5 pediatric patients. Though 3 patients achieved a CR, including 1 MRD-negative CR, all subsequently relapsed with CD22-positive disease. Postclinical translational experiments demonstrated that the short linker allowed for more enhanced immune synapse formation and downstream receptor activation, leading to a beneficial impact on T-cell effector function and ultimately more clinical activity.[18] A new CART construct using a novel CD22 scFV with a short linker is now under investigation (NCT02650414).

Additional centers
CD22-targeted CART are being optimized at other centers with preliminary data forthcoming.

CD19/CD22 Dual-antigen Chimeric Antigen Receptor T-cell

Beijing Boren hospital

Sequential CD19-and CD22-CART infusions were performed in 2 CAYA studies, one in patients with relapsed/refractory B-ALL and the other in patients with relapsed B-ALL post-HCT (ChiCTR-OIB-17013670, ChiCTRONC-17013648). These studies demonstrated the feasibility of sequential dosing. The first demonstrated 100% MRD-negative CR at 1-month postinfusion, with 12-month EFS and OS rates of 79.5% and 92.3%, respectively, without additional therapy. Patients with somatic TP53 mutations had significantly lower 12-month EFS (0% vs 93.33%, $P = .044$).[19]

The post-HCT relapse study (n = 21) showed OS and EFS rates of 88.5% (95% CI, 74.8–100) and 67.5% (95% CI, 48.6–93.6), respectively, at both 12 months and 18 months. GVHD occurred in 23% of patients,; both active GVHD ($P = .001$) and recent donor lymphocyte infusion ($P = .046$) associated with post-CART GVHD. The authors posit that this combination approach improved long-term survival in patients with B-ALL who had relapsed post-HCT.[20]

Stanford-NCI experience

A novel bivalent construct[21] manufactured on the CliniMACS Prodigy (Miltenyi Biotec) was used in 2 simultaneous trials (NCT03233854, NCT03448393). Manufacturing feasibility was attained, with most products meeting protocol-specified doses.

In the adult B-ALL cohort, the MRD-negative CR rate was 88%. The overall response rate in patients with lymphoma was 62%, with one-third of patients attaining a CR.[22]

In patients with CAYA ALL with a median age of 20.5 years (range, 5.4–34.6, [n = 20]), the rate of MRD-negative CR was 60%, with differences noted between CART-naïve and CART-exposed patients (9/12 vs 3/8; $P = .17$).[23] The 6- and 12-month EFS were 80.8% (95% CI: 42.4%–94.9%) and 57.7% (95% CI: 22.1%–81.9%), respectively (Personal communication, H. Shalabi). Relapses were associated with antigen loss and diminution, particularly against CD19. Posttranslational work demonstrated decreased cytokine production when stimulated with CD22-positive versus CD19-positive leukemia, suggesting decreased potency of the CD22 scFV.[22]

Multi-center United Kingdom trial

A bicistronic CD19/CD22-CART trial (NCT03289455) treated 15 patients with CAYA and demonstrated an MRD-negative CR rate of 86%. The 12-month OS and EFS were 60% and 32%, respectively. Nine patients subsequently relapsed. Limited CART persistence was hypothesized to be the primary cause of treatment failure; however, antigen loss and diminution were also observed.[24]

Seattle Children's Hospital

Early data using a co-transduction method for dual-antigen targeting CART (NCT03330691) have demonstrated efficacy in most of the patients treated. A new CD22-CAR construct was incorporated after initial results suggested poor CD22-CART activity, with improved bispecific activity noted with the new CD22-CART. However, despite even fractionation, final CART composition favored CD22-CART and cotransduced CD19/CD22-CART with a small minority of CD19-CART, and engraftment heavily favored the CD22-CART.[25] Longer follow-up is needed to evaluate the durability of remission and frequency of antigen escape.

TOXICITY PROFILE

Treatment with CART carries the potential for life-threatening short-term toxicities and long-term risks. Reported toxicities have been similar across various products and primarily related to immune-mediated effects during CART activation and expansion, as well as on-target engagement (**Fig. 2**). With longer duration of follow-up and continued investigation into novel CART products, careful attention and evaluation for treatment-related toxicities will be critical.

Immune Mediated

CRS is the most well-described toxicity, occurring in approximately half of the patients.[4–9,16,26,27] After infusion, CART engagement with the intended target leads to expansion and activation, resulting in the release of cytokines characteristic of a T-cell immune response.[28] CRS onset correlates with expansion kinetics, manifesting within a few days of infusion, peaking at 7 to 10 days postinfusion, and resolving with CART contraction. The hallmark of CRS is fever, followed by hypotension and/or hypoxia. Symptoms can rapidly progress over hours to days, and may include coagulopathy, vascular leak, and/or multi-organ system dysfunction/failure.[29–33] Importantly, clinical symptoms of CRS can mimic sepsis; thus, work-up and treatment should include potential infectious etiologies.[34]

Immune effector cell-associated neurotoxicity (ICANS) typically manifests during or after CRS, with ICANS rarely noted in the absence of CRS.[4–9,16,26,27] A variety of neurologic symptoms have been reported, including delirium, encephalopathy, confusion, seizure, aphasia, tremor, increased intracranial pressure and cerebral

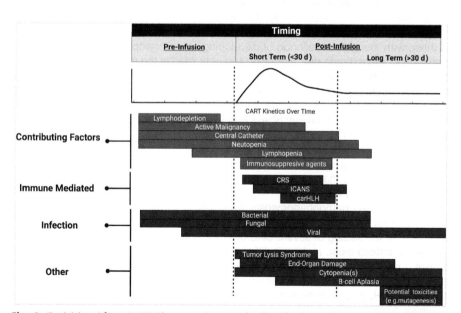

Fig. 2. Toxicities After CART Therapy. Commonly described toxicities of CART, including contributing factors. Toxicities are taken from the CD19 and CD22-CART experience. Postinfusion toxicities are subdivided into the etiology categories of immune mediated, infection, and other. Common timing of toxicities (short and long term) is denoted in relation to lymphodepleting chemotherapy, CART infusion, and CART expansion. (*Created with BioRender.com.*)

edema.[29,30,35–37] Due to seizure risk, antiepileptic prophylaxis is sometimes used, particularly in patients deemed to be at higher risk of ICANS.

Grading of CRS and ICANS is guided by symptom severity. Initial trials used a variety of grading scales incorporating a combination of symptoms, interventions, and/or laboratory abnormalities, making it difficult to compare toxicity rates across studies.[38] The American Society of Transplantation and Cellular Therapy (ASTCT) developed a Consensus Grading System, using a uniform grading approach for CRS and ICANS.[39] CRS grading includes fever (required at onset) and/or hypotension and/or hypoxia. The ICANS grading system uses an age-appropriate encephalopathy assessment tool (Immune Effector Cell-associated Encephalopathy score [$\geq$12 years old]; Cornell Assessment of Pediatric Delirium score [<12 year old]) in combination with the evaluation of other neurologic domains (level of consciousness, motor dysfunction, seizure and increased intracranial pressure/cerebral edema). Notably, these grades are not stagnant, and a patient can develop progressive symptoms requiring escalating support. Therefore, short interval reassessment is necessary.[39]

CRS and ICANS treatment includes supportive care and interruption of the cytokine storm, while minimizing CART destruction.[40] Tocilizumab, an anti-IL-6 receptor antibody, is FDA approved for the treatment of CRS and is the first-line agent for severe CRS,[41] with the addition of corticosteroids for symptom progression. ICANS is less responsive to tocilizumab, and corticosteroids are the primary intervention for severe ICANS, particularly dexamethasone due to improved penetrance of the blood–brain barrier. Other agents used in the setting of refractory CRS/ICANS include siltuximab (anti-IL-6 antibody) and anakinra (anti-IL-1 receptor antibody); however, more experience is needed to inform their utility.[31,40,42–45]

CRS and ICANS are generally treatable without long-lasting deficits, but can be life-threatening.[29,30,39,46,47] Additionally, the full extent of long-term end-organ damage is not yet known.[48–50] Given the morbidity and mortality risks of CRS/ICANS, prediction of those with increased likelihood of developing severe symptoms would help guide intervention and mitigate risk. Increased tumor burden in the marrow has consistently been associated with severe CRS/ICANS.[3,5,6,37,51] Presence of CNS disease has not been associated with increased ICANS risk,[52] although many trials excluded patients with high-burden CNS disease (CNS-3 or focal lesions).[5–7,9] Others have reported use of the Endothelial Activation and Stress Index (EASIX)[53] or modified EASIX[54] scores to predict CRS/ICANS risk using pre and postinfusion laboratory characteristics. Importantly, the use of tocilizumab for low-grade CRS has been shown to mitigate the risk of progression to high-grade CRS without impacting CART efficacy.[55,56] This has led clinicians to use tocilizumab earlier, particularly in patients at risk of severe CRS and/or associated organ dysfunction.

CAR-associated hemophagocytosis lymphohistiocytosis syndrome (carHLH) occurs in a small subset of patients.[16,57,58] Often described as a CRS-variant, carHLH can occur in the setting of severe CRS or after recovery from initial CRS. No uniform diagnostic criteria exist, making it difficult to compare clinical characteristics across patient cohorts. Commonly used criteria include hyperferritinemia, multi-organ dysfunction, and/or evidence of hemophagocytosis in the bone marrow.[59] Given similarities to HLH, proposed treatment options have included steroids and/or anakinra. However, further research is needed to elucidate the pathophysiology of and risk factors for carHLH, and to develop uniform diagnostic criteria and treatment approaches.

Infections

Infectious complications during CART therapy are common; thus, routine monitoring and prophylactic strategies are necessary.[29,30,60–63] Risk factors include prior intensive therapy, active malignancy, preinfusion lymphodepletion, pre and postinfusion cytopenias, presence of a central venous line and receipt of immunomodulators to treat immune-mediated side effects.[64] Most infections occur within 30-days post-infusion and are primarily bacterial, followed by viral and fungal etiologies.[61,65] Later onset infections are mostly viral, particularly respiratory, though bacterial and fungal infections still occur.[61]

BCA is an expected on-target, off-tumor side effect of B-cell-directed CART treatments. BCA correlates with CART persistence and may last for years.[29,66,67] Ongoing BCA results in hypogammaglobulinemia, posing an added infection risk, and patients are often supplemented with immunoglobulin. Further studies are needed to evaluate the necessity of extended supplementation in pediatrics. Additionally, preinfusion lymphodepletion results in autologous T-cell depletion. Immune reconstitution varies between patients and should be considered when evaluating a patient's infectious risk and prophylactic needs.[66] While response to vaccination is largely unknown, criteria for vaccination after CD19-CART have been proposed. Further studies are needed to further inform these recommendations.[62,68]

Other Toxicities

Cytopenias post-CART are common. Most resolve within a month of infusion, but a subset of patients experience prolonged cytopenias.[29,30] Lymphodepletion generally results in transient suppression, and pretreatment high disease burden and/or prior intensive therapies (including HCT) often contribute to a longer recovery. Additionally, cytokine-induced myelosuppression can occur in the setting of CRS[69] and/or carHLH.[57,58] Given the associated morbidity risk of prolonged cytopenias, growth factors can be used, though it is commonly recommended to avoid these agents in the initial weeks postinfusion due to added risk of inflammation.[29]

Genetic modification of cells using viral vectors carries the potential risk of a replication-competent retro/lentivirus or insertional mutagenesis leading to secondary malignancy or autoimmune phenomena; however, no events have been reported.[70–73] With current vector and manufacturing approaches, this risk is thought to be minimal, but patients receiving novel products continue to be monitored in accordance with FDA guidelines.

LIMITATIONS OF CURRENT CART THERAPIES AND STRATEGIES TO IMPROVE SUCCESS

A summary of barriers to the success of CART in B-ALL and examples of strategies to overcome these challenges, many of which are under active investigation, are depicted in **Fig. 3**.

Access to CART

The FDA approval of tisagenlecleucel substantially improved access to CART for pediatric patients, although major logistical barriers remain. A finite number of sites are authorized to administer tisagenlecleucel, and cost/insurance coverage can be prohibitive. Access to newer CART products under clinical trials is more geographically restricted, and eligibility criteria may exclude subsets of patients.

Manufacturing Challenges and Optimization Strategies

Manufacturing failures up to 25% have been reported for patient-derived CART products and are generally related to the quantity and quality of lymphocytes collected. The use of potent lymphodepleting chemotherapy agents before aphereses, such

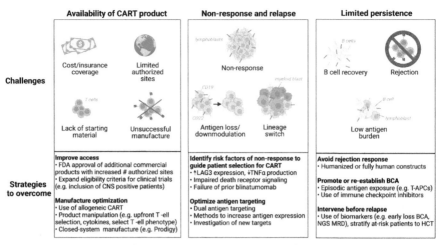

Fig. 3. Barriers to Success of CART in B-ALL. Categories of challenges include the availability of CART, nonresponse or early relapse following CART, and loss of functional CART persistence/durable remissions. Potential strategies to overcome these challenges, many under active investigation, are listed. CNS (central nervous system), T-APCs (T-cell antigen-presenting cells), BCA (B-cell aplasia), NGS (next-generation sequencing), MRD (minimal residual disease), HCT (hematopoietic stem cell transplant). (*Created with* BioRender.com)

as clofarabine and fludarabine, may inhibit successful manufacturing and should be avoided when CART is being considered.[7] For patients in whom lymphocyte collection or wait time for manufacture of an autologous product is not feasible, one possible solution is the use of donor-derived CART products, though further work is needed to optimize the efficacy and durability of these products.

Upfront T-cell selection from apheresis products has led to higher rates of manufacturing success and increased potency of the clinical product.[6,16,74] T-cell selection excludes myeloid-derived suppressor cells, which can be inhibitory to expansion in culture,[75] and excludes circulating blasts to avoid the unintentional transduction of a leukemia cell resulting in a CAR-expressing leukemic clone.[70] The addition of homeostatic cytokines to the cell culture, including IL-7 and IL-15, have been shown to rescue a poorly expanding product.[76] The specific T-cell phenotype of the product may influence downstream clinical activity. Therefore, either upfront selection of central memory or stem-cell memory T-cells, or skewing product manufacture toward these specific T-cell types, may optimize products.[76,77] Finally, novel closed-system devices such as the CliniMACS Prodigy (Miltenyi Biotec) are increasingly available for the manufacture of CART products, and their impact on product activity and availability will need to be studied closely.

Non-response to CART: Product, Leukemia, and Patient-intrinsic Factors

In addition to manufacturing challenges, other product intrinsic factors may present barriers to CART response. One report found that higher LAG-3 expression and lower TNFα production in the starting T-cell product were associated with nonresponse.[78] If further validated, this could prospectively identify patients at risk for nonresponse to autologous CART.

Investigations are underway to identify leukemic intrinsic properties, other than antigen loss, that predict non-response. One report used a CRISPR-based genome-wide loss of function screen to determine that impaired death receptor signaling in leukemia cells leads to resistance to T-cell cytotoxicity and impairment of CART function, resulting in rapidly progressive leukemia.[79] Another report, which used exomic, single-cell genomics, and epigenomic analyses, found that CREBB-P fusions, methylation-based upregulation of JUND/JUN regulation and a significant increase in open chromatin regions correlated with dysfunctional responses to CD19-CART.[80]

In a recent retrospective review of 420 patients who received CD19-CART, 77 (18.3%) had prior blinatumomab exposure. Those with a poor response to blinatumomab were more likely to fail subsequent CD19-CART, suggesting some patients may harbor an intrinsic resistance to immunotherapy.[81]

Relapse with Antigen Loss or Down Modulation

Antigen loss is a well-described barrier to the success of targeted immunotherapy. Multiple mechanisms of CD19-antigen loss have been described; however, risk factors for antigen escape have not been well-elucidated.[82–84] Recent studies have found that preinfusion high-disease burden was associated with CD19-negative relapse after CD19-CART.[81,85–87] One of these studies also found that CD19-dim disease among patients with prior blinatumomab exposure was associated with CD19-negative relapse after subsequent CD19-CART.[81]

The mechanism of escape following CD22-CART has predominately involved CD22 site density down-regulation, rather than loss of the target.[14] Of note, CD22 expression is differentially expressed at baseline in subgroups of B-ALL. BCR/ABL1 and KMT2A-rearranged B-ALL have lower CD22 site density, which may impact the ability of these subgroups to respond to CD22-targeting.[88] Interestingly, compounds such as bryostatin 1 are reported to upregulate CD22 and could possibly increase the efficacy of CD22-targeting therapy.[89]

The simultaneous targeting of multiple antigens has been the primary strategy to overcome antigen loss. Dual targeting of CD19 and CD22 is currently being explored in B-ALL. Additional targets for B-ALL are in development, including TSLPR,[90] CD123,[91] and BAFF-R.[92]

A unique category of antigen escape is lineage switch (LS), most commonly myeloid transformation, following CD19-CART. LS has most frequently been described in patients with KMT2A-rearrangements. In a multicenter review, 9/38 (23.7%) patients with B-ALL with KMT2A-r experienced LS following CD19-CART, none of which were long-term survivors.[93] Of note, no patients with KMT2A-r experienced LS following a consolidative HCT.

Loss of Functional CART Persistence and Antigen Positive Relapse

Cellular rejection and T-cell exhaustion are thought to be 2 primary mechanisms of loss of CD19-CART functional persistence, and early loss of persistence is associated with increased risk of CD19-positive relapse.[6,86,94] Immunogenicity directed against the murine derived FMC63 binder in CD19-CART products confers loss of persistence and decreases the likelihood of success with reinfusion of the same product.[95] This rejection response may be overcome by humanized or fully human scFv binders.[10] One potential strategy to overcome T-cell exhaustion is reinfusion of the same CD19-CART product. Preliminary results from a single-center review found that reinfusion for B-cell recovery/hematogone detection reestablished or maintained BCA in 33/63 (52%) patients.[96] In addition, 5/10 patients with CD19-positive relapse after CD19-CART achieved another CR with reinfusion; however, reinfusion was not successful for patients with nonresponse to initial infusion. Another strategy under investigation to overcome the loss of persistence mediated by T-cell exhaustion is the use of immune checkpoint inhibition (ICI). In one preliminary report, pembrolizumab reestablished BCA in 3/6 patients with early B-cell recovery and achieved a CR in 2/4 patients with bulky extramedullary disease not responsive to initial CART infusion.[97] Further studies are needed to determine which patients are likely to respond to ICI and the optimal timepoint for ICI administration.

In one study, low CD19-antigen burden was associated with inferior duration of CART persistence.[6] To overcome this, an ongoing pilot trial is investigating patient-derived CD19-positive T-cell antigen-presenting cells (T-APCs) to provide periodic CD19 antigen stimulation following CD19-CART (NCT03186118). Preliminary results demonstrated secondary expansion of CART in patients following T-APC infusions, without recrudescence of CRS or ICANS.[98]

Role of Transplant in Promoting Durable Remissions

In the largest study to date of CD22/4-1BB-CART, data favor consolidative HCT following remission induction.[16] The role of consolidative HCT following treatment with CD19/4-1BB-CART, however, is presently unclear. One study demonstrated improved leukemia-free survival (LFS; $P = .01$) in patients who pursued consolidative HCT, with a trend toward improved LFS with consolidative HCT among patients with no prior history of HCT, and significantly improved LFS ($P = .01$) among those who lost CART persistence before 2 months, regardless of prior history of HCT.[99]

However, given that a subset of patients has achieved durable remissions following CD19/4-1BB-CART without further therapy, there is significant interest in identifying biomarkers to predict which patients may not require consolidative HCT. In a recent report, detectable MRD by next-generation sequencing at 3 months and loss of BCA before 6 months were highly predictive of subsequent relapse after tisagenlecleucel.[86]

Extramedullary Disease

Though early pivotal trials of CART in B-ALL excluded patients with active extramedullary disease (EMD), CART were shown to traffic to the CSF and effectively clear CNS disease.[100] More recent reports of CD19-CART have described favorable outcomes for patients with CNS disease, including durable remissions[52,101,102] and less favorable outcomes for those with active non-CNS EMD.[10,102] Importantly, there has been no increased incidence of high-grade CRS or ICANS demonstrated among patients with EMD receiving CD19-CART. Challenges remain in the treatment of patients with non-CNS EMD including trafficking of CART to sites of disease, persistence of CART (eg, duration of BCA), and impact of the microenvironment on CART activity, with strategies such as immunomodulatory agents (eg, PD-1 inhibitors or radiation therapy) under investigation to help bolster efficacy.[103–111] More systematic and larger cooperative studies are needed to explore these combinatorial regimens.

BEYOND B-CELL ACUTE LYMPHOBLASTIC LEUKEMIA
B-Cell Lymphoma

Several CD19-CART products are FDA approved in adults with relapsed/refractory non-Hodgkin lymphoma (NHL); however, pediatric data are lacking, due to the rare incidence. There are several ongoing clinical trials in pediatric Hodgkin Lymphoma (HL) and NHL (**Table 2**). Preliminary data of CD30-CART have illustrated safety and efficacy in pediatric patients with HL.[112] Sequential infusions with CD19/20/22-CART have shown manufacturing feasibility and efficacy, with similar rates of toxicity compared with pediatric B-ALL data.[113] Additionally, sequential CART infusions are

Table 2
Select ongoing CART clinical trials for pediatric hematologic malignancies in the United States

Clinicaltrials.gov Identifier (Trial)	Program(s)	Phase	Product	Disease	Indications
B-cell malignancies					
Tisagenlecleucel for new indications					
NCT03876769 (CASSIOPEIA)	COG	II	Tisagenlecleucel	B-ALL	High-risk B-ALL, end of Consolidation MRD+
NCT04276870 (Basket trial)	CHOP	II	CTL019/Tisagenlecleucel	B-ALL	Cohort A: hypodiploid B-ALL Cohort B: t(17;19) B-ALL Cohort C: Very high-risk infant KMT2A-R B-ALL Cohort D: CNS relapse
NCT03610724 (BIANCA)	Multicenter/Novartis	II	Tisagenlecleucel	NHL	Relapsed/refractory mature B-cell NHL
Other CD19 CARs					
NCT04544592	CHCO	I/II	CD19/4-1BB	B-ALL, NHL	Relapsed/refractory B-ALL or NHL, age ≤ 25 y
NCT03016377	UNC	I/II	iC9-CAR19 Cells	B-ALL	Relapsed/refractory B-ALL, age 3–70 y
NCT03792633	CHOP	II	Humanized CD19 (huCART19)	B-ALL	Relapsed/refractory B-ALL, retreatment cohort includes short persistence to prior CART, age ≤29 y
CD22 CAR					
NCT04571138 (PLAT-07)	SCH[a] CHLA Riley CNMC	I/II	SCRI-CAR22v2 (CD22-targeted/4-1BB)	B-ALL	Relapsed/refractory B-ALL
NCT02650414	CHOP	I	CART22-65s (CD22-targeted/4-1BB)	B-ALL	Relapsed/refractory B-ALL

(continued on next page)

Table 2
(continued)

Clinicaltrials.gov Identifier (Trial)	Program(s)	Phase	Product	Disease	Indications
NCT02315612	NCI	I	CD22-CAR (CD22-targeted/4-1BB)	B-ALL, NHL	Relapsed/refractory B-ALL or NHL, age 3–39 y
Dual-targeted CARs					
NCT03330691 (PLAT-05)	SCH[a] CHLA CNMC Riley	I	CD19-specific CAR also expressing a HER2t and CD22-specific CAR also expressing an EGFRt	B-ALL	Relapsed/refractory B-ALL, age ≤30 y
NCT03448393	NCI Stanford	I	CD19/CD22 CAR (FMC63/m971/4-1BB)	B-ALL, NHL	Relapsed/refractory B-ALL or NHL, age 3–39 y
NCT04049383	Medical College of Wisconsin	I	CAR-20/19-T Cells	B-ALL	Relapsed/refractory B-ALL or NHL, age ≤39 y
Allogeneic CARs					
NCT04881240 (MEMCAR19)	St. Jude	I	CD19-CAR.CD45RA-negative T-cells (allogeneic memory T cells expressing a CD19-specific CAR 4-1BBz)	B-ALL	Relapsed/refractory B-ALL, age ≤21 y
NCT04150497 (BALLI-01)	UCLA University of Chicago DFCI Cornell University MDACC	I	UCART22	B-ALL	Relapsed/refractory B-ALL, age 15–70 y
CARs for Hodgkin lymphoma					
NCT02690545	UNC Lineberger	I/II	CD30 CAR T cells (ATLCAR.CD30)	HL, NHL	Relapsed/Refractory HL or NHL, age ≥3 years
NCT04268706 (CHARIOT)	City of Hope University of Chicago CHOP Sarah Cannon Research Institute MDACC	II	CD30 CAR T cells (CD30.CAR-T)	cHL	Relapsed/Refractory classic HL (cHL), age ≥12 y

CARs for acute myeloid leukemia

NCT number	Institution	Phase	CAR	Target	Indication
NCT03971799	NCI, CHOP, CHLA, CHCO, DFCI, SCH	I/II	CD33 CART (CD33-28z CAR T cells)	AML	Relapsed/refractory AML, age ≤35 y
NCT04318678 (CATCHAML)	St. Jude	I	CD123 CAR T cells	CD123+ expressing malignancies	Relapsed/refractory CD123+ disease: AML, B-ALL, T-ALL, BPDCN, age ≤ 21
NCT02159495	City of Hope	I	CD123 CAR T cells (CD28-CD3z-EGFRt CARs)	AML BPDCN	Relapsed/refractory AML, persistent or recurrent BPDCN, age ≥ 12 y
NCT04678336	CHOP	I	CART123 (Tandem TCRz and 4-1BB)	AML	Relapsed/refractory AML, age 1–29 y
NCT04219163	Baylor College of Medicine	I	CLL-1 CAR T cells (CLL-1-28z)	AML	Relapsed/refractory AML, CLL-1 positive tumor with at least 30% CLL-1 blasts by flow cytometry, age ≤ 75 y

T-cell malignancies

NCT number	Institution	Phase	CAR	Target	Indication
NCT03690011	Baylor College of Medicine, The Methodist Hospital Research Institute	I	CD7-28z CAR T cells	T-ALL T-cell lymphoma	Relapsed/refractory T-ALL or T-cell lymphoma, age ≤ 75 y
NCT030819910 (MAGENTA)	Baylor College of Medicine, The Methodist Hospital Research Institute	I	CD5-28z CAR T cells	T-ALL T-cell lymphoma	Relapsed/refractory T-ALL or T-cell lymphoma, age ≤ 75 y

Abbreviations: AML, acute myeloid leukemia; B-ALL, B cell acute lymphoblastic leukemia; BPDCN, blastic plasmacytoid dendritic cell neoplasm; CHCO, Children's Hospital of Colorado; CHLA, Children's Hospital Los Angeles; CHOP, Children's Hospital of Philadelphia; CNMC, Children's National Medical Center; CNS, central nervous system; COG, Children's Oncology Group; DFCI, Dana-Farber Cancer Institute; HL, Hodgkin lymphoma; MDACC; MD Anderson Cancer Center; MRD, minimal residual disease; NCI, National Cancer Institute; NHL, non-Hodgkin lymphoma; Riley, Riley Hospital for Children; SCH, Seattle Children's Hospital; T-ALL, T cell acute lymphoblastic leukemia; UCLA, University of California, Los Angeles; UNC Lineberger, UNC Lineberger Comprehensive Cancer Center; UNC, University of North Carolina -Chapel Hill;

[a] Trial sponsor.

being investigated in patients with concurrent secondary CNS lymphoma, demonstrating preliminary efficacy without increased incidence of neurotoxicity.[114]

T-cell Malignancies

T-cell malignancies are a heterogeneous group of diseases that can evolve at all stages of T-cell development. Implementing CART treatment of these malignancies has proven difficult due to a lack of tumor-specific antigens on the cell surface, product contamination with healthy and malignant T-cells, fratricide and limited expansion of CART products, and the potential for on-target, off-tumor toxicity of T-cell aplasia.[115] Several potential solutions are under investigation including but not limited to genome-editing of the targeted antigen, antigen selection with a limited expression on T-cells, use of NK cells, safety switches, use of CART as a bridge to HCT, and donor-derived CART products.[112,116–123]

Indeed, donor-derived CD7-CART were tested in patients with relapsed/refractory T-ALL (ChiCTR2000034762), demonstrating manufacturing feasibility and a 90% CR rate.[124] Of 18 patients who achieved a CR, 6/7 who had consolidative HCT and 9/11 who did not receive additional therapy remained in remission. Toxicity profiles were consistent with CD19-CART; however, cytopenias were present and required rhGM-CSF or infusion of CD34-positive stem cells in 5 patients for prolonged cytopenias. Additionally, 12/20 (60%) patients experienced early-onset mild GVHD. Finally, T-cell aplasia was noted. Infections were not seen at increased rates, and recovery of total T-cells and NK cells was noted at 1-month postinfusion. Additional CD7-and CD5-CART trials are ongoing (NCT03081910).[125–127]

Acute Myeloid Malignancies

There is a dearth of data regarding the utilization of CART in pediatric AML, with treatment limited to early phase clinical trials. The development and implementation of CART in this patient population have highlighted some key challenges related to both the disease and patients being treated. Antigen identification has been complicated by shared antigens between leukemia blasts and normal hematopoietic cells.[128] As such, most clinical trial eligibility criteria require patients to have a suitable HCT donor identified in case of bone marrow aplasia, a theoretic on-target, off-tumor toxicity specific to AML-targeted CART. Furthermore, due to the AML microenvironment and increased incidence of extramedullary disease sites, there is a concern for limited CART efficacy.[129] Additional key considerations for AML patients include the feasibility of apheresis and manufacturing in part due to disease burden and prior therapies, disease control/bridging chemotherapy during manufacturing often due to rapidly progressive disease, and infection risk in this heavily pretreated patient population. Several CART trials are actively accruing pediatric patients with AML (see **Table 2**), targeting CLL-1, CD33, and CD123, with limited data demonstrating manufacturing feasibility, in-vivo CAR expansion, and some clinical activity.[130]

SUMMARY AND FUTURE DIRECTIONS

Exceptional progress has been made with CART therapy in the last 2 decades, with CD19-CART therapy in pediatric B-ALL demonstrating remarkable success rates, shifting the treatment paradigm for this patient population. As the field continues to evolve, novel strategies to overcome limitations in CART therapy are emerging, with dual and novel antigen targeting demonstrating early success in clinical trials both for B-ALL as well as for new disease categories. However, long-term data are needed to fully elucidate the safety, efficacy, and long-term durability of these early responses.

As this therapy continues to advance, optimization of timing for CART administration and techniques to promote durable remissions continue to be evaluated. Additionally, efforts are ongoing to develop algorithms based on biomarkers to enhance safety profiles and treatment strategies post-CART, as well as provide clinical insight in predicting those who will have durable remissions with CART alone and those patients who may require consolidative therapy post-CART. While significant and important work has been conducted to fine-tune manufacturing, administration, and toxicity mitigation in CART for pediatric B-ALL, work remains to optimize this potent therapy for B-ALL and other pediatric hematologic malignancies.

CLINICS CARE POINTS

- Immune-mediated toxicities, most notably cytokine release syndrome (CRS) and immune effector cell neurotoxicity syndrome (ICANS), are common after CART, and can be severe or life-threatening. It is highly recommended that grading be conducted according to the American Society of Transplantation and Cellular Therapy Consensus Grading System. The primary anti-inflammatory therapies are tocilizumab and corticosteroids for CRS and ICANS, respectively.

- Patients with high bone marrow disease burden pre-CART, nonresponse to prior blinatumomab therapy, short CART persistence/early loss of autologous B-cell aplasia, and post-CART emergence of detectable minimal residual disease by next-generation sequencing have been found to be at increased risk for post-CD19-CART relapse. Therefore, these patients should be monitored particularly closely. There should also be consideration for prioritizing these patients for novel CART products and/or pursuit of relapse prevention strategies such as hematopoietic cell transplantation.

- There are numerous, exciting novel CART products and manufacturing strategies under active clinical investigation for a variety of hematologic malignancies, but a paucity of long-term efficacy data currently to guide their usage.

FUNDING SUPPORT

A.C. Talleur has funding support through American Society of Hematology (ASH). R. Myers is supported by NIH K12-CA-076931 and Alex's Lemonade Stand Foundation.

DISCLOSURE

The authors have nothing to disclose.

CONFLICTS

The authors report no conflicts of interest.

REFERENCES

1. Maus MV, June CH. Making better chimeric antigen receptors for adoptive T-cell Therapy. Clin Cancer Res 2016;22(8):1875–84.
2. Mackall CL, Merchant MS, Fry TJ. Immune-based therapies for childhood cancer. Nat Rev Clin Oncol 2014;11(12):693–703.
3. Maude SL, Frey N, Shaw PA, et al. Chimeric antigen receptor T cells for sustained remissions in leukemia. N Engl J Med 2014;371(16):1507–17.

4. Maude SL, Teachey DT, Rheingold SR, et al. Sustained remissions with CD19-specific chimeric antigen receptor (CAR)-modified T cells in children with relapsed/refractory ALL. J Clin Oncol 2016;34(15_suppl):3011.

5. Maude SL, Laetsch TW, Buechner J, et al. Tisagenlecleucel in children and young adults with B-Cell lymphoblastic leukemia. N Engl J Med 2018;378(5):439–48.

6. Gardner RA, Finney O, Annesley C, et al. Intent-to-treat leukemia remission by CD19 CAR T cells of defined formulation and dose in children and young adults. Blood 2017;129(25):3322–31.

7. Lee DW, Kochenderfer JN, Stetler-Stevenson M, et al. T cells expressing CD19 chimeric antigen receptors for acute lymphoblastic leukaemia in children and young adults: a phase 1 dose-escalation trial. Lancet 2015;385(9967):517–28.

8. Shah NN, Lee DW, Yates B, et al. Long-term follow-up of CD19-CAR T-Cell therapy in children and young adults with B-ALL. J Clin Oncol 2021;39(15):1650–9.

9. Curran KJ, Margossian SP, Kernan NA, et al. Toxicity and response after CD19-specific CAR T-cell therapy in pediatric/young adult relapsed/refractory B-ALL. Blood 2019;134(26):2361–8.

10. Myers RM, Li Y, Barz Leahy A, et al. Humanized CD19-Targeted Chimeric Antigen Receptor (CAR) T Cells in CAR-Naive and CAR-Exposed Children and Young Adults With Relapsed or Refractory Acute Lymphoblastic Leukemia. J Clin Oncol 2021;39(27):3044–55.

11. Benjamin R, Graham C, Yallop D, et al. Genome-edited, donor-derived allogeneic anti-CD19 chimeric antigen receptor T cells in paediatric and adult B-cell acute lymphoblastic leukaemia: results of two phase 1 studies. Lancet 2020;396(10266):1885–94.

12. Lee DW, Kochenderfer JN, Stetler-Stevenson M, et al. T cells expressing CD19 chimeric antigen receptors for acute lymphoblastic leukaemia in children and young adults: a phase 1 dose-escalation trial. Lancet 2015;385(9967):517–28.

13. Majzner RG, Mackall CL. Tumor antigen escape from CAR T-cell therapy. Cancer Discov 2018;8(10):1219–26.

14. Fry TJ, Shah NN, Orentas RJ, et al. CD22-targeted CAR T cells induce remission in B-ALL that is naive or resistant to CD19-targeted CAR immunotherapy. Nat Med 2018;24(1):20.

15. Haso W, Lee DW, Shah NN, et al. Anti-CD22-chimeric antigen receptors targeting B-cell precursor acute lymphoblastic leukemia. Blood 2013;121(7):1165–74.

16. Shah NN, Highfill SL, Shalabi H, et al. CD4/CD8 T-Cell Selection Affects Chimeric Antigen Receptor (CAR) T-Cell Potency and Toxicity: Updated Results From a Phase I Anti-CD22 CAR T-Cell Trial. J Clin Oncol 2020;38(17):1938–50.

17. Pan J, Niu Q, Deng B, et al. CD22 CAR T-cell therapy in refractory or relapsed B acute lymphoblastic leukemia. Leukemia 2019;33(12):2854–66.

18. Singh N, Frey NV, Engels B, et al. Antigen-independent activation enhances the efficacy of 4-1BB-costimulated CD22 CAR T cells. Nat Med 2021;27(5):842–50.

19. Pan J, Zuo S, Deng B, et al. Sequential CD19-22 CAR T therapy induces sustained remission in children with r/r B-ALL. Blood 2020;135(5):387–91.

20. Liu S, Deng B, Yin Z, et al. Combination of CD19 and CD22 CAR-T cell therapy in relapsed B-cell acute lymphoblastic leukemia after allogeneic transplantation. Am J Hematol 2021;96(6):671–9.

21. Qin H, Ramakrishna S, Nguyen S, et al. Preclinical development of bivalent chimeric antigen receptors targeting both CD19 and CD22. Mol Ther Oncolytics 2018;11:127–37.

22. Spiegel JY, Patel S, Muffly L, et al. CAR T cells with dual targeting of CD19 and CD22 in adult patients with recurrent or refractory B cell malignancies: a phase 1 trial. Nat Med 2021;1–13.

23. Shalabi H, Yates B, Shahani S, et al. Abstract CT051: Safety and efficacy of CD19/CD22 CAR T cells in children and young adults with relapsed/refractory ALL. Cancer Res 2020;80(16 Supplement):CT051.

24. Cordoba S, Onuoha S, Thomas S, et al. CAR T cells with dual targeting of CD19 and CD22 in pediatric and young adult patients with relapsed or refractory B cell acute lymphoblastic leukemia: a phase 1 trial. Nat Med 2021;27(10):1797–805.

25. Gardner RA, Annesley C, Wilson A, et al. Efficacy of SCRI-CAR19x22 T cell product in B-ALL and persistence of anti-CD22 activity. J Clin Oncol 2020;38(15_suppl):3035.

26. DiNofia AM, Maude SL. Chimeric Antigen Receptor T-Cell Therapy Clinical Results in Pediatric and Young Adult B-ALL. Hemasphere 2019;3(4):e279.

27. Pasquini MC, Hu ZH, Curran K, et al. Real-world evidence of tisagenlecleucel for pediatric acute lymphoblastic leukemia and non-Hodgkin lymphoma. Blood Adv 2020;4(21):5414–24.

28. Teachey DT, Lacey SF, Shaw PA, et al. Identification of predictive biomarkers for cytokine release syndrome after chimeric antigen receptor T-cell therapy for acute lymphoblastic leukemia. Cancer Discov 2016;6(6):664–79.

29. Maus MV, Alexander S, Bishop MR, et al. Society for Immunotherapy of Cancer (SITC) clinical practice guideline on immune effector cell-related adverse events. J Immunother Cancer 2020;8(2).

30. Shalabi H, Gust J, Taraseviciute A, et al. Beyond the storm - subacute toxicities and late effects in children receiving CAR T cells. Nat Rev Clin Oncol 2021;18(6):363–78.

31. Sheth VS, Gauthier J. Taming the beast: CRS and ICANS after CAR T-cell therapy for ALL. Bone Marrow Transpl 2020;56(3):552–66.

32. Johnsrud A, Craig J, Baird J, et al. Incidence and risk factors associated with bleeding and thrombosis following chimeric antigen receptor T-cell therapy. Blood Adv 2021;5(21):4465–75.

33. Buechner J, Grupp SA, Hiramatsu H, et al. Practical guidelines for monitoring and management of coagulopathy following tisagenlecleucel CAR T-cell therapy. Blood Adv 2021;5(2):593–601.

34. Diorio C, Shaw PA, Pequignot E, et al. Diagnostic biomarkers to differentiate sepsis from cytokine release syndrome in critically ill children. Blood Adv 2020;4(20):5174–83.

35. Shalabi H, Wolters PL, Martin S, et al. Systematic Evaluation of Neurotoxicity in Children and Young Adults Undergoing CD22 Chimeric Antigen Receptor T-Cell Therapy. J Immunother 2018;41(7):350–8.

36. Gust J, Annesley CE, Gardner RA, et al. EEG Correlates of Delirium in Children and Young Adults With CD19-Directed CAR T Cell Treatment-Related Neurotoxicity. J Clin Neurophysiol 2019;38(2):135–42.

37. Gust J, Finney OC, Li D, et al. Glial injury in neurotoxicity after pediatric CD19-directed chimeric antigen receptor T cell therapy. Ann Neurol 2019;86(1):42–54.

38. Pennisi M, Jain T, Santomasso BD, et al. Comparing CAR T-cell toxicity grading systems: application of the ASTCT grading system and implications for management. Blood Adv 2020;4(4):676–86.

39. Lee DW, Santomasso BD, Locke FL, et al. ASTCT Consensus Grading for Cytokine Release Syndrome and Neurologic Toxicity Associated with Immune Effector Cells. Biol Blood Marrow Transpl 2019;25(4):625–38.

40. Banerjee R, Fakhri B, Shah N. Toci or not toci: innovations in the diagnosis, prevention, and early management of cytokine release syndrome. Leuk Lymphoma 2021;62(11):2600–11.

41. Si S, Teachey DT. Spotlight on Tocilizumab in the Treatment of CAR-T-Cell-Induced Cytokine Release Syndrome: Clinical Evidence to Date. Ther Clin Risk Manag 2020;16:705–14.

42. Santomasso B, Bachier C, Westin J, et al. The Other Side of CAR T-Cell therapy: cytokine release syndrome, neurologic toxicity, and financial burden. Am Soc Clin Oncol Educ Book 2019;39:433–44.

43. Frey N, Porter D. Cytokine Release Syndrome with Chimeric Antigen Receptor T Cell Therapy. Biol Blood Marrow Transpl 2019;25(4):e123–7.

44. Cobb DA, Lee DW. Cytokine release syndrome biology and management. Cancer J 2021;27(2):119–25.

45. Zi FM, Ye LL, Zheng JF, et al. Using JAK inhibitor to treat cytokine release syndrome developed after chimeric antigen receptor T cell therapy for patients with refractory acute lymphoblastic leukemia: A case report. Medicine (Baltimore) 2021;100(19):e25786.

46. Fitzgerald JC, Weiss SL, Maude SL, et al. Cytokine release syndrome after chimeric antigen receptor T Cell therapy for acute lymphoblastic leukemia. Crit Care Med 2017;45(2):e124–31.

47. Shimabukuro-Vornhagen A, Boll B, Schellongowski P, et al. Critical care management of chimeric antigen receptor T-cell therapy recipients. CA Cancer J Clin 2021;72(1):78–93.

48. Shalabi H, Sachdev V, Kulshreshtha A, et al. Impact of cytokine release syndrome on cardiac function following CD19 CAR-T cell therapy in children and young adults with hematological malignancies. J Immunother Cancer 2020; 8(2):e001159.

49. Burstein DS, Maude S, Grupp S, et al. Cardiac profile of chimeric antigen receptor t cell therapy in children: a single-institution experience. Biol Blood Marrow Transpl 2018;24(8):1590–5.

50. Gutgarts V, Jain T, Zheng J, et al. Acute Kidney Injury after CAR-T Cell Therapy: Low Incidence and Rapid Recovery. Biol Blood Marrow Transpl 2020;26(6): 1071–6.

51. Gofshteyn JS, Shaw PA, Teachey DT, et al. Neurotoxicity after CTL019 in a pediatric and young adult cohort. Ann Neurol 2018;84(4):537–46.

52. Leahy AB, Newman H, Li Y, et al. CD19-targeted chimeric antigen receptor T-cell therapy for CNS relapsed or refractory acute lymphocytic leukaemia: a post-hoc analysis of pooled data from five clinical trials. Lancet Haematol 2021;8(10):e711–22.

53. Greenbaum U, Strati P, Saliba RM, et al. CRP and ferritin in addition to the EASIX score predict CAR-T-related toxicity. Blood Adv 2021;5(14):2799–806.

54. Pennisi M, Sanchez-Escamilla M, Flynn JR, et al. Modified EASIX predicts severe cytokine release syndrome and neurotoxicity after chimeric antigen receptor T cells. Blood Adv 2021;5(17):3397–406.

55. Kadauke S, Myers RM, Li Y, et al. Risk-Adapted Preemptive Tocilizumab to Prevent Severe Cytokine Release Syndrome After CTL019 for Pediatric B-Cell Acute Lymphoblastic Leukemia: A Prospective Clinical Trial. J Clin Oncol 2021;39(8): 920–30. JCO2002477.

56. Gardner RA, Ceppi F, Rivers J, et al. Preemptive mitigation of CD19 CAR T-cell cytokine release syndrome without attenuation of antileukemic efficacy. Blood 2019;134(24):2149–58.

57. Lichtenstein DA, Schischlik F, Shao L, et al. Characterization of HLH-Like Manifestations as a CRS Variant in Patients Receiving CD22 CAR T-Cells. Blood 2021;138(24):2469–84.
58. Hines MR, Keenan C, Maron Alfaro G, et al. Hemophagocytic lymphohistiocytosis-like toxicity (carHLH) after CD19-specific CAR T-cell therapy. Br J Haematol 2021;194(4):701–7.
59. Neelapu SS, Tummala S, Kebriaei P, et al. Chimeric antigen receptor T-cell therapy - assessment and management of toxicities. Nat Rev Clin Oncol 2018;15(1): 47–62.
60. Mikkilineni L, Yates B, Steinberg SM, et al. Infectious Complications of CAR T-Cell Therapy Across Novel Antigen Targets in the first 30 days. Blood Adv 2021;5(23):5312–22.
61. Vora SB, Waghmare A, Englund JA, et al. Infectious Complications Following CD19 Chimeric Antigen Receptor T-cell Therapy for Children, Adolescents, and Young Adults. Open Forum Infect Dis 2020;7(5):ofaa121.
62. Los-Arcos I, Iacoboni G, Aguilar-Guisado M, et al. Recommendations for screening, monitoring, prevention, and prophylaxis of infections in adult and pediatric patients receiving CAR T-cell therapy: a position paper. Infection 2021; 49(2):215–31.
63. Hill JA, Seo SK. How I prevent infections in patients receiving CD19-targeted chimeric antigen receptor T cells for B-cell malignancies. Blood 2020;136(8): 925–35.
64. Stewart AG, Henden AS. Infectious complications of CAR T-cell therapy: a clinical update. Ther Adv Infect Dis 2021;8. 20499361211036773.
65. Maron GM, Hijano DR, Epperly R, et al. Infectious Complications in Pediatric, Adolescent and Young Adult Patients Undergoing CD19-CAR T Cell Therapy. Frontiers in oncology 2022;12:845540.
66. Deya-Martinez A, Alonso-Saladrigues A, Garcia AP, et al. Kinetics of humoral deficiency in CART19-treated children and young adults with acute lymphoblastic leukaemia. Bone Marrow Transpl 2021;56(2):376–86.
67. Hill JA, Giralt S, Torgerson TR, et al. CAR-T - and a side order of IgG, to go? - Immunoglobulin replacement in patients receiving CAR-T cell therapy. Blood Rev 2019;38:100596.
68. Walti CS, Loes AN, Shuey K, et al. Humoral immunogenicity of the seasonal influenza vaccine before and after CAR-T-cell therapy. medRxiv 2021;9(10): e003428.
69. Juluri KR, Wu V, Voutsinas JM, et al. Severe cytokine release syndrome is associated with hematologic toxicity following CD19 CAR T-cell therapy. Blood Adv 2021;6(7):2055–68.
70. Ruella M, Xu J, Barrett DM, et al. Induction of resistance to chimeric antigen receptor T cell therapy by transduction of a single leukemic B cell. Nat Med 2018; 24(10):1499–503.
71. Laetsch TW, Maude SL, Milone MC, et al. False-positive results with select HIV-1 NAT methods following lentivirus-based tisagenlecleucel therapy. Blood 2018; 131(23):2596–8.
72. Gardner R, Wu D, Cherian S, et al. Acquisition of a CD19-negative myeloid phenotype allows immune escape of MLL-rearranged B-ALL from CD19 CAR-T-cell therapy. Blood 2016;127(20):2406–10.
73. Mo G, Wang HW, Talleur AC, et al. Diagnostic approach to the evaluation of myeloid malignancies following CAR T-cell therapy in B-cell acute lymphoblastic leukemia. J Immunother Cancer 2020;8(2):e001563.

74. Shah NN, Fry TJ. Anti-CD19 resistance can "stem" from progenitors. Blood 2017; 130(18):1961–3.

75. Stroncek DF, Ren J, Lee DW, et al. Myeloid cells in peripheral blood mononuclear cell concentrates inhibit the expansion of chimeric antigen receptor T cells. Cytotherapy 2016;18(7):893–901.

76. Singh N, Perazzelli J, Grupp SA, et al. Early memory phenotypes drive T cell proliferation in patients with pediatric malignancies. Sci Transl Med 2016;8(320): 320ra323.

77. Sabatino M, Hu J, Sommariva M, et al. Generation of clinical-grade CD19-specific CAR-modified CD8+ memory stem cells for the treatment of human B-cell malignancies. Blood 2016;128(4):519–28.

78. Finney OC, Brakke HM, Rawlings-Rhea S, et al. CD19 CAR T cell product and disease attributes predict leukemia remission durability. J Clin Invest 2019; 129(5):2123–32.

79. Singh N, Lee YG, Shestova O, et al. Impaired Death Receptor Signaling in Leukemia Causes Antigen-Independent Resistance by Inducing CAR T-cell Dysfunction. Cancer Discov 2020;10(4):552–67.

80. Masih KE, Gardner R, Gryder B, et al. Detailed Multi-Method Analysis of Bone Marrow from Pediatric Pre-B-ALL Patients Prior to CD19-CAR-T Therapy Subsequently Evidencing Overt CAR-T Resistance. Blood 2019;134(Supplement_1): 2744.

81. Myers RM, Taraseviciute A, Steinberg SM, et al. Blinatumomab Nonresponse and High-Disease Burden Are Associated With Inferior Outcomes After CD19-CAR for B-ALL. J Clin Oncol 2021;40(9):932–44. Jco2101405.

82. Orlando EJ, Han X, Tribouley C, et al. Genetic mechanisms of target antigen loss in CAR19 therapy of acute lymphoblastic leukemia. Nat Med 2018;24(10): 1504–6.

83. Bagashev A, Sotillo E, Tang CH, et al. CD19 Alterations Emerging after CD19-Directed Immunotherapy Cause Retention of the Misfolded Protein in the Endoplasmic Reticulum. Mol Cell Biol 2018;38(21):e00383-18.

84. Sotillo E, Barrett DM, Black KL, et al. Convergence of Acquired Mutations and Alternative Splicing of CD19 Enables Resistance to CART-19 Immunotherapy. Cancer Discov 2015;5(12):1282–95.

85. Dourthe ME, Rabian F, Yakouben K, et al. Determinants of CD19-positive vs CD19-negative relapse after tisagenlecleucel for B-cell acute lymphoblastic leukemia. Leukemia 2021;35(12):3383–93.

86. Pulsipher MA, Han X, Maude SL, et al. Next-generation sequencing of minimal residual disease for predicting relapse after tisagenlecleucel in children and young adults with acute lymphoblastic leukemia. Blood Cancer Discovery 2021;3(1):66–8.

87. Ravich JW, Huang S, Zhou Y, et al. Impact of high disease burden on survival in pediatric patients with B-all treated with tisagenlecleucel. Transplantation and Cell Ther 2021;28(2):73.e1–9.

88. Shah NN, Stevenson MS, Yuan CM, et al. Characterization of CD22 expression in acute lymphoblastic leukemia. Pediatr Blood Cancer 2015;62(6):964–9.

89. Ramakrishna S, Highfill SL, Walsh Z, et al. Modulation of Target Antigen Density Improves CAR T-cell Functionality and Persistence. Clin Cancer Res 2019; 25(17):5329–41.

90. Qin H, Cho M, Haso W, et al. Eradication of B-ALL using chimeric antigen receptor-expressing T cells targeting the TSLPR oncoprotein. Blood 2015; 126(5):629–39.

91. Ruella M, Barrett DM, Kenderian SS, et al. Dual CD19 and CD123 targeting prevents antigen-loss relapses after CD19-directed immunotherapies. J Clin Invest 2016;126(10):3814–26.

92. Qin H, Dong Z, Wang X, et al. CAR T cells targeting BAFF-R can overcome CD19 antigen loss in B cell malignancies. Sci Transl Med 2019;11(511):eaaw9414.

93. Lamble AJ, Myers RM, Taraseviciute A, et al. KMT2A Rearrangements Are Associated with Lineage Switch Following CD19 Targeting CAR T-Cell Therapy. Blood 2021;138(Supplement 1):256.

94. Zebley CC, Brown C, Mi T, et al. CD19-CAR T cells undergo exhaustion DNA methylation programming in patients with acute lymphoblastic leukemia. Cell Rep 2021;37(9):110079.

95. Turtle CJ, Hanafi LA, Berger C, et al. CD19 CAR-T cells of defined CD4+:CD8+ composition in adult B cell ALL patients. J Clin Invest 2016;126(6):2123–38.

96. Myers R, Devine K, Li Y, et al. Outcomes after reinfusion of CD19-specific chimeric antigen receptor (CAR)-modified T cells in children and young adults with relapsed/refractroy B-cell acute lymphoblastic leukemia. Blood 2021;138(s1):474.

97. Li AM, Hucks GE, Dinofia AM, et al. Checkpoint Inhibitors Augment CD19-Directed Chimeric Antigen Receptor (CAR) T Cell Therapy in Relapsed B-Cell Acute Lymphoblastic Leukemia. Blood 2018;132(Supplement 1):556.

98. Annesley C, Gardner R, Wilson A, et al. Novel CD19t T-Antigen Presenting Cells Expand CD19 CAR T Cells In Vivo. Blood 2019;134(Supplement_1):223.

99. Summers C, Wu QV, Annesley C, et al. Hematopoietic Cell Transplantation after CD19 Chimeric Antigen Receptor T Cell-Induced Acute Lymphoblastic Lymphoma Remission Confers a Leukemia-Free Survival Advantage. Transpl Cell Ther 2021;28(1):21–9.

100. Rheingold SR, Chen LN, Maude SL, et al. Efficient Trafficking of Chimeric Antigen Receptor (CAR)-Modified T Cells to CSF and Induction of Durable CNS Remissions in Children with CNS/Combined Relapsed/Refractory ALL. Blood 2015;126(23):3769.

101. Rubinstein JD, Krupski C, Nelson AS, et al. Chimeric Antigen Receptor T Cell Therapy in Patients with Multiply Relapsed or Refractory Extramedullary Leukemia. Biol Blood Marrow Transpl 2020;26(11):e280–5.

102. Fabrizio VA, Phillips CL, Lane A, et al. Tisagenlecleucel Outcomes in Relapsed/Refractory Extramedullary ALL: A Pediatric Real World CAR Consortium Report. Blood Adv 2021;6(2):600–10.

103. Li AM, Hucks GE, Dinofia AM, et al. Checkpoint Inhibitors Augment CD19-Directed Chimeric Antigen Receptor (CAR) T Cell Therapy in Relapsed B-Cell Acute Lymphoblastic Leukemia. Blood 2018;132:556.

104. Yoon DH, Osborn MJ, Tolar J, et al. Incorporation of Immune Checkpoint Blockade into Chimeric Antigen Receptor T Cells (CAR-Ts): Combination or Built-In CAR-T. Int J Mol Sci 2018;19(2):340.

105. Chong EA, Melenhorst JJ, Lacey SF, et al. PD-1 blockade modulates chimeric antigen receptor (CAR)-modified T cells: refueling the CAR. Blood 2017;129(8):1039–41.

106. Hill BT, Roberts ZJ, Rossi JM, et al. Marked Re-Expansion of Chimeric Antigen Receptor (CAR) T Cells and tumor regression following nivolumab treatment in a patient treated with axicabtagene ciloleucel (axi-cel; KTE-C19) for Refractory Diffuse Large B Cell Lymphoma (DLBCL). Blood 2017;130.

107. Wright CM, LaRiviere MJ, Baron JA, et al. Bridging Radiation Therapy Before Commercial Chimeric Antigen Receptor T-Cell Therapy for Relapsed or

Refractory Aggressive B-Cell Lymphoma. Int J Radiat Oncol Biol Phys 2020; 108(1):178–88.

108. DeSelm C, Palomba ML, Yahalom J, et al. Low-Dose Radiation Conditioning Enables CAR T Cells to Mitigate Antigen Escape. Mol Ther 2018;26(11):2542–52.

109. Imber BS, Sadelain M, DeSelm C, et al. Early experience using salvage radiotherapy for relapsed/refractory non-Hodgkin lymphomas after CD19 chimeric antigen receptor (CAR) T cell therapy. Br J Haematol 2020;190(1):45–51.

110. Sim AJ, Jain MD, Figura NB, et al. Radiation Therapy as a Bridging Strategy for CAR T cell therapy with axicabtagene ciloleucel in diffuse large B-Cell Lymphoma. Int J Radiat Oncol Biol Phys 2019;105(5):1012–21.

111. Holland EM, Yates B, Ling A, et al. Characterization of Extramedullary Disease in B-ALL and Response to CAR T-cell Therapy. Blood Adv 2021;6(7):2167–82.

112. Ramos CA, Ballard B, Zhang H, et al. Clinical and immunological responses after CD30-specific chimeric antigen receptor-redirected lymphocytes. J Clin Invest 2017;127(9):3462–71.

113. Liu Y, Deng B, Hu B, et al. Sequential different B cell antigen-targeted CAR T-cell therapy for pediatric refractory/relapsed Burkitt Lymphoma. Blood Adv 2021; 6(3):717–30.

114. Liu Y, Deng B, Hu B, et al. Efficacy and Safety of Sequential Different B Cell Antigen-Targeted CAR T-Cell therapy for pediatric refractory/relapsed burkitt lymphoma with secondary central nervous system involvement. Blood 2021; 138(Supplement 1):257.

115. Fleischer LC, Spencer HT, Raikar SS. Targeting T cell malignancies using CAR-based immunotherapy: challenges and potential solutions. J Hematol Oncol 2019;12(1):141.

116. Gomes-Silva D, Srinivasan M, Sharma S, et al. CD7-edited T cells expressing a CD7-specific CAR for the therapy of T-cell malignancies. Blood 2017;130(3): 285–96.

117. Cooper ML, Choi J, Staser K, et al. An "off-the-shelf" fratricide-resistant CAR-T for the treatment of T cell hematologic malignancies. Leukemia 2018;32(9): 1970–83.

118. Raikar SS, Fleischer LC, Moot R, et al. Development of chimeric antigen receptors targeting T-cell malignancies using two structurally different anti-CD5 antigen binding domains in NK and CRISPR-edited T cell lines. Oncoimmunology 2018;7(3):e1407898.

119. Sanchez-Martinez D, Baroni ML, Gutierrez-Aguera F, et al. Fratricide-resistant CD1a-specific CAR T cells for the treatment of cortical T-cell acute lymphoblastic leukemia. Blood 2019;133(21):2291–304.

120. Maciocia PM, Wawrzyniecka PA, Philip B, et al. Targeting the T cell receptor beta-chain constant region for immunotherapy of T cell malignancies. Nat Med 2017;23(12):1416–23.

121. Chen KH, Wada M, Firor AE, et al. Novel anti-CD3 chimeric antigen receptor targeting of aggressive T cell malignancies. Oncotarget 2016;7(35):56219–32.

122. Chen KH, Wada M, Pinz KG, et al. Preclinical targeting of aggressive T-cell malignancies using anti-CD5 chimeric antigen receptor. Leukemia 2017;31(10): 2151–60.

123. Ma G, Shen J, Pinz K, et al. Targeting T Cell Malignancies Using CD4CAR T-Cells and Implementing a Natural Safety Switch. Stem Cell Rev Rep 2019; 15(3):443–7.

124. Pan J, Tan Y, Wang G, et al. Donor-Derived CD7 Chimeric Antigen Receptor T Cells for T-Cell Acute Lymphoblastic Leukemia: First-in-Human, Phase I Trial. J Clin Oncol 2021;39(30):3340–51.
125. Yang J, Zhang X, Liu Y, et al. High Effectiveness and Safety of Anti-CD7 CAR T-Cell Therapy in Treating Relapsed or Refractory (R/R) T-Cell Acute Lymphoblastic Leukemia (T-ALL). Blood 2021;138(Supplement 1):473.
126. Yang J, Yang X, Liu Y, et al. A novel and successful patient or donor-derived CD7-Targeted CAR T-Cell Therapy for Relapsed or Refractory T-Cell Lymphoblastic Lymphoma (R/R T-LBL). Blood 2021;138(Supplement 1):652.
127. Rouce RH, Hill LC, Smith TS, et al. Early signals of anti-tumor efficacy and safety with autologous CD5.CAR T-Cells in patients with refractory/relapsed T-Cell Lymphoma. Blood 2021;138(Supplement 1):654.
128. Perna F, Berman SH, Soni RK, et al. Integrating proteomics and transcriptomics for systematic combinatorial chimeric antigen receptor therapy of AML. Cancer Cell 2017;32(4):506–19.e505.
129. Epperly R, Gottschalk S, Velasquez MP. A Bump in the Road: How the Hostile AML Microenvironment Affects CAR T Cell Therapy. Front Oncol 2020;10:262.
130. PEI K, Xu H, Wang P-F, et al. A comparison study of anti-CLL1 CART Cells equipped with different co-stimulatory domains in the treatment of children with refractory/relapsed acute myeloid leukemia. Blood 2021;138(Supplement 1):824.

Genome-Edited T Cell Therapies

Giorgio Ottaviano, MD, Waseem Qasim, BMedSci, MBBS, PhD*

KEYWORDS

- Genome editing • CRISPR/Cas9 • Base editor • Cytidine deamination
- T cell therapies • Chimeric antigen receptor

KEY POINTS

- Genome editing can help address allogeneic barriers for 'off-the-shelf' T cell therapies against cancer.
- First clinical applications of genome-edited T cells have provided preliminary safety and efficacy data.
- Further applications are addressing 'fratricide' effects and manipulating checkpoint pathways for enhanced cellular immunotherapy and wider applications.

INTRODUCTION

Genome editing offers the prospect of enhanced gene therapy and new therapeutic avenues beyond those envisaged by conventional 'gene-addition' strategies. The breakthrough innovation of genome editing is the ability to alter cellular DNA at very specific sites for precise and advantageous therapeutic effects.

Early emerging tools to target specific genome sequences shared a common mechanism of action: a variety of engineered DNA nuclease platforms allow recognition of specific DNA loci and can generate double-strand brakes (DSBs) that, in combination with the endogenous DNA repair pathways, result in permanent disruption of targeted genes (**Fig. 1**). For over a decade, genome editing platforms including Zinc Finger Nucleases (ZNF),[1] Transcription Activator-Like Effector Nucleases (TALENs)[2] Meganucleases (MNs)[3] and mega-TALENs[4] and Clustered Regularly Interspaced Short Palindromic Repeats (CRISPR)-based systems, have been investigated for their potential in cellular therapies. Structural differences among these tools include the modality of target site recognition, either by customized DNA-binding proteins (for ZFNs, MNs, and TALENs) or single guide RNA (sgRNA for CRISPR-based systems), and the cleavage modules that generate precise DNA DSBs (Fok-1 for ZFNs/TALENs or

Infection, Immunity & Inflammation Department, UCL Great Ormond Street Institute of Child Health, University College London Institute of Child Health, 30 Guilford Street, London WC1N 1EH, UK
* Corresponding author.
E-mail address: w.qasim@ucl.ac.uk

Hematol Oncol Clin N Am 36 (2022) 729–744
https://doi.org/10.1016/j.hoc.2022.03.006
0889-8588/22/© 2022 Elsevier Inc. All rights reserved.
hemonc.theclinics.com

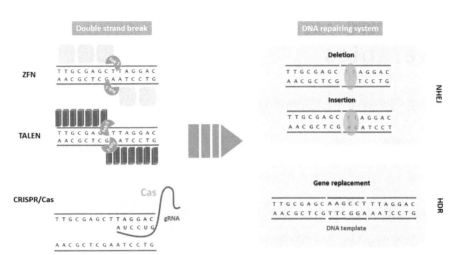

Fig. 1. Platforms for precise genome editing have already moved into clinic and include ZFN, TALEN, and CRISPR/Cas. A common strategy to deliver on-target alteration of DNA sequences relies on the generation of DNA double-strands breaks. Endogenous repair systems in the cell, such as non-homologous end-joining repairing generate insertions or deletions within the target sequence and disrupt expression. Alternatively, homologous repair can be activated, and homology flanked DNA sequences might be recruited by DNA repair machinery to incorporate a transgene into a specific locus. Abbreviation: gRNA, guide RNA; HDR, homologous direct repair; NHEJ, non-homologous end-joining.

bacterial-derived Caspase9 for CRISPR) (**Table 1**). Early designs of modular zinc-finger proteins that could recognize multiple DNA triplets provided initial proof-of-concept that specific DNA sites could be edited in mammalian cells. Increased specificity of DNA sequence recognition was obtained with TALE–DNA binding repeats delivering more flexibility than triplet-limited zinc-finger domains. Limitations of these strategies included difficulties in targeting multiple sites and laborious development and validation pathways. More recently RNA-guided engineered nucleases based on CRISPR/Cas9 or derivatives comprising alternative Cas or guide systems (such as Cas12 and Clover-Cas) have provided more cost-effective and efficient genome-editing avenues and promise simpler bench to bedside development and clinical phase testing.[5–7] Similar to previous iterations of genome editing platforms, initial applications aimed to disrupt the expression of one or more cell surface proteins through non-homologous end joining (NHEJ) at sites of targeted DNA breakage, but recently more complex strategies have included delivery of therapeutic transgene DNA templates through site-specific integration by homologous recombination (HR).[8] Further improvements, including precise nucleotide conversion using base-editing is also being advanced for multiplexed editing[9] and investigations into modifications using prime-editing are also well underway.[10]

T cells are attractive targets for such emerging technologies, with fewer hurdles and risks than following ex-vivo manipulation of hematopoietic stem cells,[11] or the immunologic and biodistribution challenges of direct in vivo approaches.[12–14] T cells are easily accessible from peripheral blood, resist transformation and can be readily manipulated and cryopreserved. They are receptive to viral and non-viral engineering, and the efficiency of the latter has been notably refined with the availability of improved electroporation devices and stabilized RNA.

Table 1
Characteristics of widely investigated strategies for genome editing and examples of investigated clinical application

	ZFN	TALEN	CRISPR/Cas9	Base-editor
Advantages	Specific editing Limited off-target effect	Highly specific and more versatile editing	Adaptable design and efficient editing of multiple targets Low costs	Precise base conversion without double-strand breaks Low risk of translocations Highly efficient
Limitations	Difficult to design for multiple editing Risk of translocations	High costs Large size Risk of translocations	DNA off-target effects Risk of translocations Possible immunogenicity from non-human components	By-stander conversions and off-target effects on DNA or RNA Possible immunogenicity from non-human components
Example of human application for T cell engineering	CCR5 ko in T cells to prevent HIV entry[66]	TCR and CD52 ko For universal CAR T[27]	PD1 ko for lung cancer TILs TCR and PD1 ko in rTCR engineered cells for cancer[49,51]	Anti CD7 universal CAR T cells (pending)

Proof of concept studies that collected T cells for ex vivo culture ahead of adoptive cell therapy for cancer have been underway since the early 1980's[15] and included trials of tumor-infiltrating lymphocytes (TILs), anticipating that the triggered cytotoxic activity could be exploited to tackle certain cancers.[16] Following initial experiences and emergence of gene transfer technologies, development of adoptive therapies employing recombinant TCR (rTCR)[17] or chimeric antigen receptor (CAR)[18] emerged as targeted immunotherapy for cancer. Autologous CAR-T cell therapies have led the way and have been amongst the first to be authorized as marketable advanced therapies and are now being developed worldwide.[19] As genome editing has become available, applications for "next generation" adoptive T cell therapies based on TILs, rTCR and CAR-T cells have aimed to improve anti-tumor activity,[8] persistence,[20] safety and accessibility.[21]

In particular, genome-edited allogeneic "universal" donor CAR T cells represent an attractive strategy to guarantee rapid availability of pre-manufactured cells for use in multiple recipients, thereby reducing costs and widening accessibility.[22] T cells from healthy donors may exhibit superior fitness compared to patient-derived T cells, especially after multiple cycles of chemotherapy or recent stem cell transplantation.[23] Pre-manufactured CAR-T cells can be stored in cell banks, with minimal discrepancies in product specification across different batches, and be readily available, avoiding treatment delays in patients with aggressive disease (**Fig. 2**). Furthermore, healthy donor cells address the risk of product contamination with unwanted leukemic blasts that could be inadvertently transduced and refractory to CAR effects.[24] Genome

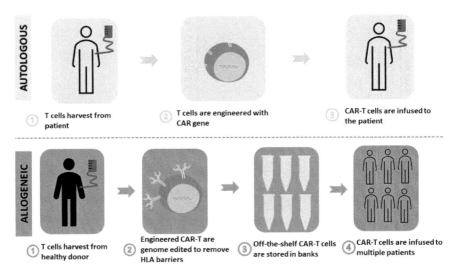

Fig. 2. Manufacturing outline of autologous and allogeneic CAR-T cells. After collection of autologous peripheral blood lymphocytes from a patient at a clinic or harvest center, the cells are usually transported to a centralized manufacturing site. T cells are engineered in a cleanroom facility, using compliant reagents and validated processes. CAR T cells are subsequently cryopreserved before release for shipping to the healthcare provider. The cells are infused back into the patient after they have received lymphodepletion. On the other hand, healthy donor PBLs are collected from a volunteer to generate allogeneic CAR-T cells and one donation can generate dozens of doses of CAR T cells for multiple recipients. Additional genome editing strategies are used to address HLA barriers and "universal" CAR-T cells are stored frozen in multi-dose cell banks.

editing of T cells has also been applied to reduce exhaustion and promote persistence by targeting checkpoint pathways such as PD1, and strategies are in development to allow targeting of other hematological lineage malignancies[9] and to tackle hurdles for cellular immunotherapy against solid tumors.

ADDRESSING HLA BARRIERS FOR 'Universal CAR T CELL THERAPY AGAINST B CELL MALIGNANCIES

HLA mismatched T cells operating in a hostile environment are prone to rejection following host immune system recognition of non-self HLA molecules and may themselves be triggered through their antigen-specific TCRαβ to cause graft versus host disease (GVHD). To overcome these obstacles, T cell manipulation through genome editing has been implemented to prevent TCRαβ expression, and strategies to remove HLA molecules or render cells insensitive to lymphodepletion drugs are being investigated (**Fig. 3**).

Autologous CAR-T cell therapies for CD19 expressing malignancies became rapidly accessible over the past 5 years, and as "real-life" data are being collected, the optimal strategies for a higher chance of success are being established. For instance, it is now clear that CAR-T cell therapies are more effective when used after preparative lymphodepletion regimens, most commonly comprising fludarabine and cyclophosphamide.[25] This strategy appears to favor homeostatic expansion of infused cells, perhaps by reducing competition of cytokines and growth factors, and possibly by disrupting constraints in immunologic niches and regulatory pathways.[25,26] In the allogeneic HLA-mismatched setting, lymphodepletion scheme must also sufficiently inhibit host immunity to prevent rapid rejection of allogeneic T cells by host immune system. Patients can be screened for pre-existing anti-HLA antibodies against incoming cells, but host cellular immunity mediated by T and NK cells requires additional intervention. In addition to chemotherapy, anti-CD52 monoclonal antibody (alemtuzumab) has been used in the allogeneic setting to deplete host cellular

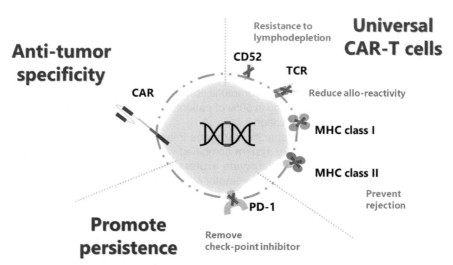

Fig. 3. Strategies for generation of CAR-T cells using genome-editing platforms. CAR: chimeric antigen receptor; CD52: cluster domain-52; MHC: major histocompatibility complex; PD-1: programmed cell death-1; TCR: T cell receptor.

immunity and allow CAR T cells edited to remove CD52 an in vivo survival advantage after infusion.[27] Suppression of host NK and T cells for 2 to 3 weeks could be sufficient to allow incoming engineered T cells to mediate potent anti-leukemic effects, and alemtuzumab may also dampen macrophage activity linked to cytokine release phenomena during CAR activity. In 2015, two infants with relapsed B-cell acute lymphoblastic leukemia (B-ALL) received single dose infusions of UCART19 cells knocked out using TALENs for TRAC and CD52 and achieved molecular remissions allowing them to proceed to allo-SCT.[27] Subsequent multi-center trials in children and adults encountered only mild GvHD and manageable CAR related side effects such as cytokine release syndrome (CRS) and neurotoxicity, though the consequences of deeper lymphodepletion in the allogeneic setting in terms of cytopenia and viral infections was noted.[21] UCART19 cells are under further investigation in adults with non-Hodgkin lymphoma (NHL),[28] and next-generation universal cells disrupted for TCR/CD52 using CRISPR/Cas9 were generated using a lentiviral system that couples TCR knockout and CAR expression and are currently used in study in children with refractory/relapsed B-ALL who failed or are ineligible to an autologous approach.[29,30] Additional data from CRISPR-edited CAR with disruption of TRAC and CD52 have been reported in 6 adults with B-ALL that received an "universal" bi-specific CD19/CD22 (CTA101).[31] CD22 has also been targeted as a single antigen in r/r B-ALL in adults as a single target by Cellectis using TALENs to disrupt TRAC and CD52.[32]

Another strategy to address host-mediated immune rejection involves disruption of HLA molecules: targeting HLA class I by editing β2-microglobulin chain (B_2M), a conserved domain across all class I molecules, has been readily achievable. The strategy aims to prevent recognition of mismatched donor HLA class I by host $CD8^+$ T cells and thereby avoid direct cytotoxic effects. Additional manipulations have been proposed to address the issue of host NK cell triggering by 'missing self' mechanisms.[33] Addressing interactions between host $CD4^+$ T cells and HLA class II molecules on activated donor CAR T cells has been investigated through disruption of CIITA, a critical transcriptional regulator of HLA class II expression in preclinical studies.[34] In the clinic, CRISPR Therapeutics have reported preliminary data of a trial where universal donor CAR19 T cells, incorporating a CAR19 cassette integrated into the TRAC locus using adeno-associated virus (AAV), were also modified at B_2M locus using CRISPR/Cas9 for class I immunologic stealth. Previously, animal studies have suggested that endogenous control of CAR gene mediated by TCR transcriptional machinery at the TRAC locus may provide improved cytotoxic activity and reduce exhaustion.[8] The study treated adults with relapsed refractory diffuse large B-cell lymphoma and preliminary data from 26 patients were communicated in 2021, reporting 38% remission rate, no GvHD, mild CRS occurring in 50% of patients, and one case of severe neurotoxicity attributed to viral reactivation.

Others are also testing site-specific transgene integration. Precision Biosciences have used a similar AAV delivery system combined with a proprietary endonuclease platform again to direct a CAR transgene expression cassette integration into the TRAC locus, although with an internal promoter rather than using TRAC transcriptional machinery.[3] Interim reports of 13 NHL patients treated showed an encouraging safety profile and overall complete response rate of 54%, with indicators favoring more intense lymphodepletion.[35,36]

Finally, as an alternative to viral delivery, Poseida biotech is developing a non-viral PiggyBac transposon platform for CAR expression and is targeting BCMA in multiple myeloma, to be combined with genome editing of TRAC and B_2M with Cas-Clover. The latter comprises inactivated Cas9 fused with dimerization dependent Clo51 endonuclease and requires two RNA guides and potentially offers enhanced editing specificity.[37] Whether disruption of HLA class I is sufficient to evade immune rejection, or if additional removal of class II antigens may also be required is an important issue still to be addressed in human studies.

Although crucial questions remain unanswered, data from the above-mentioned clinical trials investigating genome-edited CAR-T cells in B cell malignancies (summarized in **Table 2**) will contribute to optimize strategies for universal allogeneic approaches.

ENGINEERED T CELLS FOR NON-B LINEAGE HEMATOLOGICAL MALIGNANCIES

Two major reasons why CD19 is an ideal target for engineered T cells against B-cell malignancies are the consistently high expression across a variety of B cell malignancies and the limited risk of "on-target/off-tumor" toxicity other than protracted B cell aplasia. Long-term hypogammaglobulinemia might persist for years after treatment[38] and can be managed with immunoglobulin replacement therapy if required. However, a similar T-cell therapy strategy against T cell malignancies has to accommodate fratricide effects between T cells during manufacturing, and immunodeficiency caused by protracted T-cell aplasia mediated by engineered effector T cells in vivo. Suitable T-cell antigens include the TCR $\alpha\beta$/CD3 complex, CD5, and CD7 and the issue of fratricide during manufacture has been addressed by protein inhibition strategies as well as genome editing. For example, anti-CD7 CAR T cells have been generated following the expression of inhibitory proteins to restrict CD7 surface expression.[39] Trials are underway in Singapore (NCT05043571) and in China (NCT04689659), where a cohort of patients infused with CAR7 T cells derived from their hematopoietic stem cell or alternate donors achieved remission in 15/20 patients, albeit with relatively high incidence of GVHD and lymphopenia.[40]

Genome editing with TALENs against TRAC has been shown to inhibit expression of the multimeric TCR$\alpha\beta$/CD3 complex on T cell surface ahead of lentiviral transduction of an anti-CD3ε CAR transgene. CAR3 expression was followed by 'self-enrichment' of engineered T cells during culture to yield an anti-T cell product devoid of TCR (and less able to mediate GVHD) but with potent anti-T cell immunity, both in vitro and in humanized mice in vivo.[41] Similarly, CRISPR/Cas9 editing of CD7 in combination with TRAC knockout, has produced 'universal' donor CAR7 T cells,[42] and an allogeneic donor strategy may offer a "bridge to transplant", for rapid donor-derived T cell recovery once remission is secured. Similar to B-cell malignancies, an allogenic approach also avoids the risk of unintended transduction of leukemic blasts during manufacture.[24] Preclinical development and comparison of CRISPR/Cas9 and base-edited CAR7 T cells[9] found that efficient multiplexed disruption was achieved with both platforms, although low level of translocation events associated with Cas9 nuclease activity was virtually undetectable in base-edited CAR7 T cells, suggesting advantages in terms of transformation risk. First-in-human application of anti-CD7 CAR T cell therapies is emerging, with encouraging remissions in the small number of individuals with refractory T-cell malignancies treated to date. Multiplexed CD7 and TRAC-edited T cell trials using CRISPR/Cas9 in China have already reported remissions with manageable toxicities,[43] and a trial of multiplexed base-edited CAR7 T cells is planned in the UK (**Table 3**).

CAR-T cells redirected against myeloid targets in acute myeloid leukemia (AML), have also been constrained by the risk of "on-target/off-tumor" consequences against the normal hematopoietic compartment given that common myeloid markers such as CD33 and CD123 are shared between myeloid-derived blasts and healthy progenitors. Approaches to remove target antigen expression from healthy hematopoietic

Table 2
Selected active and/or enrolling clinical trials of "universal" genome-edited T cell against B cell malignancies with early clinical data available

Sponsor/Study	Product	Indication	Target Edits	Platforms	Patients (n)	Safety	Reference
Servier/Allogene NCT02808442 NCT02746952	UCART19	r/r CD19+ B-ALL	TRAC CD52	TALEN LV	Children (7) and adults (14)	Grade 3+ CRS 15%; Grade 3+ infections 39%	Benjamin, et al,[21] 2020
Allogene NCT04416984 NCT03939026	ALLO-501A ALLO-501	r/r large B cell CD19+ lymphoma	TRAC CD52	TALEN LV	Adults (47)	Grade 3+ CRS: 2%; Grade 3+ infections 24%	Neelapu et al,[28] 2020, Locke et al,[67] 2021, Neelapu, et al,[68] 2021
Cellectis NCT04150497	UCART22	r/r CD22+ B-ALL	TRAC CD52	TALEN LV	Adults (9)	No Grade 3+ infections/CRS/ICANS	Jain et al,[32] 2020, Jain et al,[69] 2020
Precision Bio NCT03666000	PBCAR0191	r/r CD19+ B cell malignancy	TRAC	Homing endonuclease AAV	Adults (21)	Grade 3+ CRS 6%; Grade 3+ infections 31%	Shah et al,[36] 2020
CRISPR Therapeutic NCT04035434	CTX110	r/r CD19+ B cell malignancy	TRAC B2M	CRISPR/Cas9 AAV	Adults (26)	No Grade 3+ CRS; Grade 3+ infections 9%; Grade 3+ ICANS 4%	Eyquem et al,[8] 2020 McGuirk et al,[70] 2021 ; sponsor communications
Great Ormond Street Hospital NCT04557436	TT52CAR19	r/r CD19+ B-ALL	TRAC CD52	CRISPR/Cas9 LV	Children (2)	No Grade 3+ CRS/ICANS; Grade 3+ infections 2/2	Ottaviano et al,[29] 2021

Nanjing Bioheng Biotech Co. NCT04227015	CTA101	CD19+CD22+ B cell malignancy	TRAC CD52	CRISPR/Cas9 LV	Adults (6)	Grade 3+ CRS 17%; Grade 3+ infections 50%	Hu et al,[31] 2021
Poseida NCT04960579	P-BCMAAllo1	r/r Multiple myeloma	TRAC B2m	Cas-Clover PiggyBac transposon	Adults	N/A	Cranert et al,[37] 2020
Caribou Biosciences NCT04637763	CB-010	CD19+ r/r B cell NHL	TRAC PDCD1	chRDNA/Cas12a AAV	Adults	N/A	Donohoue et al,[52] 2021

Abbreviations: CRS, cytokine release syndrome; ICANS, immune-effector cell-associated neurotoxicity syndrome; LV, lentivirus; AAV, adeno-associated virus; N/A, not available

Table 3
Selected clinical trials investigating allogeneic CAR-T cells for T-ALL and AML

Sponsor/Country/ Trial ref.	Indication	Target	Platform	Reference
Wugen, USA NCT04984356	CD7[+] T-ALL	CD7 TRAC	CRISPR/Cas9	Leedom et al,[71] 2021; Ghobadi et al,[72] 2021
Gracell Bio, China NCT04264078	CD7[+] T-ALL	CD7 TRAC	CRISPR/Cas9	Li et al,[43] 2021
Nanjing Bioheng Biotech Co., China	CD7[+] T-ALL	CD7 TRAC HLA-II	CRISPR/Cas9	He et al,[73] 2021
Great Ormond Street Hospital, UK (Opening in 2022)	CD7[+], CD33[+], CD123[+] AML/T-ALL	CD7 TRBC CD52	Base editor	Georgiadis et al,[9] 2021
Yake Bio, China NCT04599556	CD7[+] T-ALL	CD7	Protein expression blockers (PEBLs)	Pan et al,[40] 2021
Cellectis, USA NCT03190278	CD123[+] AML	TRAC CD52	TALEN	Roboz et al,[45] 2020

progenitors using CRISPR/Cas9 have been developed[44] although have not yet been tested in clinic. Alternatively, genome editing is being applied to generate 'universal' allogeneic CAR-T cells against such antigens, as a prelude to allo-SCT and donor-derived reconstitution once remission is achieved. For example, UCART123 are TALEN-edited donor T cells with anti-CD123 CAR that have been investigated against adult acute myeloid leukemia (NCT03190278) and blastic plasmacytoid dendritic cell leukemia (NCT03203369), with toxicities reported early in Phase 1 testing.[45] A clinical study of base-edited anti-CD33 and anti-CD123 universal CAR T cells against pediatric AML plans to use combinations of CAR T cells to address the issue of disease escape when single antigens are targeted (see **Table 3**).

ADDRESSING T CELL EXHAUSTION AND PERSISTENCE

Promoting persistence and addressing exhaustion are widely being explored through the manipulation of checkpoint pathways. PD-1-PDL-1 pathway represents an attractive target due to its role in inhibition of T cell activation, proliferation, and survival within inhibitory tumor microenvironments.[46] Anti- PD-1 and PD-L1 antibodies (eg, nivolumab, pembrolizumab) have been approved for a variety of cancers[47] and there has been extensive interest in using genome editing to disrupt expression in T cells.[48–50] The first human application of CRISPR/Cas9 involved editing autologous TILs at the PDCD1 locus (encoding PD-1) in adults with refractory lung cancer, and there were no immediate or short-term toxicities uncovered.[51] A similar engineered T cell therapy, manufactured with multiplex genome editing of TRAC, TRBC, and PDCD1 loci and lentiviral transduction of a synthetic cancer-specific rTCR against NY-ESO-1 has been used in adults with advanced cancer.[49] In both these reports, extended persistence of engineered T cells was attributed to PD-1 disruption, although no definitive conclusions could be drawn for efficacy. A similar approach has been applied to allogeneic CAR19 cells for the treatment of B-cell NHL by Caribou

Biosciences: the ANTLER trial is investigating the safety of CB-010, PD-1 disrupted allogeneic CAR19 T cells, manufactured using proprietary CRISPR hybrid RNA-DNA guides (chRDNA) in combination with Cas12a for high-efficiency gene insertions of template delivered using AAV.[52] As discussed above, as PD-1 has been reported to act as haplo-insufficient immune suppressor of T-cell lymphomagenesis,[53] one concern of using PD-1 genome-edited T cells is the potential risk of malignant T cell transformation. Although the above-mentioned reports appear reassuring to date, further monitoring will be required to better evaluate such risks and benefits.

SAFETY AND LONG-TERM MONITORING

Experience with gamma-retroviral and lentiviral transduction for gene addition to hematopoietic stem cells for the correction of inherited monogenic disorders has uncovered transformation risks following vector-mediated manipulation.[54–57] Description of transactivation effects from enhancer elements in retroviral long terminal repeats almost 20 years ago led to the development of self-inactivating configurations, advancement of lentiviral systems and long-term monitoring plans for all patients receiving gene therapies. Genetic manipulation of human T cells using retroviral vectors has not been linked to transformation,[58] although recent concerns emerged from new-onset CAR-T lymphoma in two patients following modification of T cells using piggyBac transposons for the expression of CAR19 with mechanisms yet to be defined.[59] Clonal dominance after lentiviral transduction of T cells has been described in two subjects after CAR19[60] and CAR22[61] therapy and attributed to specific integration sites. In the context of genome editing, a trial of TALEN-edited CAR19 T cells in r/r B cell lymphoma was temporarily placed on hold while regulators in the US considered possible translocation related adverse effects.[62] Pre-clinical studies and early clinical applications of genome-edited T cells quantified frequencies of translocation between chromosomes using both TALEN and CRISPR/Cas9 technology, with up to 5% abnormal karyotypes observed for the former ahead of trial applications.[27,49] In other circumstances studies with CRISPR/Cas9 in T cells have previously indicated T cell transformation could arise through disruption of PD1 checkpoint pathways.[53] Alternative genome editing strategies using base editing for precise genetic modification and single base conversion may address some concerns. Cytidine deamination mediated-based editing has demonstrated that translocations can be virtually eliminated in T cells in comparison to CRISPR/Cas9.[9,63] Nevertheless, there remains the possibility of unpredictable genome-wide off-target activity[64,65] warranting careful monitoring of patients as the technology reaches the clinical application.

SUMMARY

The first licensed gene-modified T cell products represent beginning of new opportunities to exploit the immune system to fight cancer. Emerging genome-editing applications represent efforts to extend novel therapies including pre-manufactured 'off the shelf' CAR-T cell banks that might contribute to reducing costs while widening accessibility. While the potential of the technology is rapidly evolving, watchful and continuous monitoring for longer terms effects will be part of the investigational landscape. Clinical trial observations will contribute to defining optimal strategies, including the degree of immunosuppression required, duration and persistence for anti-leukemic effects, and the role of hematopoietic stem cell transplantation to consolidate responses.

CLINICS CARE POINTS

- Genome-edited T cells are being investigated for cancer immunotherapy and could help extend the application of CAR-T cell therapy.
- Hurdles of allogeneic CAR-T cells (rejection and allo-reactivity) are being addressed using different preparative strategies and cell engineering platforms
- Long-term monitoring of safety and outcomes will be essential as treatments roll out

FUNDING & DISCLOSURES

Supported by the National Institute of Health Research (NIHR) via the Biomedical Research Centre (BRC). G. Ottaviano is supported by Medical Research Council (MRC) and WQ by NIHR, MRC & Wellcome Trust. W. Qasim has previously received research funding from Cellectis & Servier related to T cell editing. W. Qasim has filed patents related to the application of genome-edited T cells; Unrelated, W. Qasim holds stock in Autolus Therapeutics and has advised Tessa Therapeutics, Wugen, Novartis, Kite & Virocell.

REFERENCES

1. Torikai H, Reik A, Liu PQ, et al. A foundation for universal T-cell based immunotherapy: T cells engineered to express a CD19-specific chimeric-antigen-receptor and eliminate expression of endogenous TCR. Blood 2012;119(24):5697–705.
2. Poirot L, Philip B, Schiffer-Mannioui C, et al. Multiplex Genome-Edited T-cell Manufacturing Platform for "Off-the-Shelf" Adoptive T-cell Immunotherapies. Cancer Res 2015;75(18):3853–64.
3. MacLeod DT, Antony J, Martin AJ, et al. Integration of a CD19 CAR into the TCR Alpha Chain Locus Streamlines Production of Allogeneic Gene-Edited CAR T Cells. Mol Ther 2017;25(4):949–61.
4. Boissel S, Jarjour J, Astrakhan A, et al. megaTALs: a rare-cleaving nuclease architecture for therapeutic genome engineering. Nucleic Acids Res 2014;42(4):2591–601.
5. Ren J, Zhang X, Liu X, et al. A versatile system for rapid multiplex genome-edited CAR T cell generation. Oncotarget 2017;8(10):17002–11.
6. Tseng H, Zhang Y, Cranert SA, et al. Memory Phenotype in Allogeneic Anti-BCMA CAR-T Cell Therapy (P-BCMA-ALLO1) Correlates with In Vivo Tumor Control. Blood 2021;138(Supplement 1):4802.
7. Kleinstiver BP, Sousa AA, Walton RT, et al. Engineered CRISPR-Cas12a variants with increased activities and improved targeting ranges for gene, epigenetic and base editing. Nat Biotechnol 2019;37(3):276–82.
8. Eyquem J, Mansilla-Soto J, Giavridis T, et al. Targeting a CAR to the TRAC locus with CRISPR/Cas9 enhances tumour rejection. Nature 2017;543(7643):113–7.
9. Georgiadis C, Rasaiyaah J, Gkazi SA, et al. Base-edited CAR T cells for combinational therapy against T cell malignancies. Leukemia 2021;1–16.
10. Anzalone AV, Randolph PB, Davis JR, et al. Search-and-replace genome editing without double-strand breaks or donor DNA. Nature 2019;576(7785):149–57.
11. Stein S, Ott MG, Schultze-Strasser S, et al. Genomic instability and myelodysplasia with monosomy 7 consequent to EVI1 activation after gene therapy for chronic granulomatous disease. Nat Med 2010;16(2):198–204.

12. Mingozzi F, High KA. Overcoming the Host Immune Response to Adeno-Associated Virus Gene Delivery Vectors: The Race Between Clearance, Tolerance, Neutralization, and Escape. Annu Rev Virol 2017;4(1):511–34.

13. van Haasteren J, Hyde SC, Gill DR. Lessons learned from lung and liver in-vivo gene therapy: implications for the future. Expert Opin Biol Ther 2018;18(9):959–72.

14. Mendell JR, Al-Zaidy SA, Rodino-Klapac LR, et al. Current Clinical Applications of In Vivo Gene Therapy with AAVs. Mol Ther 2021;29(2):464–88.

15. Rosenberg SA, Lotze MT, Muul LM, et al. Observations on the systemic administration of autologous lymphokine-activated killer cells and recombinant interleukin-2 to patients with metastatic cancer. N Engl J Med 1985;313(23):1485–92.

16. Rosenberg SA, Packard BS, Aebersold PM, et al. Use of tumor-infiltrating lymphocytes and interleukin-2 in the immunotherapy of patients with metastatic melanoma. A preliminary report. N Engl J Med 1988;319(25):1676–80.

17. Morgan RA, Dudley ME, Wunderlich JR, et al. Cancer regression in patients after transfer of genetically engineered lymphocytes. Science 2006;314(5796):126–9.

18. Kalos M, Levine BL, Porter DL, et al. T cells with chimeric antigen receptors have potent antitumor effects and can establish memory in patients with advanced leukemia. Sci Transl Med 2011;3(95). 95ra73.

19. Maude SL, Laetsch TW, Buechner J, et al. Tisagenlecleucel in Children and Young Adults with B-Cell Lymphoblastic Leukemia. N Engl J Med 2018;378(5):439–48.

20. Chamberlain CA, Bennett EP, Kverneland AH, et al. Highly efficient PD-1-targeted CRISPR-Cas9 for tumor-infiltrating lymphocyte-based adoptive T cell therapy. Mol Ther Oncolytics 2022;24:417–28.

21. Benjamin R, Graham C, Yallop D, et al. Genome-edited, donor-derived allogeneic anti-CD19 chimeric antigen receptor T cells in paediatric and adult B-cell acute lymphoblastic leukaemia: results of two phase 1 studies. Lancet 2020;396(10266):1885–94.

22. Morgan MA, Büning H, Sauer M, et al. Use of Cell and Genome Modification Technologies to Generate Improved "Off-the-Shelf" CAR T and CAR NK Cells. Front Immunol 2020;11:1965.

23. Das RK, O'Connor RS, Grupp SA, et al. Lingering effects of chemotherapy on mature T cells impair proliferation. Blood Adv 2020;4(19):4653–64.

24.. Ruella M, Xu J, Barrett DM, et al. Induction of resistance to chimeric antigen receptor T cell therapy by transduction of a single leukemic B cell. Nat Med 2018;24(10):1499–503.

25. Hirayama AV, Gauthier J, Hay KA, et al. The response to lymphodepletion impacts PFS in patients with aggressive non-Hodgkin lymphoma treated with CD19 CAR T cells. Blood 2019;133(17):1876–87.

26. Nissani A, Lev-Ari S, Meirson T, et al. Comparison of non-myeloablative lymphodepleting preconditioning regimens in patients undergoing adoptive T cell therapy. J Immunother Cancer 2021;9(5).

27. Qasim W, Zhan H, Samarasinghe S, et al. Molecular remission of infant B-ALL after infusion of universal TALEN gene-edited CAR T cells. Sci translational Med 2017;9(374).

28. Neelapu SS, Munoz J, Locke FL, et al. First-in-human data of ALLO-501 and ALLO-647 in relapsed/refractory large B-cell or follicular lymphoma (R/R LBCL/FL): ALPHA study. J Clin Oncol 2020;38(15_suppl):8002.

29. Ottaviano G, Georgiadis C, Syed F, et al. TT52CAR19: Phase 1 Trial of CRISPR/Cas9 Edited Allogeneic CAR19 T Cells for Paediatric Relapsed/Refractory B-ALL. Blood 2021;138(Supplement 1):4838.
30. Georgiadis C, Preece R, Nickolay L, et al. Long Terminal Repeat CRISPR-CAR-Coupled "Universal" T Cells Mediate Potent Anti-leukemic Effects. Mol Ther 2018;26(5):1215–27.
31. Hu Y, Zhou Y, Zhang M, et al. CRISPR/Cas9-Engineered Universal CD19/CD22 Dual-Targeted CAR-T Cell Therapy for Relapsed/Refractory B-cell Acute Lymphoblastic Leukemia. Clin Cancer Res 2021;27(10):2764–72.
32. Jain N, Roboz GJ, Konopleva M, et al. Preliminary Results of Balli-01: A Phase I Study of UCART22 (allogeneic engineered T-cells expressing anti-CD22 Chimeric Antigen Receptor) in Adult Patients with Relapsed or Refractory (R/R) CD22+ B-Cell Acute Lymphoblastic Leukemia (B-ALL). Blood 2020;136(Supplement 1):7–8.
33. Gornalusse GG, Hirata RK, Funk SE, et al. HLA-E-expressing pluripotent stem cells escape allogeneic responses and lysis by NK cells. Nat Biotechnol 2017;35(8):765–72.
34. Kagoya Y, Guo T, Yeung B, et al. Genetic Ablation of HLA Class I, Class II, and the T-cell Receptor Enables Allogeneic T Cells to Be Used for Adoptive T-cell Therapy. Cancer Immunol Res 2020;8(7):926–36.
35. Jacobson CA, Herrera AF, Budde LE, et al. Initial Findings of the Phase 1 Trial of PBCAR0191, a CD19 Targeted Allogeneic CAR-T Cell Therapy. Blood 2019;134(Supplement_1):4107.
36. Shah BD, Jacobson C, Solomon SR, et al. Allogeneic CAR-T PBCAR0191 with Intensified Lymphodepletion Is Highly Active in Patients with Relapsed/Refractory B-Cell Malignancies. Blood 2021;138(Supplement 1):302.
37. Cranert SA, Richter M, Tong M, et al. Manufacture of an Allogeneic CAR-T Stem Cell Memory Product Candidate for Multiple Myeloma, P-Bcma-ALLO1, Is Robust, Reproducible and Highly Scalable. Blood 2019;134(Supplement_1):4445.
38. Doan A, Pulsipher MA. Hypogammaglobulinemia due to CAR T-cell therapy. Pediatr Blood Cancer 2018;65(4).
39. Png YT, Vinanica N, Kamiya T, et al. Blockade of CD7 expression in T cells for effective chimeric antigen receptor targeting of T-cell malignancies. Blood Adv 2017;1(25):2348–60.
40. Pan J, Tan Y, Wang G, et al. Donor-Derived CD7 Chimeric Antigen Receptor T Cells for T-Cell Acute Lymphoblastic Leukemia: First-in-Human, Phase I Trial. J Clin Oncol 2021;39(30):3340–51.
41. Rasaiyaah J, Georgiadis C, Preece R, et al. TCRαβ/CD3 disruption enables CD3-specific antileukemic T cell immunotherapy. JCI Insight 2018;3(13).
42. Gomes-Silva D, Srinivasan M, Sharma S, et al. CD7-edited T cells expressing a CD7-specific CAR for the therapy of T-cell malignancies. Blood 2017;130(3):285–96.
43. Li S, Wang X, Yuan Z, et al. Eradication of T-ALL Cells by CD7-targeted Universal CAR-T Cells and Initial Test of Ruxolitinib-based CRS Management. Clin Cancer Res 2021;27(5):1242–6.
44. Kim MY, Yu KR, Kenderian SS, et al. Genetic Inactivation of CD33 in Hematopoietic Stem Cells to Enable CAR T Cell Immunotherapy for Acute Myeloid Leukemia. Cell 2018;173(6):1439–1453 e19.
45. Roboz GJ, DeAngelo DJ, Sallman DA, et al. Ameli-01: Phase I, Open Label Dose-Escalation and Dose-Expansion Study to Evaluate the Safety, Expansion,

Persistence and Clinical Activity of UCART123 (allogeneic engineered T-cells expressing anti-CD123 chimeric antigen receptor), Administered in Patients with Relapsed/Refractory Acute Myeloid Leukemia. Blood 2020;136(Supplement 1):41–2.

46. Jiang X, Wang J, Deng X, et al. Role of the tumor microenvironment in PD-L1/PD-1-mediated tumor immune escape. Mol Cancer 2019;18(1):10.

47. Vaddepally RK, Kharel P, Pandey R, et al. Review of Indications of FDA-Approved Immune Checkpoint Inhibitors per NCCN Guidelines with the Level of Evidence. Cancers (Basel). 2020;12(3).

48. Su S, Hu B, Shao J, et al. CRISPR-Cas9 mediated efficient PD-1 disruption on human primary T cells from cancer patients. Scientific Rep 2016;6:20070.

49. Stadtmauer EA, Fraietta JA, Davis MM, et al. CRISPR-engineered T cells in patients with refractory cancer. Science 2020;367(6481).

50. Ren J, Liu X, Fang C, et al. Multiplex Genome Editing to Generate Universal CAR T Cells Resistant to PD1 Inhibition. Clin Cancer Res 2017;23(9):2255–66.

51. Lu Y, Xue J, Deng T, et al. Safety and feasibility of CRISPR-edited T cells in patients with refractory non-small-cell lung cancer. Nat Med 2020;26(5):732–40.

52. Donohoue PD, Pacesa M, Lau E, et al. Conformational control of Cas9 by CRISPR hybrid RNA-DNA guides mitigates off-target activity in T cells. Mol Cell 2021; 81(17):3637–49, e5.

53. Wartewig T, Kurgyis Z, Keppler S, et al. PD-1 is a haploinsufficient suppressor of T cell lymphomagenesis. Nature 2017;552:121–5.

54. Hacein-Bey-Abina S, Von Kalle C, Schmidt M, et al. A serious adverse event after successful gene therapy for X-linked severe combined immunodeficiency. N Eng J Med 2003;348(3):255–6.

55. Ott MG, Schmidt M, Schwarzwaelder K, et al. Correction of X-linked chronic granulomatous disease by gene therapy, augmented by insertional activation of MDS1-EVI1, PRDM16 or SETBP1. Nat Med 2006;12(4):401–9.

56. Howe SJ, Mansour MR, Schwarzwaelder K, et al. Insertional mutagenesis combined with acquired somatic mutations causes leukemogenesis following gene therapy of SCID-X1 patients. JClinInvest 2008;118(9):3143–50.

57. Braun CJ, Boztug K, Paruzynski A, et al. Gene therapy for wiskott-Aldrich syndrome–long-term efficacy and genotoxicity. Sci Transl Med 2014;6(227):227ra33.

58. Newrzela S, Cornils K, Li Z, et al. Resistance of mature T cells to oncogene transformation. Blood 2008;112(6):2278–86.

59. Bishop DC, Clancy LE, Simms R, et al. Development of CAR T-cell lymphoma in 2 of 10 patients effectively treated with piggyBac-modified CD19 CAR T cells. Blood 2021;138(16):1504–9.

60. Fraietta JA, Nobles CL, Sammons MA, et al. Disruption of TET2 promotes the therapeutic efficacy of CD19-targeted T cells. Nature 2018;558(7709):307–12.

61. Shah NN, Qin H, Yates B, et al. Clonal expansion of CAR T cells harboring lentivector integration in the CBL gene following anti-CD22 CAR T-cell therapy. Blood Adv 2019;3(15):2317–22.

62. Sheridan C. Off-the-shelf, gene-edited CAR-T cells forge ahead, despite safety scare. Nat Biotechnol 2022;40(1):5–8.

63. Billon P, Bryant EE, Joseph SA, et al. CRISPR-Mediated Base Editing Enables Efficient Disruption of Eukaryotic Genes through Induction of STOP Codons. Mol Cell 2017;67(6):1068–79, e4.

64. Grunewald J, Zhou R, Garcia SP, et al. Transcriptome-wide off-target RNA editing induced by CRISPR-guided DNA base editors. Nature 2019;569(7756):433–7.

65. Grunewald J, Zhou R, Iyer S, et al. CRISPR DNA base editors with reduced RNA off-target and self-editing activities. Nat Biotechnol 2019;37(9):1041–8.

66. Tebas P, Stein D, Tang WW, et al. Gene editing of CCR5 in autologous CD4 T cells of persons infected with HIV. N Engl J Med 2014;370(10):901–10.

67. Locke FL, Malik S, Tees MT, et al. First-in-human data of ALLO-501A, an allogeneic chimeric antigen receptor (CAR) T-cell therapy and ALLO-647 in relapsed/refractory large B-cell lymphoma (R/R LBCL): ALPHA2 study. J Clin Oncol 2021;39(15_suppl):2529.

68. Neelapu SS, Nath R, Munoz J, et al. ALPHA Study: ALLO-501 Produced Deep and Durable Responses in Patients with Relapsed/Refractory Non-Hodgkin's Lymphoma Comparable to Autologous CAR T. Blood 2021;138:3878.

69. Jain N, Roboz GJ, Konopleva M, et al. Preliminary Results from the Flu/Cy/Alemtuzumab Arm of the Phase I BALLI-01 Trial of UCART22, an Anti-CD22 Allogeneic CAR-T Cell Product, in Adult Patients with Relapsed or Refractory (R/R) CD22+ B-Cell Acute Lymphoblastic Leukemia (B-ALL). Blood 2021;138(Supplement 1):1746.

70. McGuirk J, Bachier CR, Bishop MR, et al. A phase 1 dose escalation and cohort expansion study of the safety and efficacy of allogeneic CRISPR-Cas9–engineered T cells (CTX110) in patients (Pts) with relapsed or refractory (R/R) B-cell malignancies (CARBON). J Clin Oncol 2021;39(15_suppl). TPS7570-TPS.

71. Leedom T, Hamil AS, Pouyanfard S, et al. Characterization of WU-CART-007, an Allogeneic CD7-Targeted CAR-T Cell Therapy for T-Cell Malignancies. Blood 2021;138(Supplement 1):2772.

72. Ghobadi A, Aldoss I, Locke FL, et al. A Phase 1/2 Dose-Escalation and Dose-Expansion Study of the Safety and Efficacy of Anti-CD7 Allogeneic CAR-T Cells (WU-CART-007) in Patients with Relapsed or Refractory T-Cell Acute Lymphoblastic Leukemia (T-ALL)/Lymphoblastic Lymphoma (LBL). Blood 2021;138(Supplement 1):4829.

73. He H, Yongxian H, Yali Z, et al. Efficacy-enhanced and cytokine release syndrome-attenuated anti-CD7 universal chimeric antigen receptor-T cell therapy for relapsed/refractory CD7-positive hematological malignancies: A phase I clinical study. Res Square 2021. https://doi.org/10.21203/rs.3.rs-514812/v1.

Gene-Based Natural Killer Cell Therapies for the Treatment of Pediatric Hematologic Malignancies

Ruyan Rahnama, MD, MSc[a,b], Ilias Christodoulou, MD[a], Challice L. Bonifant, MD, PhD[a,b],*

KEYWORDS

- NK cell • Immunotherapy • Blood cancer • Genetic engineering

KEY POINTS

- NK cells are lymphocytes of the innate immune system with powerful intrinsic cytotoxic mechanisms that can be further enhanced by genetic engineering.
- NK cells for therapeutic use are derived from numerous sources, including peripheral blood, cord blood, pluripotent stem cells, embryonic stem cells, and transformed NK cell lines.
- Genetic modification of NK cells has been studied using viral and nonviral vectors for nontargeted and targeted genomic editing. Retroviral vectors have been optimized for safety and efficiency and are the preferred vehicle for ex vivo genetic engineering.
- NK cell activity can be enhanced through the modification of cell surface receptors, manipulation of the inflammatory and suppressive cytokine milieu, and directed evasion of regulatory mechanisms.
- Combination with small molecular engagers can strengthen NK cell targeting and activation.

BACKGROUND

Pediatric leukemias and lymphomas comprise the most common subset of pediatric cancers.[1,2] The diagnosis of pediatric leukemia encompasses diverse clinical and biological diseases. While patients with pediatric acute lymphoblastic leukemia (ALL) have a greater than 80% chance of cure,[3] other blood cancers have poorer prognoses. Novel therapies for acute myeloid leukemia (AML), infant ALL, adolescent/young

[a] The Sidney Kimmel Comprehensive Cancer Center, Johns Hopkins University School of Medicine, 1650 Orleans Street, Baltimore, MD 21287, USA; [b] Department of Pediatrics, Johns Hopkins University School of Medicine, Baltimore, MD, USA
* Corresponding author. The Sidney Kimmel Comprehensive Cancer Center, Johns Hopkins University School of Medicine, 1650 Orleans Street, Baltimore, MD 21287.
E-mail address: cbonifa2@jh.edu

Hematol Oncol Clin N Am 36 (2022) 745–768
https://doi.org/10.1016/j.hoc.2022.03.007
0889-8588/22/© 2022 Elsevier Inc. All rights reserved.

hemonc.theclinics.com

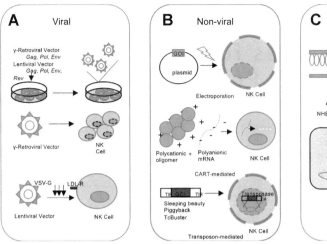
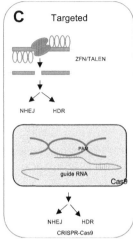

Fig. 1. Methods of Genetic Engineering in NK Cells. (*A*) Viral-mediated, including γ-retroviral and lentiviral vectors. (*B*) Nonviral mediated, including electroporation, Charge-altering releasable transporters, and transposon systems. (*C*) Targeted knockdown and knock-in, including zinc-finger nucleases (ZFN), transcription activator-like nucleases (TALENs), and CRISPR/Cas9 systems as NK cell engineering methods.

adult ALL, and relapsed or refractory ALL are urgently needed. With advanced genetic and molecular profiling of these diseases, there is now the opportunity to develop targeted therapies with more favorable safety profiles and improved efficacy.

T-cell adoptive transfer is one type of targeted therapy that has had great success in the treatment of high-risk ALL. A multicenter clinical trial of treatment with the anti-CD19 chimeric antigen receptor (CAR) T-cell therapy, tisagenlecleucel, demonstrated an overall remission rate within 3 months of 81%,[4] leading to FDA-approval for therapy of relapsed pre-B ALL.[5] Though this clinical success suggests promise for all pediatric blood cancers, expanded use of CAR-T cell therapy also has clear limitations. Treatment with CAR-T cells has the risk of severe toxicities including Cytokine Release Syndrome (CRS), Immune Effector Cell Associated Neurotoxicity Syndrome (ICANS), and CAR-associated Hemophagocytic Lymphohistiocytosis (carHLH).[6,7] Further, tisagenlecleucel and all other commercial CAR-T cell products are derived from autologous hematopoietic cell collections, which can be challenging to perform in heavily pretreated patients with active disease. Per-patient CAR-T cell manufacture is also time-consuming and costly.[8] While the collection of healthy donor T cells can be considered, the use of human leukocyte antigen (HLA)-mismatched allogeneic products carries the serious risk of graft-versus-host disease (GVHD).[9] Natural Killer (NK) cells are alternate lymphocyte effector cells that are also potent killers. NK cells have the potential for *ex vivo* expansion and storage as an "off the shelf" therapy. While activated NK cells secrete cytokines that contribute to the inflammatory milieu, they do not directly cause graft versus host disease[9,10] and have an overall less severe side effect profile than allogeneic T-cell products.[11–15] Because of these favorable characteristics, there is expanded focus on the study and development of NK cells as immunotherapeutics targeted to cancer.

Natural Killer Cell Biology

NK cells are lymphocytes of the innate immune system that serve a critical function in host defense against viral infections and malignancy.[16] They constitute 5% to 15% of

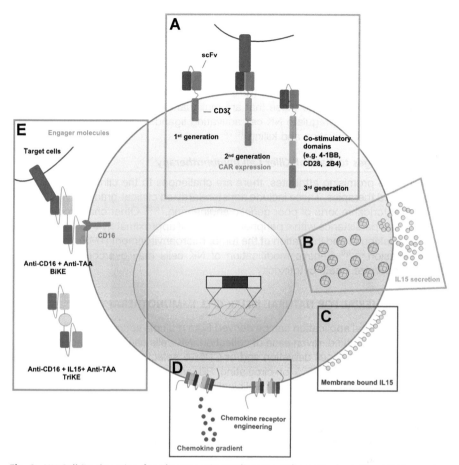

Fig. 2. NK Cell Engineering for Therapeutic Application. Schematic depicting (*A*) Expression of CARs targeting TAA to enhance cytotoxicity and NK cell activation. (*B*) Constitutive secretion or (*C*) membrane-tethered cytokine can sustain NK cell activation and persistence. (*D*) Enhanced surface expression of chemokine receptors can mediate NK cell localization to tumor along chemokine gradients. (*E*) Engager molecules (BiKEs or TriKEs) can be combined with engineered CD16 to direct powerful ADCC of tumor cells. Incorporation of IL15 in the small molecule can further support persistence.

circulating lymphocytes and are found in the peripheral blood as well as lymphoid and nonlymphoid organs such as the spleen, lung, and liver.[15,17,18] NK cells arise from CD34+ hematopoietic stem cells and progress through developmental stages defined by the expression of surface receptors in response to cytokines including Interleukin (IL)-2, IL-7, and IL-15.[15,19] NK cells in the peripheral blood are subdivided into two primary categories: CD56[bright]CD16[dim/-] cells are phenotypically less mature with the capability to produce higher levels of inflammatory cytokines, while CD56[dim]CD16[+] NK cells are more mature with greater cytotoxic potential.[15,18,19] Most NK cells in peripheral circulation fit the latter CD56[dim] profile, with the CD56[bright] subset representing <15% of the total circulating cell population,[15,18] though recent single cell analyses have revealed additional diversity.[20,21] NK cells perform their immune function through four major pathways: (1) secretion of cytokines and chemokines, (2) direct cytotoxicity,

(3) target killing through induced apoptosis, and (4) antibody-dependent cellular cyto-toxicity.[22] NK cells are activated following the integration of stimulatory and inhibitory signals without the need for antigen processing and presentation or HLA match-ing.[22,23] Major histocompatibility complex class I (MHC I) molecules are found on all healthy nucleated cells and provide protection from NK cell targeting through the liga-tion of the killer immunoglobulin-like (KIR) family of inhibitory NK cell receptors.[15,24] Cells infected with virus and those that are malignant typically downregulate MHC I expression[25–27] and upregulate NK cell activating ligands, thereby tipping the scale in favor of NK cell activation and killing.[15,28]

Unique Challenges to Natural Killer Cell Immunotherapy

Despite these promising attributes, there are challenges to the clinical translation of NK cell-based therapies. These include nonstandardized clinical-grade ex vivo expan-sion and historical reports of poor genetic engineering.[15,29] Other challenges include limited *in vivo* persistence with a peripheral half-life of approximately 7 to 10 days,[30–32] limited trafficking to and infiltration of the tumor microenvironment (TME),[33] and tumor immunoevasion.[34–36] Genetic modification of NK cells may overcome these chal-lenges to optimize innate cytotoxicity.

STARTING MATERIAL FOR NATURAL KILLER CELL IMMUNOTHERAPY

NK cells for clinical application can be derived from multiple sources. Peripheral blood (PB) is the best-studied, given ease of collection. NK cells can be purified after blood apheresis with CD3+ cell depletion and/or CD56+ selection.[37,38] Because NK cells represent only 10% to 15% of circulating PB cells, the expansion of peripheral blood-derived NK cells (PB-NKs) on a clinical scale is achieved by culture with supple-mental cytokine and/or feeder cells.[39–41] NK cell expansion using feeder cells was first described by Campana and colleagues,[42] and consists of K562 cells engineered to express ligands that trigger NK cell activation (ex. membrane-bound IL15, IL21, and 4-1BBL).[40,43,44] PB-NKs highly express a repertoire of activating receptors and are functionally mature, with cytotoxic capacity.[45] PB-NKs also express higher levels of KIRs than other sources. This is particularly important for NK cell functionality, since KIR expression has a central role in NK cell education and licensing.[46–48] One of the theoretic limitations to the use of PB-NKs as cancer immunotherapy is reportedly poor success with genetic modification.[49,50] However, we and others have shown high levels of vector transduction of PB-NKs.[37,38,51]

NK cells can also be differentiated from induced pluripotent stem cells (iPSCs) un-der standardized culture conditions.[52,53] The production of NK cells from iPSCs (iPSC-NKs) requires more expertise than peripheral blood NK cell selection.[53] The iPSC platform produces a homogeneous NK cell population. NK cell iPSC derivation allows for multiple genetic modifications while cells are relatively undifferentiated, including CAR-engineering and genetic deletion.[54,55] iPSC-NKs have a similar, but more imma-ture phenotypic profile to PB-NKs, with higher expression of the inhibitory receptor NKG2A.[52] Moreover, iPSC-NKs exhibit lower KIR expression.[52] Nevertheless, iPSC-NKs have promise as anticancer immunotherapy[54–56] and can be developed as "off-the-shelf" cellular banks, with well-defined NK cell therapy products generated on large scale, readily available for adoptive transfer.

Cancerous NK cell lines have also been established over the years as sources of NK cell therapy products (NK-92,[57] NK-101,[58] NK-YS,[59] NKL,[60] NKG,[61] KHYG-1,[62] and others). The NK-92 lymphoma cell line has been most widely used as a platform for genetic modification and subsequent adoptive transfer. NK-92 produce high levels of granzymes, perforins, and other death-inducing molecules (FAS-L, TRAIL) that exert potent cytotoxicity against cancer cells.[63] NK-92 adoptive transfer (with or without CAR modification) has been shown to be safe, but with limited efficacy in the context of both hematologic[64–66] and solid tumors.[67,68] The use of aneuploid transformed cells with multiple cytogenetic abnormalities as anticancer therapy mandates preinfusion irradiation, which has the expected deleterious effect on *in vivo* expansion, persistence, and thus efficacy.[69] Moreover, while NK-92 cells generally share a receptor repertoire with PB-NK cells, they lack CD16 (FcγRIII) and thus the capacity for antibody-dependent cellular cytotoxicity (ADCC).[57,70] NK-92 also lack activating receptors, for example, NKp44 and almost all of the KIRs, with the exception of KIR2DL4.[63]

Umbilical cord blood (UCB) is another source for the generation of "off-the-shelf" NK cell products. UCB is relatively easy to isolate[71] and contains a similar percentage of NK cells as PB.[48,72] However, the small total blood volume in each CB unit makes acquiring satisfactory NK cell numbers for clinical use challenging. Similar to PB, UCB is heterogeneous, and NK cell purification is needed. Freshly isolated UCB-NKs are characterized by an immature immune phenotype with lower surface expression of NKG2C, CD57, adhesion molecules (CD2, CD11α, CD18, DNAM-1),[73] CD62 L (LN homing receptor), and KIRs (CD158a, CD158b, and others) and higher expression of 2B4, CXCR4 (BM homing receptor), and NKG2A, compared to PB counterparts.[48,74,75] Studies comparing granzyme and perforin expression in UCB- and PB-NK cells have reported contradictory results.[75,76] The cytotoxic capacity of UCB-NK is lower than PB-NK, yet this difference can be partially mitigated with cytokine stimulation.[48,75,76] Clinical trials testing adoptive transfer of unmodified or CAR-expressing UCB-NK as hematologic malignancy treatment have shown that this approach is safe, without GVHD or other toxicities, but with limited antitumor effect.[77,78]

METHODS OF GENETIC ENGINEERING IN NATURAL KILLER CELLS

Though simple in concept, efficient genetic modification of NK cells is a challenge. Early attempts at NK cell engineering have reported low gene transfer efficiency using both viral-based and nonviral methods.[29] Recent optimization of gene transfer strategies has been more successful with an improved safety profile (**Fig. 1**).[79]

Viral-mediated natural killer cell engineering

NK cell modification with viral vectors is now associated with high-efficiency gene transfer. Viral vectors are readily manufactured and can stably integrate genetic material into the host genome.[80] The *Retroviridae* family are the most commonly used vectors for gene therapy applications, including NK cell genetic modification.[79] The *Retroviridae* family includes seven members: α-, β-, γ-, δ-, and ε-retroviruses, spumaviruses, and lentiviruses.[79] Of these, γ-retroviruses and lentiviruses are most often used in cellular gene transfer for clinical application.[79,80] Retroviral genetic modification includes the reverse transcription of the viral RNA genome into double-stranded DNA and permanent integration into the host genome facilitated by viral protein integrase encoded by the *pol* gene. Retroviral transduction has evolved to use replication-incompetent retroviruses as a safety mechanism to limit self-replication and infectivity.[80]

In γ-retrovirus vectors, the γ retroviral coding sequences are replaced by the transgene of interest and this recombinant plasmid as well as helper plasmids encoding viral capsid proteins, replication enzymes, and envelope glycoproteins (*gag, pol,* and *env*) are cotransfected into a virus packaging cell line where the recombinant plasmid is synthesized and packaged into viral particles. A limitation of successful γ-retroviral transduction is the requirement for a disrupted nuclear membrane in actively dividing target cells.[80,81] Despite this obstacle, γ-retroviral vectors have demonstrated high rates of transduction and persistence of transgene expression in gene therapy applications, including the use of NK cells.

Lentivirus-based vectors similarly involve the replacement of essential viral genes with the transgene of interest and also use helper plasmids to encode *gag, pol,* and *env.* Unlike γ-retroviral vectors, lentivirus-based vectors additionally require the incorporation of the *rev* gene, which encodes the Rev protein and enhances nuclear export and expression of gag-pol transcripts through the binding of the rev responsive element (RRE).[80,82] Lentivirus-based vectors further contain a central polypurine tract (cPTT)/central termination signal (CTS) that functions to facilitate nuclear import of the preintegration complex after target cell uptake of the virion.[80,83] As a result, lentiviral vector transduction is not dependent on active cellular division, which notably expands the repertoire of potential target cells. Despite this reach, the use of lentiviral-based vectors for NK and other hematopoietic cell transduction has not resulted in high percentages of transduced cells, largely because of limited cellular entry. Lentivirus is standardly pseudotyped with vesicular stomatitis virus g-protein (VSV-G), which binds LDL-R on human cells. NK cells express LDL-R at low levels, making transduction efficiency low.[84] The use of lineage-specific promotors and cell-type-specific lentiviral vectors using envelope proteins from viruses such as RD114 or baboon retrovirus are potential ways to improve the efficacy and specificity of lentiviral vectors.[85–87]

Though viral-based cell engineering can effectively achieve stable transgenic expression, without genomic targeting this method is inherently nonspecific and therefore associated with the risk of insertional mutagenesis. γ-retroviral vectors integrate with proximity to cellular gene promoters, transcription start sites, and CpG islands. This can result in neoplastic transformation if genomic insertion occurs at a proto-oncogenic site.[80,88,89]

Nonviral natural killer cell engineering

Nonviral NK cell modification can circumvent some potential pitfalls of viral engineering. The most used nonviral gene delivery method is electroporation, which is a simple and cost-effective strategy that can introduce nucleic acid into a target cell with high efficiency. Electroporation generates small, temporary pores in the cell and nuclear membrane by electrical pulsing, which allows for the transfer of charged nucleic acid molecules.[90,91] The primary downside to electroporation is the toxicity that can lead to high rates of cell death.[92] Successful NK cell transfection via electroporation has been described using primary NK cells with resultant efficient gene transfer.[90,91,93]

Alternative methods for the delivery of charged nucleotides across a nonpolar cell membrane include the use of cationic polymers, lipid nanoparticles, and more recently charge-altering releasable transporters. Charge-altering releasable transporters are multiblock polycationic oligomers that noncovalently complex with polyanionic mRNA to facilitate its delivery across the cellular membrane.[94] Charge-altering releasable transporters have been used to transfect resting primary NK cells with mRNA to generate cytotoxic human anti-CD19-CAR NK cells with efficient transfection, viability, and preservation of the NK cell phenotype.[95] A primary limitation to the use of charge-altering releasable transporter-mediated gene delivery is the transient nature of mRNA mediated cellular modification.95.

Another method for stable, nonviral genomic modification involves the use of DNA transposons, which are naturally occurring repetitive DNA sequences that can jump from one location in the genome to another.[91,96] This natural phenomenon can be harnessed for gene editing by using a transposon vector containing the gene of interest flanked by terminal inverted repeats (TIRs), and a transposase enzyme that targets the TIRs to excise the gene of interest from the original site and stably reintegrate into chromosomal sites.[91,97] DNA transposons have been effectively used to engineer human cells, including NK cells.[91,97,98] The most extensively studied transposon systems for clinical gene transfer are Sleeping Beauty (SB), piggyback (PB), and TcBuster, which have been used as platforms for delivery of CARs into hematopoietic cells.[91] Human iPSC-derived NK cells have been successfully engineered to express CARs using the PB transposon system with enhanced antigen-specific NK cell activity observed against mesothelin-expressing tumors in vitro and in vivo.[55] PB and SB systems have also been used to successfully express a panel of mesothelin directed CARs in NK-92 cells.[55] As with any nonspecific gene transfer, transposon-mediated chromosomal integration has the risk of causing insertional mutagenesis. A recent phase I clinical trial of donor-derived CD19-targeting CAR T-cells engineered using the PB transposon system reported the development of malignant CAR-expressing CD4+ T-cell lymphomas in 2 out of 10 treated patients.[99,100] Transcriptomic analysis of malignant tissue confirmed transgene promoter-driven transcriptional upregulation of surrounding regions, background genomic copy number variations, and high transgene copy number per cell.[100] This outcome highlights the need for careful surveillance and monitoring of patients receiving novel engineered cell therapy products, particularly when nontargeted gene engineering methodology is used.

Targeted knockdown and knock-in gene modification strategies

Targeted gene editing can also be achieved using zinc-finger nucleases (ZFN), transcription activator-like nucleases (TALENs), and (CRISPR)/CRISPR-associated protein 9 (Cas-9) systems, often in combination with adeno-associated virus (AAV) vectors. ZFN and TALEN manipulate protein–DNA interactions to target specific genomic loci for editing and require expertise in protein engineering.[101] CRISPR-Cas9 uses RNA-guided DNA recognition, with guide RNA designed with homology to the genetic locus of interest.[101] CRISPR-Cas9 can be used to reliably knockout target genes or to knock-in genetic modifications with targeted integration of a homologous recombination repair template.[91,102] Efficient CRISPR-Cas9 mediated knockout of inhibitory signaling pathways in primary NK cells was recently described with efficiency reaching 90%.[93] The CRISPR-Cas9 system was subsequently used in combination with recombinant AAV serotype 6 (rAAV6) for delivery of a homologous recombination template DNA for an efficient knock-in strategy.[93] As an alternative, other groups have packaged Cas9 and guide RNAs into ribonucleoprotein (RNP) complexes for high gene-editing efficiency in NK cells.[91,103] Related gene-editing techniques include Base editors (BEs) that fuse a catalytically inactive Cas9 protein to a DNA deaminase domain with the goal of precise introduction of a targeted single nucleotide change without double-strand breaks or DNA donor molecules.[91,104]

The development of successful NK cell gene-based therapies is rooted in an effective gene-editing strategy. Research investigating viral and nonviral delivery platforms with or without targeted knockdown or knock-in mechanisms aims to optimize the efficiency and safety profile of genetic engineering of NK cells. Regardless of the platform selected, each described genetic modification strategy has evidence of successful NK Cell modification and thus, can be considered to engineer enhanced effector cell function and immunotherapeutic efficacy.

THERAPEUTIC APPLICATIONS OF GENETICALLY MODIFIED NATURAL KILLER CELLS
Modulation of surface receptor expression

Chimeric antigen receptor-natural killer cells demonstrate target-specific activation

CAR-T cell therapy has revolutionized the treatment landscape for pediatric hematologic malignancies and broadened the developmental scope to include alternate tumor types and effector cell starting materials. NK cell CARs can be designed to target diverse antigens for specific NK cell activation by using unique extracellular single-chain variable fragments (scFvs) linked to combinations of intracellular costimulatory domains (**Fig. 2A**). A robust body of preclinical work demonstrates that NK cells can effectively be engineered to express CARs, and this has been comprehensively reviewed elsewhere.[105–110] These preclinical investigations have laid the ground for clinical translation, and a number of CAR-NK cell therapy trials are underway. As of November 2021, 26 CAR-NK cell cancer treatment trials are registered on *clinicaltrials.gov* (**Table 1**). Two of these have published results. One example is an actively recruiting phase I/II trial (NCT03056339) led by the University of Texas MD Anderson Cancer Center. In this ongoing study, HLA-mismatched anti-CD19 UCB CAR-NK cells are administered to patients with relapsed or refractory CD19-positive hematologic malignancies. In a report describing the initial cohort of 11 patients, the treatment was well-tolerated without the development of CRS, ICANS, or GVHD. Lymphodepleting chemotherapy was given prior to CAR-NK cell infusion (1×10^5, 1×10^6, or 1×10^7 CAR-NK cells per kilogram of body weight), with 7 of 11 patients achieving a complete remission.[78] A separate phase I clinical trial conducted in Suzhou, Jiangsu, China evaluated the safety of CD33 CAR-NK cells in patients with relapsed and refractory AML (NCT02944162). A third-generation lentiviral CAR construct (αCD33.CD28.4-1BB) was used for NK-92 cell transduction in this study. Three patients with relapsed and refractory AML treated with salvage chemotherapy were infused with three escalating doses of irradiated CD33-CAR NK-92 cells. No adverse effects or durable clinical efficacy were recorded.[66]

Downregulation of inhibitory receptors enhances natural killer cell activation

An alternative approach to cell surface receptor modulation is the downregulation of innate NK inhibitory receptors to bias NK cells toward activation. Cancer cells can block immune responses by targeting inhibitory receptors on the surface of NK cells. NKG2A is one such receptor that dimerizes with CD94 to bind HLA-E molecules on tumor cells, which dampens NK cell activity.[111] Consequently, RNAi-mediated inhibition of NKG2A expression has improved NK cell activity in the preclinical study. NKG2A silencing can enhance NK cell cytotoxicity by up to 40%.[112] Silencing of inhibitory receptors using CRISPR/Cas9, ZFN, or TALEN is likely to result in similarly amplified NK cell antitumor functionality.

Enhancing natural killer cell activity through the modulation of cytokine signaling

Natural killer cell in vivo persistence can be sustained with cytokine stimulation

The success of adoptive NK cell transfer relies to a great extent on the persistence of the cells.[11] Mature adoptively transferred NK cells have a limited lifespan in *vivo* with a peripheral half-life of about 7 to 10 days.[30,32] This short lifespan has certain advantages including: decreased risk of prolonged on target, off-tumor effects,[45] decreased immunogenicity, reduced risk of cytokine release syndrome and neurotoxicity,[110] and the opportunity to safely redose NK cells for continued effect. Even so, clinical studies have demonstrated the important role of persistence and expansion for clinical efficacy.[11,113–115] In order to prolong NK cell survival, exogenous cytokine administration with recombinant IL2, IL15, or IL15 "superagonists" has been used in clinical

Table 1

Clinical trials testing the use of CAR-NK cells as anticancer immunotherapy

Target	Agent	NCT	Year Posted	Phase	Status	Tumor	NK Source	Sponsor	Vector
CD19	CAR-NK019	NCT04887012	2021	I	Recruiting	B-cell NHL	iPSC	Second Affiliated Hospital, School of Medicine, Zhejiang University, China	Lentiviral
CD19	Anti-CD19 CAR NK Cells	NCT04639739	2020	Early I	Planned	• NHL	Unknown	Xinqiao Hospital of Chongqing, China	Unknown
CD22	Anti-CD22 CAR-NK Cells	NCT03692767	2018	Early I	Unknown	• Refractory B-cell Lymphoma	Unknown	Allife Medical Science and Technology Co., Ltd., China	Unknown
CD19	Anti-CD19 CAR NK Cells	NCT03690310	2018	Early I	Unknown	• Refractory B-cell Lymphoma	Unknown	Allife Medical Science and Technology Co., Ltd., China	Unknown
CD33	Anti-CD33 CAR NK Cells	NCT05008575	2021	I	Planned	• AML	Unknown	Xinqiao Hospital of Chongqing, China	Unknown
Mesothelin	Anti-Mesothelin CAR-NK Cells	NCT03692637	2018	Early I	Unknown	• Epithelial Ovarian Cancer	Unknown	Allife Medical Science and Technology Co., Ltd., China	Unknown
NKG2D	CAR-NK cells targeting NKG2D ligands	NCT03415100	2018	I	Unknown	• Metastatic Solid Tumors	PB-NK	The Third Affiliated Hospital of Guangzhou Medical University, China	mRNA electroporation
PSMA	Anti-PSMA CAR NK Cells	NCT03692663	2018	Early I	Planned	Castration-Resistant Prostate Cancer	Unknown	Allife Medical Science and Technology Co., Ltd., China	Unknown
BCMA	Anti-BCMA CAR-NK Cells	NCT05008536	2021	Early I	Planned	Refractory Multiple Myeloma	UCB-NK	Xinqiao Hospital of Chongqing, China	Unknown

(continued on next page)

Table 1
(continued)

Target	Agent	NCT	Year Posted	Phase	Status	Tumor	NK Source	Sponsor	Vector
ROBO1	ROBO1 CAR-NK Cells	NCT03940820	2019	I/II	Recruiting	Solid Tumors	NK-92	Asclepius Technology Company Group (Suzhou) Co., Ltd., China	Lentiviral
BCMA	BCMA CAR-NK 92 Cells	NCT03940833	2019	I/II	Planned	Multiple Myeloma	NK-92	Asclepius Technology Company Group (Suzhou) Co., Ltd., China	Lentiviral
PD-L1	PD-L1 t-haNK	NCT04847466	2021	II	Planned	Gastroesophageal Junction Cancers; Advanced HNSCC	NK-92	National Cancer Institute, United States	Unknown
CD19, CD22	Anti-CD19/CD22 CAR NK CElls	NCT03824964	2019	Early I	Unknown	Refractory B-Cell Lymphoma	Unknown	Allife Medical Science and Technology Co., Ltd., China	Unknown
CD19	CAR-NK-CD19 Cells	NCT04796675	2021	I	Recruiting	ALL, CLL, NHL	CB-NK	Wuhan Union Hospital, China	Retroviral
CD19	NKX019	NCT05020678	2021	I	Recruiting	B-ALL, CLL, NHL	PB-NK	Nkarta Inc., United States	Unknown
CD33	Anti-CD33 CAR-NK cells	NCT02944162	2016	I/II	Unknown	AML	NK-92	PersonGen BioTherapeutics (Suzhou) Co., Ltd., China	Lentiviral
CD19	PCAR-119	NCT02892695	2016	I/II	Unknown	Leukemia, Lymphoma	NK-92	PersonGen BioTherapeutics (Suzhou) Co., Ltd., China	Lentiviral

Target	Name	NCT Number	Year	Phase	Status	Indication	Cell Source	Sponsor	Vector
NKG2D	NKX101	NCT04623944	2021	I	Recruiting	AML, MDS	PB-NK	Nkarta Inc., United States	Unknown
ROBO1	BiCAR-NK cells	NCT03941457	2019	I/II	Recruiting	Pancreatic Cancer	NK-92	Asclepius Technology Company Group (Suzhou) Co., Ltd., China	Lentiviral
CD19	CAR.CD19-CD28-zeta-2A-iCasp9-IL15-transduced CB-NK cells	NCT03579927	2018	I/II	Withdrawn	B-cell lymphoma	UCB, CB-NK	M.D. Anderson Cancer Center	Retroviral
CD19	iC9/CAR.19/IL15-Transduced CB-NK Cells	NCT03056339	2017	I/II	Active	B-Lymphoid Malignancies, ALL, CLL, NHL	UCB, CB-NK	M.D. Anderson	Retroviral
CD70	CAR.70/IL15-transduced CB-NK cells	NCT05092451	2021	I/II	Recruiting	B-cell Lymphoma, MDS, AML	CB-NK	M.D. Anderson	Retroviral
CD19	FT596	NCT04555811	2020	I	Recruiting	NHL	iPSC	Masonic Cancer Center, University of Minnesota	Lentiviral
CD19	FT596	NCT04245722	2020	I	Recruiting	B-cell lymphoma, CLL	iPSC	Fate Therapeutics	Lentiviral
ErbB2	NK-92/5.28.z	NCT03383978	2017	I	Recruiting	HER2-positive Glioblastoma	NK-92	Johann Wolfgang Goethe University Hospital	Lentiviral
CD19	CAR-ITNK	NCT04747093	2021	I/II	Recruiting	B cell leukemia/lymphoma	T-cells	Nanfang Hospital of Southern Medical University, China	Unknown

Abbreviations: ALL, acute lymphoblastic leukemia. acute lymphocytic leukemia; AML, acute myeloid leukemia; CLL, chronic lymphocytic leukemia; iPSC, induced pluripotent stem cells; MDS, myelodysplastic syndrome; NHL, Non-Hodgkin lymphoma; PB-NK, Peripheral blood-derived NK cells; UCB, CB-NK, umbilical, cord blood-derived CAR-engineered NK cells.

trials.[116–121] However, cytokine infusion is associated with systemic toxicities that are dose- and therapeutic route-dependent.[118–121] Localized cytokine delivery to support NK cell persistence may be safer, as first studied using NK-92 (**Fig. 2B**). An animal model of liver metastases paired with NK-92 treatment was used to show that NK-92 stably expressing and secreting IL2 had better antitumor control than NK-92 alone.[122] Similarly, UCB CAR-NK cells engineered to secrete IL15 prolonged the survival of mice engrafted with CD19 positive tumors.[123] Safety of IL15-secreting CAR-NK cells was tested in human patients in the MD Anderson phase I clinical trial (NCT03056339) using UCB-derived CD19-CAR.IL15 NK cells described above.[78] The trial found that patients who had a response to therapy had a significantly higher early expansion of CAR-NK cells and that early expansion and low-level persistence of CAR-NK cells for at least 12 months after infusion was related to the inclusion of IL-15 in the CAR construct.[78] Our group has also investigated transgenic IL15 in PB-NK cells designed for the treatment of hematological malignancies. As expected, constitutive IL15 secretion enhances NK and CAR-NK cell activation and supports *in vivo* persistence. However, we found that treatment with IL15-secreting NK cells caused lethal toxicity in one AML xenograft model.[38] Membrane-bound IL15 or the IL15/IL15 R complex can as well augment NK cell persistence and may be a safer alternative to soluble IL15 (**Fig. 2C**).[43] To illustrate, oncolytic virus-mediated local IL15/IL15 Rα (OV-IL15 C) secretion has been used to enhance PB-CAR-NK persistence and *in vivo* functionality.[124] Similarly, the IL15/IL15 Rα fusion protein, a CD19-CAR, and a high-affinity, noncleavable CD16 (hnCD16) have together been expressed in iPSC-NKs, resulting in enhanced functionality in preclinical CD19+ malignancy models.[125] This product, FT596, is now being investigated in a phase 1 clinical trial for the treatment of B-cell lymphoma and chronic lymphocytic leukemia (NCT04245722).

Natural killer cell modification can direct tumor site homing

Surface expression of chemokine receptors has been tested as a method to enhance NK cell tumor trafficking (**Fig. 2D**). CXCR2 expression in the YTS NK cell line and CXCR4 in PB-NKs can promote NK cell trafficking to renal cell carcinoma (RCC) and CXCL12-secreting glioblastoma (GB), respectively.[126,127] Electroporation of primary human NK cells with gain-of-function $CXCR4_{R334X}$ mRNA upregulated CXCR4 on the NK cell surface and supported NK cell trafficking to bone marrow in a xenograft model.[128] Engineered CCR7 expression on NK cells can promote migration toward CCL19 in lymph nodes.[129] Primary NK cells transfected with mRNAs encoding for CXCR1 and an NKG2D-CAR can be efficiently directed toward IL8-secreting cancers.[130] Moreover, combinational immunotherapy utilizing an oncolytic virus encoding CCL5 and NK cells engineered to express the CCR5 receptor can improve NK cell tumor infiltration.[131]

Manipulating natural killer cell interaction with small molecule engagers

BiKEs enhance natural killer cell activation and antibody-dependent cellular cytotoxicity

Preclinical and clinical studies support the use of bispecific small molecular engagers to stabilize the NK cell-target cell immunologic synapse and improve antitumor cytolysis (**Fig. 2E**). BiKEs that simultaneously target a tumor-specific antigen and CD16 (FcγRIII), the low-affinity Fc receptor,[132,133] are capable of stimulating ADCC. For example, a CD16xCD33 BiKE tested in patients with myelodysplastic syndromes (MDS) can successfully activate primary patient NK cells with specific degranulation and cytokine production against CD33+ MDS targets and can reverse myeloid-derived suppressor cell (MDSC)-mediated immunosuppression of NK cells through

Table 2
Therapeutic applications for genetically modified NK cells

Therapeutic Modality	Mechanism of Action	Clinical Translation
Modulation of Surface Receptor Expression		
CAR-NK	CARs with specificity for tumor antigens are genetically introduced via viral or nonviral vectors for stable NK cell surface expression.	Several[105–110] (see **Table 1**)
NKG2A Silencing	RNAi-mediated inhibition of NKG2A expression, an innate inhibitory NK cells receptor. Other applicable methods of gene silencing include CRISPR/Cas9, ZFN, and TALEN.	Preclinical[112]
Modulation of Cytokine Signaling		
IL2-secreting NK cells	NK-92 cells genetically engineered to stably secrete IL2, an important stimulatory cytokine for NK cell proliferation and functionality.	Preclinical[122]
IL15-secreting CAR-NK cells	UCB CAR-NK cells genetically engineered to secrete IL15, an important stimulatory cytokine for NK cell proliferation and functionality. PB-NK cells genetically engineered to constitutively secrete transgenic IL15 to enhance NK cell activation and persistence.	UCB-derived CD19-CAR.IL15 NK cells, phase I/II clinical trial (NCT03056339)[78,123] Preclinical[38]
IL15/IL15 R complex expressing CAR-NK cells	PB-NK cells genetically engineered to locally secrete IL15/IL15 Rα to enhance NK cell persistence and functionality. iPSC-NK cells genetically engineered to express the IL15/IL15 Rα fusion protein, a CD19-targeting CAR, and a high-affinity, noncleavable CD16 for enhanced functionality in CD19+ malignancies.	Preclinical[124] iPSC-derived CD19 CAR NK cell with a high-affinity, noncleavable CD16, and recombinant fusion of IL15 and IL15RF (FT596) as monotherapy or in combination with rituximab or obinutuzumab, phase I clinical trial (NCT04245722)[125]

(continued on next page)

Table 2
(continued)

Therapeutic Modality	Mechanism of Action	Clinical Translation
Chemokine receptor expression on NK cells (ex. CXCR2, CXCR4, CCR7, CXCR1, CCR5)	NK cells are engineered to express gain of function chemokine receptors to support NK cell tumor trafficking.	Preclinical[126-131]
Small Molecule Engagers		
BiKEs	Genetically modified NK cells engineered to express high-affinity CD16 Fc receptor isoform to enhance ADCC used in combination with BiKEs, targeting CD16 on NK cells and tumor antigens on target cells.	iPSC-derived CD19 CAR NK cell with a high-affinity, noncleavable CD16 (FT516) in combination with rituximab, phase I clinical trial (NCT04023071)[138-143]
TriKEs	TriKEs incorporating IL-15 cytokine for enhanced NK cells function used together with NK cells genetically modified to express high-affinity CD16 Fc receptors, for further enhanced specify and persistence of antitumor NK cell activation.	Preclinical[144]

Abbreviations: ADCC, antibody-dependent cellular cytotoxicity; BiKE, bispecific killer engager; iPSC, induced pluripotent stem cell; PB, peripheral blood; TALEN, transcription activator-like nucleases; TriKE, trispecific killer engager; UCB, umbilical cord blood; ZFN, zinc-finger nucleases.

targeted CD33+ MDSC lysis.[134] Secondly, the use of a CD30xCD16 A BiKE (AFM13) targeting CD30 on tumor cells and the CD16 A isoform on NK cells has been extensively tested in patients with CD30+ malignancies with notable antitumor responses, a good safety profile, and dose-dependent NK cell CD69 upregulation.[135–137]

With these encouraging results, optimizing ADCC by combining BiKEs with genetically modified NK cells holds promise. Engineered expression of high-affinity Fc receptor isoforms to enhance ADCC is being studied by multiple groups.[138–142] For example, FT516 is a CD19-targeted CAR-NK cell product derived from a clonal iPSC line, further engineered to include a high-affinity, noncleavable CD16.[141] Preliminary results from a phase I trial of FT516 (NCT04023071) used in patients with relapsed/refractory B-cell lymphoma evaluated the safety of infusion in combination with the monoclonal CD20 antibody, rituximab. Patients received 3 days of lymphodepleting chemotherapy, followed by 1 dose of rituximab, and 3 weekly infusions of FT516 administered with systemic IL-2. Six patients with a median age of 65.5 years enrolled in the trial, all heavily pretreated, 5 of whom completed the therapy. Escalating doses were evaluated including 3 million cells/dose (2 patients), 90 million cells/dose (3 patients), and 300 million cells/dose (1 patients). No CRS, ICANS, GVHD, or other serious side effect were observed in 5 treated patients. Three patients treated at > 90 million cells/dose achieved an objective response.[143]

Trispecific killer engagers can complement antibody-dependent cellular cytotoxicity with cytokine driven stimulation

Similar to BiKEs, trispecific killer engagers (TriKEs) are composed of an antigen-specific scFv linked to the scFvs of two other antibodies of different specificities or to the scFv of one other antibody and a cytokine. TriKEs have also been designed to augment ADCC by engaging CD16 along with tumor-specific antigens.[144] Newer generations of TriKEs incorporate the IL-15 cytokine to augment NK cell function. This, coupled with CD16 engineering modalities described above may further enhance the specificity and persistence of antitumor NK cell activation. Additional NK cell manipulations discussed above such as the downregulation of inhibitory receptors can be employed to further enhance TriKE immunotherapy, and combinatorial manipulation remains an area of active study.

SUMMARY

NK cells are a powerful tool for targeted immunotherapy. They harbor a range of innate cytotoxic mechanisms and can be genetically engineered to enhance their function. This can be conducted by modulating cell surface receptor expression, by manipulating stimulatory cytokines and chemokines, and by optimizing engagement with targeted small molecules (**Table 2**). NK cells are subject to genetic modification using viral and nonviral vectors and can be isolated or derived from different primary sources. This diversity leaves much option for further study and discovery. While early clinical experiences underline their promise, the clinical development of engineered NK cell therapy remains in its infancy with current reports limited to small cohorts of treated patients. There is a need for further discovery and subsequent translation into large-scale clinical trials to truly detail the role of these effector cells in the expanding armamentarium of immunotherapies for blood cancers. The success of genetically engineered NK cell therapy is dependent on the complete understanding of the factors that drive NK cell activation, immune synapse formation, and target cell killing. There remains much to be discovered given the potential for these remarkable innate effector cells to be effective anticancer immunotherapeutics.

CLINICS CARE POINTS

- NK cells are an option for "off-the-shelf" cellular therapy with a favorable safety profile and limited risk of graft-versus-host disease with allogeneic products.

- NK cells can be genetically modified using both genomic targeted and nontargeted techniques. There is a risk of insertional mutagenesis without targeting, thus there is a need for close patient monitoring following engineered NK cell infusion.

- NK-cell-based immunotherapy is made more effective by the presence of a tumor antigen for CAR or BiKE/TriKE targeting and mechanisms that promote NK cell persistence and activation.

DISCLOSURE

C.L. Bonifant and I. Christodoulou have pending patent applications describing the use of CAR-NK cells as therapeutics. C.L. Bonifant and I. Christodoulou have received research support from Merck Sharp and Dohme, Bristol-Myers Squibb, and Kiadis Pharma.

REFERENCES

1. Madhusoodhan PP, Carroll WL, Bhatla T. Progress and prospects in pediatric leukemia. Curr Probl Pediatr Adolesc Health Care 2016;46(7):229–41.
2. Ward E, DeSantis C, Robbins A, et al. Childhood and adolescent cancer statistics. CA Cancer J Clin 2014;64(2):83–103.
3. Gaynon PS, Angiolillo AL, Carroll WL, et al. Long-term results of the children's cancer group studies for childhood acute lymphoblastic leukemia 1983-2002: a children's oncology group report. Leukemia 2010;24(2):285–97.
4. Maude SL, Laetsch TW, Buechner J, et al. Tisagenlecleucel in children and young adults with b-cell lymphoblastic leukemia. N Engl J Med 2018;378(5):439–48.
5. O'Leary MC, Lu X, Huang Y, et al. FDA approval summary: tisagenlecleucel for treatment of patients with relapsed or refractory b-cell precursor acute lymphoblastic leukemia. Clin Cancer Res 2019;25(4):1142–6.
6. Lee DW, Santomasso BD, Locke FL, et al. ASTCT consensus grading for cytokine release syndrome and neurologic toxicity associated with immune effector cells. Biol Blood Marrow Transplant 2019;25(4):625–38.
7. Hines MR, Keenan C, Maron Alfaro G, et al. Hemophagocytic lymphohistiocytosis-like toxicity (carHLH) after CD19-specific CAR T-cell therapy. Br J Haematol 2021; 194(4):701–7.
8. Wang X, Riviere I. Clinical manufacturing of CAR T cells: foundation of a promising therapy. Mol Ther Oncolytics 2016;3:16015.
9. Ferrara JL, Levine JE, Reddy P, et al. Graft-versus-host disease. Lancet 2009; 373(9674):1550–61.
10. Reddy P. Pathophysiology of acute graft-versus-host disease. Hematol Oncol 2003;21(4):149–61.
11. Miller JS, Soignier Y, Panoskaltsis-Mortari A, et al. Successful adoptive transfer and in vivo expansion of human haploidentical NK cells in patients with cancer. Blood 2005;105(8):3051–7.
12. Rubnitz JE, Inaba H, Ribeiro RC, et al. NKAML: a pilot study to determine the safety and feasibility of haploidentical natural killer cell transplantation in childhood acute myeloid leukemia. J Clin Oncol 2010;28(6):955–9.

13. Ruggeri L, Capanni M, Casucci M, et al. Role of natural killer cell alloreactivity in HLA-mismatched hematopoietic stem cell transplantation. Blood 1999;94(1): 333–9.

14. Ruggeri L, Capanni M, Urbani E, et al. Effectiveness of donor natural killer cell alloreactivity in mismatched hematopoietic transplants. Science 2002; 295(5562):2097–100.

15. Liu S, Galat V, Galat Y, et al. NK cell-based cancer immunotherapy: from basic biology to clinical development. J Hematol Oncol 2021;14(1):7.

16. Mace EM, Orange JS. Emerging insights into human health and NK cell biology from the study of NK cell deficiencies. Immunol Rev 2019;287(1):202–25.

17. Bjorkstrom NK, Ljunggren HG, Michaelsson J. Emerging insights into natural killer cells in human peripheral tissues. Nat Rev Immunol 2016;16(5):310–20.

18. Freud AG, Mundy-Bosse BL, Yu J, et al. The Broad spectrum of human natural killer cell diversity. Immunity 2017;47(5):820–33.

19. Abel AM, Yang C, Thakar MS, et al. Natural killer cells: development, maturation, and clinical utilization. Front Immunol 2018;9:1869.

20. Smith SL, Kennedy PR, Stacey KB, et al. Diversity of peripheral blood human NK cells identified by single-cell RNA sequencing. Blood Adv 2020;4(7):1388–406.

21. Yang C, Siebert JR, Burns R, et al. Heterogeneity of human bone marrow and blood natural killer cells defined by single-cell transcriptome. Nat Commun 2019;10(1):3931.

22. Knorr DA, Bachanova V, Verneris MR, et al. Clinical utility of natural killer cells in cancer therapy and transplantation. Semin Immunol 2014;26(2):161–72.

23. Liu D, Tian S, Zhang K, et al. Chimeric antigen receptor (CAR)-modified natural killer cell-based immunotherapy and immunological synapse formation in cancer and HIV. Protein Cell 2017;8(12):861–77.

24. Handgretinger R, Lang P, Andre MC. Exploitation of natural killer cells for the treatment of acute leukemia. Blood 2016;127(26):3341–9.

25. Algarra I, Cabrera T, Garrido F. The HLA crossroad in tumor immunology. Hum Immunol 2000;61(1):65–73.

26. Diefenbach A, Jamieson AM, Liu SD, et al. Ligands for the murine NKG2D receptor: expression by tumor cells and activation of NK cells and macrophages. Nat Immunol 2000;1(2):119–26.

27. Cerwenka A, Bakker AB, McClanahan T, et al. Retinoic acid early inducible genes define a ligand family for the activating NKG2D receptor in mice. Immunity 2000;12(6):721–7.

28. Smyth MJ, Cretney E, Kelly JM, et al. Activation of NK cell cytotoxicity. Mol Immunol 2005;42(4):501–10.

29. Carlsten M, Childs RW. Genetic manipulation of NK cells for cancer immunotherapy: techniques and clinical implications. Front Immunol 2015;6:266.

30. Prlic M, Blazar BR, Farrar MA, et al. In vivo survival and homeostatic proliferation of natural killer cells. J Exp Med 2003;197(8):967–76.

31. Ranson T, Vosshenrich CA, Corcuff E, et al. IL-15 is an essential mediator of peripheral NK-cell homeostasis. Blood 2003;101(12):4887–93.

32. Yokoyama WM, Kim S, French AR. The dynamic life of natural killer cells. Annu Rev Immunol 2004;22:405–29.

33. Vitale M, Cantoni C, Pietra G, et al. Effect of tumor cells and tumor microenvironment on NK-cell function. Eur J Immunol 2014;44(6):1582–92.

34. Cekic C, Day YJ, Sag D, et al. Myeloid expression of adenosine A2A receptor suppresses T and NK cell responses in the solid tumor microenvironment. Cancer Res 2014;74(24):7250–9.

35. Li H, Han Y, Guo Q, et al. Cancer-expanded myeloid-derived suppressor cells induce anergy of NK cells through membrane-bound TGF-beta 1. J Immunol 2009;182(1):240–9.

36. Trzonkowski P, Szmit E, Mysliwska J, et al. CD4+CD25+ T regulatory cells inhibit cytotoxic activity of T CD8+ and NK lymphocytes in the direct cell-to-cell interaction. Clin Immunol 2004;112(3):258–67.

37. Christodoulou I, Rahnama R, Ravich JW, et al. Glycoprotein Targeted CAR-NK Cells for the Treatment of SARS-CoV-2 Infection. Original Research. Front Immunol 2021;12:5349.

38. Christodoulou I, Ho WJ, Marple A, et al. Engineering CAR-NK cells to secrete IL-15 sustains their anti-AML functionality but is associated with systemic toxicities. J Immunother Cancer 2021;9(12).

39. Ciurea SO, Schafer JR, Bassett R, et al. Phase 1 clinical trial using mbIL21 ex vivo-expanded donor-derived NK cells after haploidentical transplantation. Blood 2017;130(16):1857–68.

40. Fujisaki H, Kakuda H, Shimasaki N, et al. Expansion of highly cytotoxic human natural killer cells for cancer cell therapy. Cancer Res 2009;69(9):4010–7.

41. Gomez Garcia LM, Escudero A, Mestre C, et al. Phase 2 Clinical Trial of Infusing Haploidentical K562-mb15-41BBL-Activated and Expanded Natural Killer Cells as Consolidation Therapy for Pediatric Acute Myeloblastic Leukemia. Clin Lymphoma Myeloma Leuk 2021. https://doi.org/10.1016/j.clml.2021.01.013. Jan 25.

42. Imai C, Iwamoto S, Campana D. Genetic modification of primary natural killer cells overcomes inhibitory signals and induces specific killing of leukemic cells. Blood 2005;106(1):376–83.

43. Imamura M, Shook D, Kamiya T, et al. Autonomous growth and increased cytotoxicity of natural killer cells expressing membrane-bound interleukin-15. Blood 2014;124(7):1081–8.

44. Denman CJ, Senyukov VV, Somanchi SS, et al. Membrane-bound IL-21 promotes sustained ex vivo proliferation of human natural killer cells. PLoS One 2012;7(1):e30264.

45. Marofi F, Saleh MM, Rahman HS, et al. CAR-engineered NK cells; a promising therapeutic option for treatment of hematological malignancies. Stem Cell Res Ther 2021;12(1):374.

46. Kim S, Poursine-Laurent J, Truscott SM, et al. Licensing of natural killer cells by host major histocompatibility complex class I molecules. Nature 2005; 436(7051):709–13.

47. Saetersmoen ML, Hammer Q, Valamehr B, et al. Off-the-shelf cell therapy with induced pluripotent stem cell-derived natural killer cells. Semin Immunopathol 2019;41(1):59–68.

48. Luevano M, Daryouzeh M, Alnabhan R, et al. The unique profile of cord blood natural killer cells balances incomplete maturation and effective killing function upon activation. Hum Immunol 2012;73(3):248–57.

49. Boissel L, Betancur M, Lu W, et al. Comparison of mRNA and lentiviral based transfection of natural killer cells with chimeric antigen receptors recognizing lymphoid antigens. Leuk Lymphoma 2012;53(5):958–65.

50. Muller S, Bexte T, Gebel V, et al. High cytotoxic efficiency of lentivirally and alpharetrovirally engineered cd19-specific chimeric antigen receptor natural killer cells against acute lymphoblastic leukemia. Front Immunol 2019;10:3123.

51. Herrera L, Santos S, Vesga MA, et al. Adult peripheral blood and umbilical cord blood NK cells are good sources for effective CAR therapy against CD19 positive leukemic cells. Sci Rep 2019;9(1):18729.

52. Knorr DA, Ni Z, Hermanson D, et al. Clinical-scale derivation of natural killer cells from human pluripotent stem cells for cancer therapy. Stem Cells Transl Med 2013;2(4):274–83.

53. Ni Z, Knorr DA, Kaufman DS. Hematopoietic and nature killer cell development from human pluripotent stem cells. Methods Mol Biol 2013;1029:33–41.

54. Zhu H, Blum RH, Bernareggi D, et al. Metabolic Reprograming via deletion of CISH in human iPSC-derived NK cells promotes in vivo persistence and enhances anti-tumor activity. Cell Stem Cell 2020;27(2):224–237 e6.

55. Li Y, Hermanson DL, Moriarity BS, et al. Human iPSC-Derived Natural Killer Cells Engineered with Chimeric Antigen Receptors Enhance Anti-tumor Activity. Cell Stem Cell 2018;23(2):181–92, e5.

56. Hermanson DL, Bendzick L, Pribyl L, et al. Induced pluripotent stem cell-derived natural killer cells for treatment of ovarian cancer. Stem Cells 2016; 34(1):93–101.

57. Gong JH, Maki G, Klingemann HG. Characterization of a human cell line (NK-92) with phenotypical and functional characteristics of activated natural killer cells. Leukemia 1994;8(4):652–8.

58. Yang HG, Kang MC, Kim TY, et al. Discovery of a novel natural killer cell line with distinct immunostimulatory and proliferative potential as an alternative platform for cancer immunotherapy. J Immunother Cancer 2019;7(1):138.

59. Tsuchiyama J, Yoshino T, Mori M, et al. Characterization of a novel human natural killer-cell line (NK-YS) established from natural killer cell lymphoma/leukemia associated with Epstein-Barr virus infection. Blood 1998;92(4):1374–83.

60. Robertson MJ, Cochran KJ, Cameron C, et al. Characterization of a cell line, NKL, derived from an aggressive human natural killer cell leukemia. Exp Hematol 1996;24(3):406–15.

61. Cheng M, Ma J, Chen Y, et al. Establishment, characterization, and successful adaptive therapy against human tumors of NKG cell, a new human NK cell line. Cell Transpl 2011;20(11–12):1731–46.

62. Yagita M, Huang CL, Umehara H, et al. A novel natural killer cell line (KHYG-1) from a patient with aggressive natural killer cell leukemia carrying a p53 point mutation. Leukemia 2000;14(5):922–30.

63. Maki G, Klingemann HG, Martinson JA, et al. Factors regulating the cytotoxic activity of the human natural killer cell line, NK-92. J Hematother Stem Cell Res 2001;10(3):369–83.

64. Boyiadzis M, Agha M, Redner RL, et al. Phase 1 clinical trial of adoptive immunotherapy using "off-the-shelf" activated natural killer cells in patients with refractory and relapsed acute myeloid leukemia. Cytotherapy 2017;19(10):1225–32.

65. Williams BA, Law AD, Routy B, et al. A phase I trial of NK-92 cells for refractory hematological malignancies relapsing after autologous hematopoietic cell transplantation shows safety and evidence of efficacy. Oncotarget 2017;8(51): 89256–68.

66. Tang X, Yang L, Li Z, et al. First-in-man clinical trial of CAR NK-92 cells: safety test of CD33-CAR NK-92 cells in patients with relapsed and refractory acute myeloid leukemia. Am J Cancer Res 2018;8(6):1083–9.

67. Arai S, Meagher R, Swearingen M, et al. Infusion of the allogeneic cell line NK-92 in patients with advanced renal cell cancer or melanoma: a phase I trial. Cytotherapy 2008;10(6):625–32.

68. Tonn T, Schwabe D, Klingemann HG, et al. Treatment of patients with advanced cancer with the natural killer cell line NK-92. Cytotherapy 2013;15(12):1563–70.

69. Tam YK, Maki G, Miyagawa B, et al. Characterization of genetically altered, interleukin 2-independent natural killer cell lines suitable for adoptive cellular immunotherapy. Hum Gene Ther 1999;10(8):1359–73.

70. Matsuo Y, Drexler HG. Immunoprofiling of cell lines derived from natural killer-cell and natural killer-like T-cell leukemia-lymphoma. Leuk Res 2003;27(10): 935–45.

71. Munoz J, Shah N, Rezvani K, et al. Concise review: umbilical cord blood transplantation: past, present, and future. Stem Cells Transl Med 2014;3(12): 1435–43.

72. Kotylo PK, Baenziger JC, Yoder MC, et al. Rapid analysis of lymphocyte subsets in cord blood. Am J Clin Pathol 1990;93(2):263–6.

73. Tanaka H, Kai S, Yamaguchi M, et al. Analysis of natural killer (NK) cell activity and adhesion molecules on NK cells from umbilical cord blood. Eur J Haematol 2003;71(1):29–38.

74. Veluchamy JP, Heeren AM, Spanholtz J, et al. High-efficiency lysis of cervical cancer by allogeneic NK cells derived from umbilical cord progenitors is independent of HLA status. Cancer Immunol Immunother 2017;66(1):51–61.

75. Wang Y, Xu H, Zheng X, et al. High expression of NKG2A/CD94 and low expression of granzyme B are associated with reduced cord blood NK cell activity. Cell Mol Immunol 2007;4(5):377–82.

76. Dalle JH, Menezes J, Wagner E, et al. Characterization of cord blood natural killer cells: implications for transplantation and neonatal infections. Pediatr Res 2005;57(5 Pt 1):649–55.

77. Shah N, Li L, McCarty J, et al. Phase I study of cord blood-derived natural killer cells combined with autologous stem cell transplantation in multiple myeloma. Br J Haematol 2017;177(3):457–66.

78. Liu E, Marin D, Banerjee P, et al. Use of CAR-transduced natural killer cells in CD19-positive lymphoid tumors. N Engl J Med 2020;382(6):545–53.

79. Matosevic S. Viral and nonviral engineering of natural killer cells as emerging adoptive cancer immunotherapies. J Immunol Res 2018;2018:4054815.

80. Morgan RA, Boyerinas B. Genetic modification of T cells. Biomedicines 2016; 4(2). https://doi.org/10.3390/biomedicines4020009.

81. Kay MA, Glorioso JC, Naldini L. Viral vectors for gene therapy: the art of turning infectious agents into vehicles of therapeutics. Nat Med 2001;7(1):33–40.

82. Matrai J, Chuah MK, VandenDriessche T. Recent advances in lentiviral vector development and applications. Mol Ther 2010;18(3):477–90.

83. Zennou V, Petit C, Guetard D, et al. HIV-1 genome nuclear import is mediated by a central DNA flap. Cell 2000;101(2):173–85.

84. Bari R, Granzin M, Tsang KS, et al. A Distinct Subset of Highly Proliferative and Lentiviral Vector (LV)-Transducible NK Cells Define a Readily Engineered Subset for Adoptive Cellular Therapy. Front Immunol 2019;10:2001.

85. Colamartino ABL, Lemieux W, Bifsha P, et al. Efficient and Robust NK-Cell Transduction With Baboon Envelope Pseudotyped Lentivector. Front Immunol 2019; 10:2873.

86. Sandrin V, Boson B, Salmon P, et al. Lentiviral vectors pseudotyped with a modified RD114 envelope glycoprotein show increased stability in sera and augmented transduction of primary lymphocytes and CD34+ cells derived from human and nonhuman primates. Blood 2002;100(3):823–32.

87. Chockley P, Patil SL, Gottschalk S. Transient blockade of TBK1/IKKepsilon allows efficient transduction of primary human natural killer cells with vesicular

stomatitis virus G-pseudotyped lentiviral vectors. Cytotherapy 2021;23(9): 787–92.

88. Lewinski MK, Bushman FD. Retroviral DNA integration–mechanism and consequences. Adv Genet 2005;55:147–81.

89. Wu X, Li Y, Crise B, et al. Transcription start regions in the human genome are favored targets for MLV integration. Science 2003;300(5626):1749–51.

90. Deipolyi AR, Golberg A, Yarmush ML, et al. Irreversible electroporation: evolution of a laboratory technique in interventional oncology. Diagn Interv Radiol 2014;20(2):147–54.

91. Robbins GM, Wang M, Pomeroy EJ, et al. Nonviral genome engineering of natural killer cells. Stem Cell Res Ther 2021;12(1):350.

92. Schmidt P, Raftery MJ, Pecher G. Engineering NK cells for CAR therapy-recent advances in gene transfer methodology. Front Immunol 2020;11:611163.

93. Pomeroy EJ, Hunzeker JT, Kluesner MG, et al. A genetically engineered primary human natural killer cell platform for cancer immunotherapy. Mol Ther 2020; 28(1):52–63.

94. McKinlay CJ, Vargas JR, Blake TR, et al. Charge-altering releasable transporters (CARTs) for the delivery and release of mRNA in living animals. Proc Natl Acad Sci U S A 2017;114(4):E448–56.

95. Wilk AJ, Weidenbacher NL, Vergara R, et al. Charge-altering releasable transporters enable phenotypic manipulation of natural killer cells for cancer immunotherapy. Blood Adv 2020;4(17):4244–55.

96. Munoz-Lopez M, Garcia-Perez JL. DNA transposons: nature and applications in genomics. Curr Genomics 2010;11(2):115–28.

97. Tipanee J, VandenDriessche T, Chuah MK. Transposons: moving forward from preclinical studies to clinical trials. Hum Gene Ther 2017;28(11):1087–104.

98. Tipanee J, Chai YC, VandenDriessche T, et al. Preclinical and clinical advances in transposon-based gene therapy. Biosci Rep 2017;37(6). https://doi.org/10.1042/BSR20160614.

99. Schambach A, Morgan M, Fehse B. Two cases of T cell lymphoma following Piggybac-mediated CAR T cell therapy. Mol Ther 2021;29(9):2631–3.

100. Micklethwaite KP, Gowrishankar K, Gloss BS, et al. Investigation of productderived lymphoma following infusion of piggyBac-modified CD19 chimeric antigen receptor T cells. Blood 2021;138(16):1391–405.

101. Morgan MA, Buning H, Sauer M, et al. Use of cell and genome modification technologies to generate improved "Off-the-Shelf" CAR T and CAR NK Cells. Front Immunol 2020;11:1965.

102. Naeimi Kararoudi M, Tullius BP, Chakravarti N, et al. Genetic and epigenetic modification of human primary NK cells for enhanced antitumor activity. Semin Hematol 2020;57(4):201–12.

103. Liang X, Potter J, Kumar S, et al. Rapid and highly efficient mammalian cell engineering via Cas9 protein transfection. J Biotechnol 2015;208:44–53.

104. Komor AC, Badran AH, Liu DR. CRISPR-based technologies for the manipulation of eukaryotic genomes. Cell 2017;169(3):559.

105. Rafei H, Daher M, Rezvani K. Chimeric antigen receptor (CAR) natural killer (NK)-cell therapy: leveraging the power of innate immunity. Br J Haematol 2021;193(2):216–30.

106. Xia J, Minamino S, Kuwabara K. CAR-expressing NK cells for cancer therapy: a new hope. Biosci Trends 2020;14(5):354–9.

107. Wang L, Dou M, Ma Q, et al. Chimeric antigen receptor (CAR)-modified NK cells against cancer: opportunities and challenges. Int Immunopharmacol 2019;74: 105695.

108. Daher M, Rezvani K. Outlook for new CAR-based therapies with a focus on CAR NK Cells: what lies beyond CAR-engineered T cells in the race against cancer. Cancer Discov 2021;11(1):45–58.

109. Wang W, Jiang J, Wu C. CAR-NK for tumor immunotherapy: Clinical transformation and future prospects. Cancer Lett 2020;472:175–80.

110. Xie G, Dong H, Liang Y, et al. CAR-NK cells: a promising cellular immunotherapy for cancer. EBioMedicine 2020;59:102975.

111. Kamiya T, Seow SV, Wong D, et al. Blocking expression of inhibitory receptor NKG2A overcomes tumor resistance to NK cells. J Clin Invest 2019;129(5): 2094–106.

112. Figueiredo C, Seltsam A, Blasczyk R. Permanent silencing of NKG2A expression for cell-based therapeutics. J Mol Med (Berl) 2009;87(2):199–210.

113. Bachanova V, Cooley S, Defor TE, et al. Clearance of acute myeloid leukemia by haploidentical natural killer cells is improved using IL-2 diphtheria toxin fusion protein. Blood 2014;123(25):3855–63.

114. Grzywacz B, Moench L, McKenna D Jr, et al. Natural killer cell homing and persistence in the bone marrow after adoptive immunotherapy correlates with better leukemia control. J Immunother 2019;42(2):65–72.

115. Woan KV, Miller JS. Harnessing natural killer cell antitumor immunity: from the bench to bedside. Cancer Immunol Res 2019;7(11):1742–7.

116. Margolin K, Morishima C, Velcheti V, et al. Phase I Trial of ALT-803, a novel recombinant IL15 complex, in patients with advanced solid tumors. Clin Cancer Res 2018;24(22):5552–61.

117. Romee R, Cooley S, Berrien-Elliott MM, et al. First-in-human phase 1 clinical study of the IL-15 superagonist complex ALT-803 to treat relapse after transplantation. Blood 2018;131(23):2515–27.

118. Conlon KC, Lugli E, Welles HC, et al. Redistribution, hyperproliferation, activation of natural killer cells and CD8 T cells, and cytokine production during first-in-human clinical trial of recombinant human interleukin-15 in patients with cancer. J Clin Oncol 2015;33(1):74–82.

119. Conlon KC, Potter EL, Pittaluga S, et al. IL15 by continuous intravenous infusion to adult patients with solid tumors in a phase i trial induced dramatic NK-cell subset expansion. Clin Cancer Res 2019;25(16):4945–54.

120. Cooley S, He F, Bachanova V, et al. First-in-human trial of rhIL-15 and haploidentical natural killer cell therapy for advanced acute myeloid leukemia. Blood Adv 2019;3(13):1970–80.

121. Miller JS, Morishima C, McNeel DG, et al. A First-in-human phase I study of subcutaneous outpatient recombinant human IL15 (rhIL15) in adults with advanced solid tumors. Clin Cancer Res 2018;24(7):1525–35.

122. Nagashima S, Mailliard R, Kashii Y, et al. Stable transduction of the interleukin-2 gene into human natural killer cell lines and their phenotypic and functional characterization in vitro and in vivo. Blood 1998;91(10):3850–61.

123. Liu E, Tong Y, Dotti G, et al. Cord blood NK cells engineered to express IL-15 and a CD19-targeted CAR show long-term persistence and potent antitumor activity. Leukemia 2018;32(2):520–31.

124. Ma R, Lu T, Li Z, et al. An oncolytic virus expressing IL15/IL15ralpha combined with off-the-shelf EGFR-CAR NK cells targets glioblastoma. Cancer Res 2021; 81(13):3635–48.

125. Goodridge JP, Mahmood S, Zhu H, et al. FT596: translation of first-of-kind multi-antigen targeted off-the-shelf CAR-NK cell with engineered persistence for the treatment of B cell malignancies. Blood 2019;134(Supplement_1):301.
126. Muller N, Michen S, Tietze S, et al. Engineering NK Cells Modified With an EGFRvIII-specific Chimeric Antigen Receptor to Overexpress CXCR4 Improves Immunotherapy of CXCL12/SDF-1alpha-secreting Glioblastoma. J Immunother 2015;38(5):197–210.
127. Kremer V, Ligtenberg MA, Zendehdel R, et al. Genetic engineering of human NK cells to express CXCR2 improves migration to renal cell carcinoma. J Immunother Cancer 2017;5(1):73.
128. Levy E, Reger R, Segerberg F, et al. Enhanced bone marrow homing of natural killer cells following mRNA transfection with gain-of-function variant CXCR4(R334X). Front Immunol 2019;10:1262.
129. Carlsten M, Levy E, Karambelkar A, et al. Efficient mRNA-based genetic engineering of human NK cells with high-affinity CD16 and CCR7 augments rituximab-induced ADCC against lymphoma and targets NK cell migration toward the lymph node-associated chemokine CCL19. Front Immunol 2016;7:105.
130. Ng YY, Tay JCK, Wang S. CXCR1 expression to improve anti-cancer efficacy of intravenously injected CAR-NK cells in mice with peritoneal xenografts. Mol Ther Oncolytics 2020;16:75–85.
131. Li F, Sheng Y, Hou W, et al. CCL5-armed oncolytic virus augments CCR5-engineered NK cell infiltration and antitumor efficiency. J Immunother Cancer 2020;8(1). https://doi.org/10.1136/jitc-2019-000131.
132. Felices M, Lenvik TR, Davis ZB, et al. Generation of BiKEs and TriKEs to improve NK cell-mediated targeting of tumor cells. Methods Mol Biol 2016;1441:333–46.
133. Anegon I, Cuturi MC, Trinchieri G, et al. Interaction of Fc receptor (CD16) ligands induces transcription of interleukin 2 receptor (CD25) and lymphokine genes and expression of their products in human natural killer cells. J Exp Med 1988;167(2):452–72.
134. Gleason MK, Ross JA, Warlick ED, et al. CD16xCD33 bispecific killer cell engager (BiKE) activates NK cells against primary MDS and MDSC CD33+ targets. Blood 2014;123(19):3016–26.
135. Rothe A, Sasse S, Topp MS, et al. A phase 1 study of the bispecific anti-CD30/CD16A antibody construct AFM13 in patients with relapsed or refractory Hodgkin lymphoma. Blood 2015;125(26):4024–31.
136. Sasse SM J, Plütschow A, Hüttmann A, et al. AFM13 in patients with relapsed or refractory Hodgkin lymphoma: final results of an open-label, randomized, multicenter phase II trial. Blood 2020;136(Supplement 1):31–2. https://doi.org/10.1182/blood-2020-141250. Available at.
137. Affimed announces presentation at AACR highlighting initial data from phase 1 study of cord blood-derived natural killer cells pre-complexed with innate cell engager AFM13. 2021. Available at: https://bit.ly/3m0nzJ9. Accessed September 26, 2021.
138. Repp R, Kellner C, Muskulus A, et al. Combined Fc-protein- and Fc-glyco-engineering of scFv-Fc fusion proteins synergistically enhances CD16a binding but does not further enhance NK-cell mediated ADCC. J Immunol Methods 2011;373(1–2):67–78.
139. Chen Y, You F, Jiang L, et al. Gene-modified NK-92MI cells expressing a chimeric CD16-BB-zeta or CD64-BB-zeta receptor exhibit enhanced cancer-killing ability in combination with therapeutic antibody. Oncotarget 2017;8(23):37128–39.

140. Snyder KM, Hullsiek R, Mishra HK, et al. Expression of a recombinant high affinity IgG Fc receptor by engineered NK cells as a docking platform for therapeutic mAbs to Target cancer cells. Front Immunol 2018;9:2873.

141. Zhu H, Blum RH, Bjordahl R, et al. Pluripotent stem cell-derived NK cells with high-affinity noncleavable CD16a mediate improved antitumor activity. Blood 2020;135(6):399–410.

142. Jing Y, Ni Z, Wu J, et al. Identification of an ADAM17 cleavage region in human CD16 (FcgammaRIII) and the engineering of a non-cleavable version of the receptor in NK cells. PLoS One 2015;10(3):e0121788.

143. Strati P, Bachanova V, Goodman A, et al. Preliminary results of a phase I trial of FT516, an off-the-shelf natural killer (NK) cell therapy derived from a clonal master induced pluripotent stem cell (iPSC) line expressing high-affinity, non-cleavable CD16 (hnCD16), in patients (pts) with relapsed/refractory (R/R) B-cell lymphoma (BCL). J Clin Oncol 2021;39(15_suppl):7541.

144. Davis ZB, Vallera DA, Miller JS, et al. Natural killer cells unleashed: checkpoint receptor blockade and BiKE/TriKE utilization in NK-mediated anti-tumor immunotherapy. Semin Immunol 2017;31:64–75.

Gene Therapy for Hemoglobinopathies
Beta-Thalassemia, Sickle Cell Disease

Alexis Leonard, MD[a], John F. Tisdale, MD[a],*, Melissa Bonner, PhD[b]

KEYWORDS

- Sickle cell disease • Beta-thalassemia • Gene therapy • Gene editing
- Lentiviral vector

KEY POINTS

- The two most common monogenic diseases, sickle cell disease and β-thalassemia, are both β-globin gene disorders that are potentially curable after allogeneic hematopoietic stem cell transplantation (HSCT) or autologous HSCT after genetic modification.
- Autologous genetic therapies are promising and have the potential to overcome barriers associated with allogeneic HSCT, such as donor availability and graft-vs-host disease.
- Gene addition and gene-editing strategies are in development; specific modalities and status of ongoing trials are reviewed herein.

INTRODUCTION

Sickle cell disease (SCD) and β-thalassemia are the most common monogenic disorders in the world. Their incidence is expected to increase over time, primarily in low- or middle-income countries, thereby representing a growing burden on global health resources.[1] Treatment options that aim to reduce the burden of disease, particularly for the more severe forms of SCD and transfusion-dependent β-thalassemia (TDT), are needed.

SCD and TDT represent qualitative and quantitative changes to the β-globin gene, respectively. In both, there is a spectrum of clinical phenotypes; in SCD, HbSS and HbSβ0 constitute the most severe forms of disease; in β-thalassemia, severe disease occurs with mutations resulting in minimal to no β-globin synthesis (β0) and consequently little to no HbA (TDT). The phenotypic diversity is partially explained by genetic variants controlling the expression of HbF, and coinheritance of α-thalassemia mutations. In SCD, the presence of HbF can have profound impacts on the rate of polymerization of HbS, whereas in TDT, elevated HbF can compensate for reduced β-globin

[a] Cellular and Molecular Therapeutics Branch, National Heart, Lung, and Blood Institute, National Institutes of Health, Bethesda, MD, USA; [b] bluebird bio, Inc, Cambridge, MA, USA
* Corresponding author.
E-mail address: johntis@mail.nih.gov

Hematol Oncol Clin N Am 36 (2022) 769–795
https://doi.org/10.1016/j.hoc.2022.03.008
0889-8588/22/© 2022 Elsevier Inc. All rights reserved.

hemonc.theclinics.com

levels, decrease globin chain imbalance, and minimize toxic-free intracellular α-globin. This phenomenon is consistent with what is observed clinically; (i) newborns are protected from SCD and TDT complications in the first 6 months of life when HbF levels are naturally elevated[2] and (ii) patients who coinherit large deletions, small insertions/deletions (INDELs) or point mutations within the HBB gene cluster resulting in persistently elevated HbF [hereditary persistence of fetal hemoglobin (HPFH)] are relatively asymptomatic.[3–6]

Allogeneic Hematopoietic Stem Cell Transplantation

Despite a significant increase in survival for patients with SCD through newborn screening, penicillin prophylaxis, and vaccinations, and an increase in survival for patients with TDT with regular blood transfusions, iron chelation therapy (ICT), evidence-based practice guidelines, splenectomy, and antibiotic prophylaxis, current disease-modifying therapies do not fully eliminate disease manifestations.

Hematopoietic stem cell transplantation (HSCT) offers patients with SCD and TDT a curative option, although broad use of this option is significantly limited by donor availability and transplant-related mortality and morbidity, specifically graft rejection, graft-versus-host disease (GVHD), infertility, and other treatment-related toxic effects.[7,8] HSCT is considered standard clinical practice in children and adolescents with TDT before the development of iron overload and iron-related tissue damage. Symptomatic SCD is not well defined and therefore there are no universally adopted indications for HSCT in SCD. History of stroke, however, is an undisputed indication for HSCT, whereas other "severe" disease complications mostly reflect expert opinion due to the absence of the sound evidence base. The risk/benefit ratio of HSCT in SCD is, therefore, age, disease, and donor based. HSCT is an established therapeutic option in SCD when a patient has a severe disease complication and a human leukocyte antigen (HLA)-identical sibling donor. In both TDT and SCD, age at transplantation is an important predictor of outcome in part due to the chronic nature of SCD and TDT and the accumulation of end-organ damage over time.[9] Multicenter, cohort study data from the Center for International Blood and Marrow Transplant Research report age as an important predictor in outcome, with age $\leq$12 years in SCD and $\leq$6 years in TDT reporting higher event-free survival (EFS).[10,11] When there is an indication for HSCT but no matched sibling donor, alternative donor transplantation is considered as an experimental approach to be conducted only on a clinical trial given inferior outcomes to the standard HLA-matched sibling transplantation.

Gene Therapy

Given the lack of universally beneficial disease-modifying therapies, the lack of available HLA-identical sibling donors, and the increased risks of complications with alternate donor HSCT, autologous HSCT after gene therapy is a theoretic universal cure for SCD and TDT that could eliminate major limitations of allogeneic transplantation. Autologous gene therapies in development for SCD and TDT are similar in that they aim to address the underlying genetic cause of disease either by increasing the expression of nonsickling β-globin (β^A), expressing an antisickling β-like globin, or increasing endogenous HbF expression using gene addition or gene-editing strategies. Antisickling β-like globins include γ-globin, δ-globin, and β-like globins with engineered mutations that confer antisickling properties: namely inhibition of polymer formation with mutations that disrupt axial and lateral contacts of the HbS polymers (ie, β^{A-E22A} and β^{A-T87Q}) or a competitive advantage to binding α-globin compared with β^S-globin (ie, β^{A-G16D}).[12,13] Gene therapy may result in the restored capacity of the patient's own HSCs to generate red blood cells (RBCs) with functional and nonpathogenic Hb while overcoming specific limitations associated with allogeneic HSCT.[14] Whereas limitations surrounding donor availability, GVHD, and graft rejection are nearly eliminated with autologous therapy, allogeneic HSCT and gene therapy share a common risk of toxicity associated with conditioning reagents, such as busulfan. Additional considerations specific to gene therapy include the risks of onco-genesis from vector-related toxicity, off-target editing, or deleterious on-target edit-ing.[15,16] Significant advances over the last several decades have brought multiple gene therapies for TDT and SCD into preclinical and clinical development, with limited available long-term data to address safety concerns. Here we review current gene therapies in clinical development for SCD or TDT including gene addition strategies with viral vectors, gene-editing strategies to upregulate endogenous HbF, or gene-editing strategies to repair the β-globin gene at its endogenous locus.

Gene Addition Using Viral Vectors

Gene addition therapy uses lentiviral vectors (LVVs) for semirandom stable integration of a transgene in a target cell. LVVs are considered nonpathogenic and nonimmuno-genic, can deliver large DNA payloads allowing for the incorporation of key regulatory elements such as cell-type-specific promoters, and can transduce both dividing and nondividing cells such as quiescent HSCs.[17–20] Because LVVs are reverse transcribed and integrated into the host cell genome, therapeutic transgene expression is ex-pected to be stable and durable whereby transduced cells contain both the endoge-nous gene and a stably integrated copy of a therapeutic transgene. Additionally, this genetic barcoding allows for unique traceability of transduced HSCs and their progeny enabling deeper understanding of clonal dynamics post-HSCT, during both stress and steady-state hematopoiesis, including observations of clonal hematopoiesis, both transient and persistent, and determination of potential vector involvement in cases of suspected insertional oncogenesis.[21–25]

Multiple viral-mediated gene addition strategies for TDT and SCD are in clinical development and are summarized in **Table 1**. As of 22 December 2021, there were 17 clinical trials listed on clinicaltrials.gov using gene addition therapy for the treat-ment of TDT (n = 10) and SCD (n = 8). General strategies include delivery of either γ-globin (n = 2) or a β-like globin (n = 13), including the nonsickling wild-type adult β-globin ($β^A$) or antisickling variants of β-globin.

The most studied gene therapy products in development for hemoglobinopathies are LentiGlobin BB305 for TDT (betibeglogene autotemcel) and LentiGlobin BB305 for SCD (bb1111, lovotibeglogene autotemcel). Two trials have been completed (NCT01745120 and NCT02151526) with early data published as a proof-of-concept in 1 SCD patient and 22 patients with TDT.[26,27] In both studies, there was stable and durable engraftment of gene-modified cells leading to the stable production of the therapeutic antisickling hemoglobin (HbA^{T87Q}). In the SCD patient, HbA^{T87Q} was present at 48% of total hemoglobin 15 months posttreatment and there was a subse-quent decrease in HbS to 49%. At this 15-month time point, the patient had discon-tinued all prior medications, including pain medication, and had no SCD-related clinical events or hospitalizations. In the TDT patient population, gene therapy reduced or eliminated the need for RBC transfusions in all 22 patients. Importantly, this study demonstrated different outcomes in patients with $β^0/β^0$ TDT or patients with homozy-gosity for the IVS-I-110 mutation compared with patients with non-$β^0/β^0$ TDT. In 13 pa-tients with non-$β^0/β^0$ TDT, 12 were able to stop RBC transfusions and at last study visit, the median HbA^{T87Q} was 6.0 g/dL with median total hemoglobin of 11.2 g/dL. Contrastingly, of the 9 $β^0/β^0$ or homozygosity for patients with IVS-I-110 TDT, 6 remained on transfusions and had a median HbA^{T87Q} of 4.2 g/dL. There was a median

Table 1
Gene therapy clinical trials using gene addition for TDT and SCD

ClinicalTrials.gov Identifier	Start Date	Title	Disease	Phase (Status)	Age	Study Size (N)	Agent	Vector/Transgene (Non/Antisickling)	Sponsoring Institution	Location
NCT01639690	2012	A Phase I Clinical Trial for the Treatment of β-Thalassemia Major With Autologous CD34+ Hematopoietic Progenitor Cells Transduced With TNS9.3.55 a Lentiviral Vector Encoding the Normal Human β-Globin Gene	TDT	1 (Active, not recruiting)	Adults ($\geq$18)	10	Thalagen	TNS9.3.55 LVV/β^A (Nonsickling)	Memorial Sloan Kettering Cancer Center	New York, USA
NCT01745120	2013	A Phase 1/2 Open-Label Study Evaluating the Safety and Efficacy of Gene Therapy in Subjects With β-Thalassemia Major by Transplantation of Autologous CD34+ Cells	TDT	1/2 (Completed)	Children and Adults (12-35)	19	LentiGlobin BB305 for TDT	BB305 LVV/β^{A-T87Q} (Antisickling)	bluebird bio	USA, multicenter; Sydney, Australia; Bangkok, Thailand

NCT	Year	Title	Conditions	Phase	Status	Population	N	Product	Vector	Sponsor	Location
		Transduced Ex Vivo With a Lentiviral βA-T87Q-Globin Vector (LentiGlobin® BB305 Drug Product)									
NCT02151526	2013	A Phase 1/2 Open-Label Study Evaluating the Safety and Efficacy of Gene Therapy for the β-Hemoglobinopathies (Sickle Cell Anemia and β-Thalassemia Major) by Transplantation of Autologous CD34+ Stem Cells Transduced Ex Vivo With a Lentiviral β-A-T87Q Globin Vector (LentiGlobin BB305 Drug Product)	TDT, SCD	1/2	(Completed)	Children and Adults (5-35)	7	LentiGlobin BB305 for TDT and for SCD	BB305 LVV/β^{A-T87Q} (Anti-Sickling)	bluebird bio	Paris, France

(continued on next page)

Table 1
(continued)

ClinicalTrials.gov Identifier	Start Date	Title	Disease	Phase (Status)	Age	Study Size (N)	Agent	Vector/Transgene (Non/Antisickling)	Sponsoring Institution	Location
NCT02140554	2014	A Phase 1/2 Study Evaluating Gene Therapy by Transplantation of Autologous CD34+ Stem Cells Transduced Ex Vivo With the LentiGlobin BB305 Lentiviral Vector in Subjects With Severe Sickle Cell Disease	SCD	1/2 (Active, not recruiting)	Children and Adults (12–50)	50	LentiGlobin BB305 for SCD (bb1111)	BB305 LVV/β^{A-T87Q} (Anti-Sickling)	bluebird bio	USA, multicenter
NCT02186418	2014	Gene Transfer for Patients With SCD Using a Gamma Globin Lentivirus Vector: An Open-Label Phase 1/2 Pilot Study	SCD	1/2 (Recruiting)	Adults (18–45)	10	ARU-1801	LVV/γ-globin (G16D) (Antisickling)	Aruvant Sciences GmbH	USA, multicenter and Jamaica

NCT02247843	2014	Clinical Research Study of Autologous Stem Cell Transplantation for SCD Using Peripheral Blood CD34+ Cells Modified With the Lenti/G-bAS3-FB Lentiviral Vector	SCD	1/2 (Recruiting)	Adults (≥18)	6	Lenti/β^{AS3}-FB	LVV/G-β^{AS3}-FB (Anti-Sickling)	UCLA	USA, California
NCT02453477	2015	A Phase I/II Study Evaluating Safety and Efficacy of Autologous Hematopoietic Stem Cells Genetically Modified With GLOBE Lentiviral Vector Encoding for the Human Beta-globin Gene for the Treatment of Patients Affected by Transfusion-Dependent Beta-thalassemia	TDT	1/2 (Unknown)	Children and Adults (3-64)	10	OTL-300	GLOBE LVV/β^A (Nonsickling)	IRCCS San Raffaele & Orchard Therapeutics	Milano, Italy

(continued on next page)

Table 1
(continued)

ClinicalTrials.gov Identifier	Start Date	Title	Disease	Phase (Status)	Age	Study Size (N)	Agent	Vector/Transgene (Non/Antisickling)	Sponsoring Institution	Location
NCT02906202	2016	A Phase 3 Single-Arm Study Evaluating the Efficacy and Safety of Gene Therapy in Subjects With Transfusion-dependent β-Thalassemia, Who do Not Have a β0/β0 Genotype, by Transplantation of Autologous CD34+ Stem Cells Transduced Ex Vivo With a Lentiviral βA-T87Q-Globin Vector in Subjects ≤50 y of Age	TDT	3 (Active, not recruiting)	Children and Adults (<50)	23	LentiGlobin BB305 for TDT	BB305 LVV/β^{A-T87Q} (Antisickling)	bluebird bio	USA, multicenter; Marseille, France; Hannover, Germany; Rome, Italy; London, UK; Bangkok, Thailand

NCT / Year	Title	Condition	Phase (Status)	Ages	Enrollment	Intervention	Vector	Sponsor	Location
NCT03207009 2017	A Phase 3 Single-Arm Study Evaluating the Efficacy and Safety of Gene Therapy in Subjects With Transfusion-dependent β-Thalassemia by Transplantation of Autologous CD34+ Stem Cells Transduced Ex Vivo With a Lentiviral βA-T87Q-Globin Vector in Subjects ≤50 y of Age	TDT	3 (Active, not recruiting)	Children and Adults (<50)	18	LentiGlobin BB305 for TDT	BB305 LVV/βA−T87Q (Antisickling)	bluebird bio	USA, multicenter; Marseille, France; Germany, multicenter; Thessaloniki, Greece; Rome, Italy; London, UK
NCT03351829 2017	Gene Therapy of Beta Thalassemia Using a Self-inactivating Lentiviral Vector	TDT	1/2 (Unknown)	Children and Adults (4–69)	20	Undisclosed	LVV/Undisclosed (Undisclosed)	Shenzhen Geno-Immune Medical Institute	Guangdong, China
NCT03276455 2017	Evaluation of Safety and Efficacy of Transplantation of Autologous Hematopoietic Stem Cell Genetically Modified in Beta-Thalassemia Major	TDT	1/2 (Unknown)	Children and Adults (≥8)	10	Undisclosed	LVV/βA (Nonsickling)	Nanfang Hospital of Southern Medical University	Guangdong, China

(continued on next page)

Table 1
(continued)

ClinicalTrials.gov Identifier	Start Date	Title	Disease	Phase (Status)	Age	Study Size (N)	Agent	Vector/Transgene (Non/Antisickling)	Sponsoring Institution	Location
NCT03282656	2018	Pilot and Feasibility Study of Hematopoietic Stem Cell Gene Transfer for Sickle Cell Disease	SCD	1 (Recruiting)	Children and Adults (3,40)	15	BCH-BB694 BCL11 A shmiR Drug Product	LVV/shRNA targeting BCL11 A (Antisickling[b])	Boston Children's Hospital	USA, multicenter
NCT04091737	2019	A Phase 1 Pilot Study to Evaluate the Safety and Feasibility of Gene Therapy With CSL200 (Autologous Enriched CD34+ Cell Fraction That Contains CD34+ Cells Transduced With Lentiviral Vector Encoding Human γ-GlobinG16D and Short-Hairpin RNA734) in Adult Subjects With Severe Sickle Cell Disease	SCD	1 (Terminated)	Adults (18-45)	1[a]	CSL200	LVV/γ-globin (G16D) and shRNA734 (Antisickling)	CSL Behring	USA, California

NCT03964792	2019	A Phase 1/2 Open-Label Study Evaluating the Safety and Efficacy of Gene Therapy of the Sickle Cell Disease by Transplantation of an Autologous CD34+ Enriched Cell Fraction That Contains CD34+ Cells Transduced ex Vivo With the GLOBE1 Lentiviral Vector Expressing the βAS3 Globin Gene (GLOBE1 βAS3 Modified Autologous CD34+ Cells) in Patients With Sickle Cell Disease (SCD) (DREPAGLOBE)	SCD	1/2 (Recruiting)	Children and Adults (12-20)	10	DREPAGLOBE	GLOBE 1 LVV/βAS3 (Antisickling)	Assistance Publique – Hopitaux de Paris	Paris, France

(continued on next page)

Table 1
(*continued*)

ClinicalTrials.gov Identifier	Start Date	Title	Disease	Phase (Status)	Age	Study Size (N)	Agent	Vector/Transgene (Non/Antisickling)	Sponsoring Institution	Location
NCT04293185	2020	A Phase 3 Study Evaluating Gene Therapy by Transplantation of Autologous CD34+ Stem Cells Transduced Ex Vivo With the BB305 Lentiviral Vector in Subjects With Sickle Cell Disease	SCD	3 (Recruiting)	Children and Adults (2-50)	35	LentiGlobin BB305 for SCD (bb1111)	BB305 LVV/β^{A-T87Q} (Antisickling)	bluebird bio	USA, multicenter
NCT04592458	2020	A Single-Center, Open-Label Study to Evaluate the Safety and Efficacy of β-globin Restored Autologous Hematopoietic Stem Cells in β-Thalassemia Major Patients	TDT	1 (Not yet recruiting)	Children (8-16)	10	LentiHBBT87Q	LVV/β^{A-T87Q} (Antisickling)	BGI-research & Shenzhen Children's Hospital	Guangdong, China

| NCT05015920 | 2021 | A Phase 1 Open-Label Study Evaluating the Safety and Efficacy of Gene Therapy in Subjects With β-Thalassemia Major by Transplantation of Autologous CD34+Stem Cells Transduced With a Lentiviral Vector Encoding βA-T87Q-Globin | TDT | 1 (Enrolling by invitation) | Children and Adults (5-35) | 10 | BD211 Drug Product | LVV/βA−T87Q (Antisickling) | Shanghai BDgene Co., Ltd. | Yunnan, China |

Abbreviations: HSCT, hematopoietic stem cell transplantation; SCD, sickle cell disease; TDT, transfusion-dependent thalassemia.

[a] Actual number of enrolled patients.

[b] Uniquely does not add exogenous antisickling β-like globin; induces endogenous γ-globin with simultaneous reduction of $β^S$-globin.

Data assessed from clinicaltrials.gov on 22 December 2021.

reduction of 74% in the annualized number of transfusions and a 73% reduction in transfusion volume compared with the 2 years before treatment. In the 3 patients who were able to discontinue transfusions, HbA^{T87Q} ranged from 6.6 to 8.2 g/dL and total hemoglobin ranged from 8.3 to 10.2 g/dL.

Following positive proof-of-concept data, a large, multicenter study (NCT02140554) was initiated for the evaluation of LentiGlobin BB305 in SCD. Data from the first cohort of patients (Group A, n = 7) demonstrated lower peripheral blood vector copy number (VCN) and HbA^{T87Q} production than seen in the initial SCD patient from the earlier study. Improvements were subsequently made to the manufacturing process resulting in higher VCN values in Group B (n = 2), and later to the collection of a peripherally mobilized stem cell source with plerixafor, which has been demonstrated to be safe and effective in patients with SCD[28–31], rather than bone marrow harvest in Group C (n = 35).[32] Such improvements now demonstrate high and sustained near-pancellular expression of HbA^{T87Q} that is greater than 40% of total hemoglobin by 6-months posttreatment. Clinically there is a reduction in HbS, reduction in the propensity of RBCs to sickle, near-normalization of hemolysis markers, and resolution of severe vaso-occlusive events (VOEs). LentiGlobin BB305 for SCD is being evaluated in a phase 3 study (NCT04293185) in both children and adults.

Two Phase 3 studies (NCT02906202 and NCT03207009) evaluating LentiGlobin BB305 for TDT in both children and adults are ongoing. Key manufacturing improvements made in LentiGlobin BB305 for SCD to increase gene modification efficiency were also made in LentiGlobin BB305 for TDT. Following treatment in these Phase 3 studies, 89% of evaluable patients across ages and genotypes achieved transfusion independence.[33] Additionally, these patients have been transfusion independent for a median duration of 25 months with a median weighted hemoglobin of 11.6 g/dL. Of the 27 pediatric patients treated 91% of evaluable patients achieved transfusion independence. Results from patients with non-β^0/β^0 TDT have been recently published and demonstrate transfusion independence in 91% of evaluable patients with an average transfusion-free hemoglobin of 11.7 g/dL.[34]

LVV delivery of the wild-type β^A-globin is being evaluated in 3 studies (NCT01639690, NCT02453477, NCT03276455). OTL-300 was evaluated in TDT subjects and demonstrated reduced or eliminated need for transfusions in 8 of 9 treated subjects (n = 5 children; n = 3 adults) at 12-months posttreatment.[35] However, it was announced in May 2020 that the development of this program will be deprioritized.[36] A second study evaluating a different LVV delivering wild-type β^A-globin, Thalagen, demonstrated a 33% and 48% reduction in blood transfusions in 2 of 3 patients with treated TDT with follow-ups of 4 and 7 years, respectively.[37]

Drepaglobe, LVV delivery of a β^{AS3} antisickling globin, is being evaluated (NCT03964792) and data presented from 3 patients with 8 to 18 months of follow-up demonstrate mixed results.[38] Two patients are no longer on transfusions and seem to produce 20% to 30% HbAS3. Of these patients, one initiated hydroxyurea 7-months postgene therapy for 9 months and is currently on crizanlizumab and iron chelation treatment. They have both had hospitalizations due to vaso-occlusive crisis (VOC). The third patient restarted transfusions 3-months posttreatment.

LVV delivery of γ-globin is being evaluated in 2 studies. One study evaluating CSL200 (NCT04091737) was terminated due to enrollment difficulties. Data from a different ongoing study (NCT02186418) evaluating ARU-1801, autologous HSCs transduced with an LVV encoding a γ-globin gene with a single amino acid substitution (G16D) allowing for the distinction of the gene therapy derived antisickling HbF^{G16D} from endogenous HbF, has been presented.[39] Four patients have been treated with ARU-1801, all using a modestly reduced intensity melphalan conditioning regimen. The first 2 patients have greater than 36 months of follow-up. Low peripheral blood VCN values and production of HbF^{G16D} led to protocol refinements and development of a predictive model for targeted melphalan conditioning.[40] In the first patient, 31% of hemoglobin was antisickling hemoglobin; 20% was specifically HbF^{G16D}. The second patient had lower hemoglobin values with 22% comprised of antisickling hemoglobin. The third and fourth patients were treated using a refined manufacturing process; at 18 months posttreatment patient 3 was making 38% HbF, 27% was specifically HbF^{G16D} and at 12-months posttreatment patient 4 was making 18% HbF, 15% was specifically HbF^{G16D}.

One therapy in clinical development (NCT03282656) is unique as its LVV does not deliver a globin gene and instead delivers a transgene that results in erythroid-specific expression of a short hairpin RNA targeting *BCL11 A* leading to knockdown of the critical repressor of HbF.[41,42] A theoretic advantage of this approach of forcing endogenous hemoglobin switching is the concomitant upregulation of HbF and downregulation of HbS; whereas, transgenic expression of a β-like globin evokes competition with β^S for hemoglobin tetramer formation. Initial results in 6 patients with follow-up ranging from 7 to 29 months demonstrated increased total hemoglobin over baseline values and median 30.4% HbF in untransfused patients (n = 5).[43] At the most recent visit for all patients, median percentage of F-cells among untransfused red cells was 70.8%, a robust increase from a median 14% at baseline. Despite vector copy number (VCN) in the drug products ranging from 1.8 to 6.9 copies per diploid genome (c/dg), VCN in whole blood at the most recent time point ranged from 0.30 to 1.61 c/dg. VCNs in CD34+ bone marrow 6 months posttreatment ranged from 0.53 to 1.52 c/dg. Of the 3 patients who were noted to have prestudy severe SCD clinical events such as VOC, acute chest syndrome, and priapism requiring an emergency department visit or admission, 2 have not had any posttreatment. The patient who had the most prestudy events (n = 13) had 5 within the first 5-months posttreatment; the most recent severe event as of the publication occurred 8-months posttherapy and this patient was 20-months posttherapy.

Two cases of AML were reported following gene addition therapy for SCD; importantly, in both cases, it was determined that AML was unrelated to LVV.[24,25] The two patients who developed AML were treated in Group A (NCT02140554) with LentiGlobin BB305 for SCD produced from bone marrow-harvested HSCs using an earlier version of the drug product manufacturing process. Current theories suggest the stress of switching from homeostatic to regenerative hematopoiesis by transplanted cells drives the clonal expansion and leukemogenic transformation of preexisting premalignant clones, eventually resulting in AML/myelodysplastic syndrome (MDS).[44] Bone marrow harvests as the cell source resulted in lower cell doses with fewer CD34$^{hi/+}$ long-term HSCs, likely increasing proliferative stress on the repopulating cells. Low drug product VCNs for these patients resulted in modest transgene expression and an inadequate therapeutic response. These patients continued to experience hemolysis and persistent anemia, resulting in transplanted and endogenous bone marrow cells to continue experiencing hematopoietic stress posttreatment, providing a further opportunity for the accumulation of mutations. To date, no cases of insertional oncogenesis have been reported in gene addition trials using LVV for TDT or SCD. There are no reports of leukemia in patients with 63 β-thalassemia who received drug products manufactured with the identical BB305 LVV used for the manufacture of LentiGlobin for SCD in separate clinical trials (NCT01745120, NCT02151526, NCT03207009, and NCT02906202), suggesting a uniqueness to the pathophysiology of SCD. Constant erythropoietic stress with dysregulated hematopoiesis, chronic inflammation, repeat bony infarction, and preexisting clonal hematopoiesis of indeterminant potential (CHIP)-related mutations compound the already known risks associated with genotoxic conditioning, autologous HSCT, and an increased relative but low absolute risk of AML/MDS.[45–48]

In totality, the reported data from the completed or ongoing trials encompassing gene addition therapies using LVVs support this mode of treatment to be a potentially safe and efficacious option for patients with TDT or SCD. To date, no cases of GVHD or immune rejection have been reported, no cases of insertional oncogenesis, and the overall safety profiles of the ongoing and completed studies are generally consistent with that of HSCT requiring myeloablative conditioning and of underlying disease.

Gene Editing

While the specific strategies of gene-editing therapies in development for TDT and SCD differ, all rely on site-specific DNA nucleases creating a double-stranded DNA break (DSB) that is repaired by cellular machinery either by an error-prone process, nonhomologous end joining (NHEJ) or microhomology-mediated end joining (MMEJ), or a more precise process, homology-directed repair (HDR) which necessitates the use of a donor template in conjunction with the nuclease to facilitate a directed and specific genomic alteration. Using these different repair mechanisms results in either the creation of insertions or deletions (INDELs), which can effectively knockout a gene regulatory region and lead to knockdown and/or knockout of a gene, or a precise genomic repair. The potential adverse consequences of gene editing on HSCs have been recently and comprehensively reviewed.[49] Potential risks of gene editing include off-target editing effects,[50] deleterious on-target editing effects such as translocations[51] or chromothripsis,[52] preexisting immune responses, consequences of the activation of the DSB repair pathway, and p53 activation.[53–55] While early clinical data are promising, the small sample sizes and limited clinical experience overall, specifically in long-term follow-up of patients treated with gene-edited HSC products, warrants caution in data interpretation, particularly as many of the identified potential risks of gene addition strategies targeting HSCs were only evident with time.

Multiple gene-editing therapies for TDT and SCD are currently in clinical development and are summarized in **Table 2**. As of 22 December 2021, there were 9 clinical trials listed on clinicaltrials.gov using gene editing for the treatment of TDT (n = 3) and SCD (n = 6) using either zinc finger nuclease (ZFN) products or CRISPR/Cas9 products. In 7 of the 9 studies, the goal of the edit is to increase endogenous fetal hemoglobin expression and in most of those studies, this is achieved by knockdown of *BCL11 A*. Two studies (NCT04819841 and NCT04774536) aim to correct the underlying β^S glutamate to valine amino acid substitution at position 6 (E6V) in SCD by editing the β-globin gene and achieving repair via HDR by providing template DNA. Data from these studies are not currently available.

ST-400 and SAR445136 (formerly BIVV003) are autologous cell therapies in development that use ZFNs to disrupt the *BCL11 A* erythroid enhancer to increase endogenous HbF. SAR445136 is being evaluated in one study (NCT03653247, PRECIZN-1 study) for SCD. Thus far, 4 patients have been treated with SAR445136 with follow-up ranging from 26 to 91 weeks.[56] European Medicines Agency minutes suggest increases in HbF expression concordant with the assumed mechanism of action and supportive of orphan designation.[57,58] Recent data demonstrate on-target editing resulted in 61% to 78% INDELs in the drug products though there was a mean 25% INDELs in BM from the 4 subjects. At most recent visit, the HbF level ranged from 14% to 38%. ST-400 was being evaluated in one study (NCT03432364; Thales study) for TDT. Five patients with TDT have been treated and data presented demonstrated peak HbF levels of 23.5 $\pm$ 11.4% that were not sustained and patients

Table 2
Gene therapy clinical trials using gene editing for TDT and SCD

ClinicalTrials.gov Identifier	Start Date	Title	Disease	Phase (Status)	Age	Study Size (N)	Agent	Nuclease/Edit (Non/Antisickling)	Sponsoring Institution	Location
NCT03745287	2018	A Phase 1/2/3 Study to Evaluate the Safety and Efficacy of a Single Dose of Autologous CRISPR-Cas9 Modified CD34+ Human Hematopoietic Stem and Progenitor Cells (CTX001) in Subjects With Severe Sickle Cell Disease	SCD	2/3 (Active, Not recruiting)	Children and Adults (12-35)	45	CTX001	CRISPR-Cas9/ *BCL11A* erythroid enhancer (Antisickling)	Vertex Pharmaceuticals Incorporated	USA, multicenter; Toronto, Canada; Rome, Italy; London, UK; Brussels, Belgium; Germany, multicenter; Paris, France
NCT03655678	2018	A Phase 1/2/3 Study of the Safety and Efficacy of a Single Dose of Autologous CRISPR-Cas9 Modified CD34+ Human Hematopoietic Stem and Progenitor Cells (hHSPCs) in Subjects With Transfusion-Dependent β-Thalassemia	TDT	2/3 (Active, Not recruiting)	Children and Adults (12-35)	45	CTX001	CRISPR-Cas9/ *BCL11A* erythroid enhancer (Antisickling)	Vertex Pharmaceuticals Incorporated	USA, multicenter; Canada, multicenter; Germany, multicenter; Rome, Italy; UK, multicenter

(continued on next page)

Table 2
(continued)

ClinicalTrials.gov Identifier	Start Date	Title	Disease	Phase (Status)	Age	Study Size (N)	Agent	Nuclease/Edit (Non/Antisickling)	Sponsoring Institution	Location
NCT03432364	2018	A Phase 1/2, Open-label, Single-arm Study to Assess the Safety, Tolerability, and Efficacy of ST-400 Autologous Hematopoietic Stem Cell Transplant for Treatment of Transfusion-Dependent Beta-thalassemia (TDT)	TDT	1/2 (Active, not recruiting)	Adults (18-40)	6	ST-400	ZFN/*BCL11 A* erythroid enhancer (Antisickling)	Sangamo Therapeutics & Sanofi	USA, multicenter
NCT03653247	2019	A Phase 1/2, Open-Label, Multicenter, Single-Arm Study to Assess the Safety, Tolerability, and Efficacy of BIVV003 for Autologous Hematopoietic Stem Cell Transplantation in Patients With Severe Sickle Cell Disease	SCD	1/2 (Recruiting)	Adults (18-40)	8	BIVV003 (Now called SAR445136)	ZFN/ *BCL11 A* erythroid enhancer (Antisickling)	Sangamo Therapeutics & Sanofi[a]	USA, multicenter

NCT Number	Year	Title	Condition	Phase (Status)	Population	N	Product	Approach	Company	Location
NCT04211480	2020	An Open-Label Trial of Evaluation of the Safety and Efficacy of Treatment With γ-globin Reactivated Autologous Hematopoietic Stem Cells in Subjects With β-thalassemia Major	TDT	1/2 (Recruiting)	Children (5-15)	12	Undisclosed	CRISPR-Cas9/ Undisclosed (Antisickling)	Bioray Laboratories	Shanghai, China
NCT04443907	2020	A first-in-patient Phase I/II Clinical Study to Investigate the Safety, Tolerability, and Efficacy of Genome-edited Hematopoietic Stem and Progenitor Cells in Subjects With Severe Complications of Sickle Cell Disease	SCD	1/2 (Recruiting)	Children and Adults (2-40)	30	OTQ923/ HIX763	CRISPR-Cas9/ BCL11 A (Antisickling)	Novartis Pharmaceuticals	USA, multicenter

(continued on next page)

Table 2
(continued)

ClinicalTrials.gov Identifier	Start Date	Title	Phase (Status)	Disease	Age	Study Size (N)	Agent	Nuclease/Edit (Non/Antisickling)	Sponsoring Institution	Location
NCT04819841	2021	A Phase I/II Study of the Correction of a Single-Nucleotide Mutation (Adenosine–>Thymine [A–>T]) in Autologous CD34+ Hematopoietic Stem Cells to Convert HbS to HbA for Treating Severe Sickle Cell Disease	1/2 (Recruiting)	SCD	Children and Adults (12–40)	15	GPH101	CRISPR-Cas9/β^S -> β^A (Nonsickling)	Graphite Bio, Inc.	USA, multicenter
NCT04853576	2021	A Phase 1/2 Study to Evaluate the Safety and Efficacy of a Single Dose of Autologous Clustered Regularly Interspaced Short Palindromic Repeats Gene-edited CD34+ Human Hematopoietic Stem and Progenitor Cells (EDIT-301) in Subjects With Severe Sickle Cell Disease	1/2 (Recruiting)	SCD	Adults (18–50)	40	EDIT-301	CRISPR-Cas9/HGB1/2 (Antisickling)	Editas Medicine, Inc.	USA, multicenter

| NCT04774536 | 2021 | Transplantation of CRISPRCas9 Corrected Hematopoietic Stem Cells (CRISPR_SCD001) in Patients With Severe Sickle Cell Disease | SCD | 1/2 (Not yet recruiting) | Children and Adults (12-35) | 9 | CRISPR_SCD001 | CRISPR-Cas9/β^S -> β^A (Nonsickling) | UCSF Benioff Children's Hospital Oakland | USA, multicenter |

Abbreviations: HSCT, hematopoietic stem cell transplantation; SCD, sickle cell disease; TDT, transfusion-dependent thalassemia.

[a] Program transitioning back to Sangamo through first half of 2022(77).

Data assessed from clinicaltrials.gov on 22 December 2021.

resumed transfusions by 3-months posttreatment.[59] Interestingly, a significant drop in long-term HSCs was observed in process development runs using the same manufacturing scale process performed during the clinical trial manufacturing. Of note, following these observations of the only transient increase in HbF and challenges with the manufacturing process development of this program has been terminated.[60]

CTX001 is an investigational autologous cell therapy that uses CRISPR/Cas9 to disrupt the *BCL11 A* erythroid enhancer to increase endogenous HbF. CTX001 is being evaluated in 2 studies (NCT03655678 and NCT03745287) for TDT and SCD, respectively. In one reported TDT subject (β^0/β^+ (IVS-I-110)) stable engraftment was achieved with rapid increase in HbF to 13.1 g/dL by 18 months posttreatment with nearly 100% of RBCs containing detectable levels of HbF (F+ cells).[61] This patient was able to discontinue RBC transfusions. In one reported SCD patient stable engraftment was achieved with HbF reaching 43.2% of total hemoglobin 15 months posttreatment and nearly 100% of F+ cells. HbF increase corresponded to a decrease of HbS to 52.3% 15 months posttreatment and total hemoglobin rose from a baseline of 7.2 g/dL to 12 g/dL. Beyond the publication, additional data have been presented.[62,63] In patients with TDT (n = 15) with a median of 8.7 months (4.0–26.2 months) of follow-up, HbF comprised 10.3 g/dL of total hemoglobin at 6-months posttreatment (n = 11) and all patients have discontinued transfusions. One patient did experience 4 severe adverse events potentially related to CTX001, all in the context of hemophagocytic lymphohistiocytosis (HLH). In patients with SCD (n = 7) with a median 5.5 (2.5–9.5) months of follow-up HbF comprised 45% of total hemoglobin 6 months posttreatment (n = 5). In patients with more than 6 months of follow-up (n = 5) median total hemoglobin was 13.7 (11–15.9) g/dL with 96% F+ cells reported in 4 patients.

To date, cumulative data from the ongoing gene-editing clinical trials for SCD and TDT suggest gene editing of the *BCL11 A* erythroid enhancer could be an effective mechanism to induce HbF expression, compensating for the lack of HbA production in TDT and, due to the mechanism of hemoglobin switching, resulting in the compensatory decrease of HbS in SCD. While promising, these studies are early and the field would benefit from longer term follow-up.

Future Directions

Future iterations of gene therapies are currently in preclinical development and focus on overcoming the existing barriers of current *ex vivo* strategies. Critical areas of understanding and improvement of gene therapy for hemoglobinopathies are 3-fold; safe collection of an adequate quantity of long-term HSCs; safe, efficient, and cost-effective manufacturing techniques enabling equitable access to therapies; and long-term expression with adequate engraftment of gene-modified cells with minimal toxicity to patients. Data suggest plerixafor mobilization is safe, efficient, and capable of yielding sufficient HSC quantities in most patients for clinical gene therapy applications,[28–31] though expanded options are urgently needed for those who do not mobilize sufficiently with plerixafor alone[64] given the inability to use granulocyte colony stimulating factor in patients with SCD.[65,66] Concerns regarding toxic conditioning, infertility, and secondary malignancy remain significant, leading to the development of multiple reduced toxicity conditioning strategies, largely antibody based.[67–69] Early preclinical work in mouse models demonstrated promise of improved safety profiles with comparable efficacy to standard conditioning regimens, but large animal models have not yet replicated this data.[70,71] Initial data from one newly diagnosed severe combined immunodeficiency (SCID) patient treated with JSP191, a humanized monoclonal antibody targeting CD117, as a conditioning reagent before allogeneic HSCT resulted in peripheral myeloid chimerism of 8% and bone marrow CD34+ chimerism of 25% 12 weeks posttransplant.[72] A larger dataset evaluating JSP191 (previously called AMG 191) in patients with transplant nonnaïve SCID demonstrated lower levels of peripheral myeloid chimerism in 6 of 7 reported patients.[73] Additionally, the totality of data across both the gene addition and gene-editing clinical experience suggests low VCN or editing rates may not be sufficient to be disease ameliorative, challenging the dogma of 20% chimerism[74] in a gene therapy setting as an efficacy threshold and reenforcing the need for high engraftment efficiencies of gene-modified cells. While initial results of antibody-based conditioning strategies are promising, additional strategies including the clinical development of antibody–drug conjugates (ADCs) will be necessary to achieve the higher-level engraftment necessary to revert the hemoglobinopathies. Lastly, the overall projected costs of and equitable access to *ex vivo* gene therapies have fueled the ongoing preclinical development of *in vivo* gene therapies,[75,76] which could prove to be more portable and require less infrastructure, thus expanding access to these critical therapies.

SUMMARY

Gene therapy for both TDT and SCD has the potential to be curative, with preliminary data showing small successes that have improved over time. The term "cure" from the scientific perspective involves the engraftment of HSCs capable of lifelong hematopoietic potential expressing stable, erythroid-specific expression capable of overcoming the pathogenic phenotype; improvement in patient-related outcomes, remaining disease free, and not substituting one disease process for another is a more likely definition from the patient's perspective. Early data in both gene addition and gene-editing trials for TDT and SCD suggest the possibility of a future free from transfusions, near-complete resolution of VOE/acute chest syndrome, and clinically meaningful improvements in patient outcomes. Data are limited by the small number of patients treated, a relatively short follow-up period, and concerns regarding long-term safety; however, hope remains for a large population of patients with hemoglobinopathies in need of curative therapeutic options.

CONFLICT OF INTEREST

M. Bonner is an employee and shareholder of bluebird bio, Inc.

REFERENCES

1. Modell B, Darlison M. Global epidemiology of haemoglobin disorders and derived service indicators. Bull World Health Organ 2008;86(6):480–7.
2. Watson J. The significance of the paucity of sickle cells in newborn Negro infants. Am J Med Sci 1948;215(4):419–23.
3. Jacob GF, Raper AB. Hereditary persistence of foetal haemoglobin production, and its interaction with the sickle-cell trait. Br J Haematol 1958;4(2):138–49.
4. Forget BG. Molecular basis of hereditary persistence of fetal hemoglobin. Ann N Y Acad Sci 1998;850:38–44.
5. Weber L, Frati G, Felix T, et al. Editing a gamma-globin repressor binding site restores fetal hemoglobin synthesis and corrects the sickle cell disease phenotype. Sci Adv 2020;6(7).
6. Cui S, Engel JD. Reactivation of Fetal Hemoglobin for Treating beta-Thalassemia and Sickle Cell Disease. Adv Exp Med Biol 2017;1013:177–202.

7. Gragert L, Eapen M, Williams E, et al. HLA match likelihoods for hematopoietic stem-cell grafts in the U.S. registry. N Engl J Med 2014;371(4):339–48.

8. Walters MC, Patience M, Leisenring W, et al. Barriers to bone marrow transplantation for sickle cell anemia. Biol Blood Marrow Transplant 1996;2(2):100–4.

9. Kanter J, Liem RI, Bernaudin F, et al. American Society of Hematology 2021 guidelines for sickle cell disease: stem cell transplantation. Blood Adv 2021; 5(18):3668–89.

10. Eapen M, Brazauskas R, Walters MC, et al. Effect of donor type and conditioning regimen intensity on allogeneic transplantation outcomes in patients with sickle cell disease: a retrospective multicentre, cohort study. Lancet Haematol 2019; 6(11):e585–96.

11. Li C, Mathews V, Kim S, et al. Related and unrelated donor transplantation for β-thalassemia major: results of an international survey. Blood Adv 2019;3(17): 2562–70.

12. Levasseur DN, Ryan TM, Reilly MP, et al. A recombinant human hemoglobin with anti-sickling properties greater than fetal hemoglobin. J Biol Chem 2004;279(26): 27518–24.

13. McCune SL, Reilly MP, Chomo MJ, et al. Recombinant human hemoglobins designed for gene therapy of sickle cell disease. Proc Natl Acad Sci U S A 1994; 91(21):9852–6.

14. Sheth S, Licursi M, Bhatia M. Sickle cell disease: time for a closer look at treatment options? Br J Haematol 2013;162(4):455–64.

15. Hacein-Bey-Abina S, Von Kalle C, Schmidt M, et al. LMO2-associated clonal T cell proliferation in two patients after gene therapy for SCID-X1. Science 2003;302(5644):415–9.

16. Hacein-Bey-Abina S, Garrigue A, Wang GP, et al. Insertional oncogenesis in 4 patients after retrovirus-mediated gene therapy of SCID-X1. J Clin Invest 2008; 118(9):3132–42.

17. Morgan RA, Gray D, Lomova A, et al. Hematopoietic Stem Cell Gene Therapy: Progress and Lessons Learned. Cell Stem Cell 2017;21(5):574–90.

18. White M, Whittaker R, Gandara C, et al. A Guide to Approaching Regulatory Considerations for Lentiviral-Mediated Gene Therapies. Hum Gene Ther Methods 2017;28(4):163–76.

19. Schambach A, Zychlinski D, Ehrnstroem B, et al. Biosafety features of lentiviral vectors. Hum Gene Ther 2013;24(2):132–42.

20. Ferrari G, Thrasher AJ, Aiuti A. Gene therapy using haematopoietic stem and progenitor cells. Nat Rev Genet 2021;22(4):216–34.

21. Biasco L, Pellin D, Scala S, et al. In Vivo Tracking of Human Hematopoiesis Reveals Patterns of Clonal Dynamics during Early and Steady-State Reconstitution Phases. Cell Stem Cell 2016;19(1):107–19.

22. Cavazzana-Calvo M, Payen E, Negre O, et al. Transfusion independence and HMGA2 activation after gene therapy of human beta-thalassaemia. Nature 2010;467(7313):318–22.

23. Six E, Guilloux A, Denis A, et al. Clonal tracking in gene therapy patients reveals a diversity of human hematopoietic differentiation programs. Blood 2020;135(15): 1219–31.

24. Goyal S, Tisdale J, Schmidt M, et al. Acute Myeloid Leukemia Case after Gene Therapy for Sickle Cell Disease. N Engl J Med 2022;386:138–47.

25. Hsieh MM, Bonner M, Pierciey FJ, et al. Myelodysplastic syndrome unrelated to lentiviral vector in a patient treated with gene therapy for sickle cell disease. Blood Adv 2020;4(9):2058–63.

26. Ribeil JA, Hacein-Bey-Abina S, Payen E, et al. Gene Therapy in a Patient with Sickle Cell Disease. N Engl J Med 2017;376(9):848–55.
27. Thompson AA, Walters MC, Kwiatkowski J, et al. Gene Therapy in Patients with Transfusion-Dependent beta-Thalassemia. N Engl J Med 2018;378(16):1479–93.
28. Uchida N, Leonard A, Stroncek D, et al. Safe and efficient peripheral blood stem cell collection in patients with sickle cell disease using plerixafor. Haematologica 2020;105(10):e497.
29. Boulad F, Shore T, van Besien K, et al. Safety and efficacy of plerixafor dose escalation for the mobilization of CD34(+) hematopoietic progenitor cells in patients with sickle cell disease: interim results. Haematologica 2018;103(5):770–7.
30. Esrick EB, Manis JP, Daley H, et al. Successful hematopoietic stem cell mobilization and apheresis collection using plerixafor alone in sickle cell patients. Blood Adv 2018;2(19):2505–12.
31. Lagresle-Peyrou C, Lefrere F, Magrin E, et al. Plerixafor enables safe, rapid, efficient mobilization of hematopoietic stem cells in sickle cell disease patients after exchange transfusion. Haematologica 2018;103(5):778–86.
32. Kanter J, Walters MC, Krishnamurti L, et al. Biologic and clinical efficacy of lentiglobin for sickle cell disease. N Engl J Med 2022;386:617–28.
33. Andreas E. Kulozik IT, Janet L. Kwiatkowski, Alexis A. Thompson, et al. Interim results of betibeglogene autotemcel gene therapy in pediatric patients with transfusion-dependent β-thalassemia (tdt) treated IN The phase 3 NORTHSTAR-2 and NORTHSTAR-3 studies. 06/09/212021. p. EP1301.
34. Locatelli F, Thompson AA, Kwiatkowski JL, et al. Betibeglogene Autotemcel Gene Therapy for Non-beta(0)/beta(0) Genotype beta-Thalassemia. N Engl J Med 2022;386:415–27.
35. Marktel S, Scaramuzza S, Cicalese MP, et al. Intrabone hematopoietic stem cell gene therapy for adult and pediatric patients affected by transfusion-dependent ss-thalassemia. Nat Med 2019;25(2):234–41.
36. Orchard therapeutics Unveils New strategic plan and reports First Quarter 2020 Financial Results [press release]. May 07, 2020 2020.
37. Aurelio Maggio MS, Isabelle Riviere, Xiuyan Wang, et al. Gene therapy with the lentiviral vector TNS9.3.55 PRODUCES long-term improvement IN severe ß-THALASSEMIA. European Hematology Association; 06/12/202020. p. EP1497.
38. Magrin E, Magnani A, Semeraro M, et al. Clinical Results of the Drepaglobe Trial for Sickle Cell Disease Patients. Blood 2021;138(Supplement 1):1854.
39. Grimley M, Asnani M, Shrestha A, et al. Safety and Efficacy of Aru-1801 in Patients with Sickle Cell Disease: Early Results from the Phase 1/2 Momentum Study of a Modified Gamma Globin Gene Therapy and Reduced Intensity Conditioning. Blood 2021;138(Supplement 1):3970.
40. Brendan Johnson TH, Christopher Lo, Courtney Little, et al. Towards patient-specific DOSING OF melphalan conditioning for ARU-1801, a NOVEL gene therapy for treatment OF sickle cell disease. European Hematology Association; 2021. p. EP745.
41. Brendel C, Guda S, Renella R, et al. Lineage-specific BCL11A knockdown circumvents toxicities and reverses sickle phenotype. J Clin Invest 2016;126(10):3868–78.
42. Brendel C, Negre O, Rothe M, et al. Preclinical Evaluation of a Novel Lentiviral Vector Driving Lineage-Specific BCL11A Knockdown for Sickle Cell Gene Therapy. Mol Ther Methods Clin Dev 2020;17:589–600.
43. Esrick EB, Lehmann LE, Biffi A, et al. Post-Transcriptional Genetic Silencing of BCL11A to Treat Sickle Cell Disease. N Engl J Med 2021;384(3):205–15.

44. Jones RJ, DeBaun MR. Leukemia after gene therapy for sickle cell disease: insertional mutagenesis, busulfan, both, or neither. Blood 2021;138(11):942–7.

45. Leonard A, Tisdale JF. A pause in gene therapy: Reflecting on the unique challenges of sickle cell disease. Mol Ther 2021;29(4):1355–6.

46. Seminog OO, Ogunlaja OI, Yeates D, et al. Risk of individual malignant neoplasms in patients with sickle cell disease: English national record linkage study. J R Soc Med 2016;109(8):303–9.

47. Brunson A, Keegan THM, Bang H, et al. Increased risk of leukemia among sickle cell disease patients in California. Blood 2017;130(13):1597–9.

48. Pincez T, Lee SSK, Ilboudo Y, et al. Clonal hematopoiesis in sickle cell disease. Blood 2021 Nov 25;138(21):2148–52.

49. Lee BC, Lozano RJ, Dunbar CE. Understanding and overcoming adverse consequences of genome editing on hematopoietic stem and progenitor cells. Mol Ther 2021 Nov 3;29(11):3205–18.

50. Cradick TJ, Fine EJ, Antico CJ, et al. CRISPR/Cas9 systems targeting beta-globin and CCR5 genes have substantial off-target activity. Nucleic Acids Res 2013; 41(20):9584–92.

51. AlJanahi AA, Lazzarotto CR, Chen S, et al. Prediction and validation of hematopoietic stem and progenitor cell off-target editing in transplanted rhesus macaques. Mol Ther 2022 Jan 5;30(1):209–22.

52. Leibowitz ML, Papathanasiou S, Doerfler PA, et al. Chromothripsis as an on-target consequence of CRISPR-Cas9 genome editing. Nat Genet 2021;53(6):895–905.

53. Schiroli G, Conti A, Ferrari S, et al. Precise Gene Editing Preserves Hematopoietic Stem Cell Function following Transient p53-Mediated DNA Damage Response. Cell Stem Cell 2019;24(4):551–565 e8.

54. Haapaniemi E, Botla S, Persson J, et al. CRISPR-Cas9 genome editing induces a p53-mediated DNA damage response. Nat Med 2018;24(7):927–30.

55. Enache OM, Rendo V, Abdusamad M, et al. Cas9 activates the p53 pathway and selects for p53-inactivating mutations. Nat Genet 2020;52(7):662–8.

56. Alavi A, Krishnamurti L, Abedi M, et al. Preliminary Safety and Efficacy Results from Precizn-1: An Ongoing Phase 1/2 Study on Zinc Finger Nuclease-Modified Autologous CD34+ HSPCs for Sickle Cell Disease (SCD). Blood 2021;138(Supplement 1):2930.

57. Agency EM. Committee for Orphan Medicinal Products (COMP). 2021.

58. News GEB. Sangamo, Sanofi Show Positive Early Data for SCD Gene-Edited Cell Therapy. 2021. Available at: https://www.genengnews.com/news/sangamo-sanofi-show-positive-early-data-for-scd-gene-edited-cell-therapy/.

59. Walters MC, Smith AR, Schiller GJ, et al. Updated Results of a Phase 1/2 Clinical Study of Zinc Finger Nuclease-Mediated Editing of BCL11A in Autologous Hematopoietic Stem Cells for Transfusion-Dependent Beta Thalassemia. Blood 2021;138(Supplement 1):3974.

60. Sangamo Therapeutics Reports Recent Business and Clinical Highlights and Third Quarter 2021 Financial Results [press release]. 2021.

61. Frangoul H, Altshuler D, Cappellini MD, et al. CRISPR-Cas9 Gene Editing for Sickle Cell Disease and beta-Thalassemia. N Engl J Med 2021;384(3):252–60.

62. Stephan Grupp NB, Charis Campbell, Clinton Carroll, et al, Haydar Frangoul. CTX001 for sickle cell disease: safety and efficacy results from the ongoing CLIMB SCD-121 study OF autologous CRISPR-CAS9-MODIFIED CD34+ hematopoietic stem and PROGENITOR cells. European Hematology Association; 2021.

63. Franco Locatelli SA-L, Yael Bobruff, Maria Domenica Cappellini, et al. CTX001 for transfusion-dependent β-thalassemia: safety and efficacy results from the ongoing CLIMB THAL-111 study OF autologous CRISPR-CAS9-MODIFIED CD34+ hematopoietic stem and PROGENITOR cells. European Hematology Association; 2021. p. EP733.

64. Leonard A, Sharma A, Uchida N, et al. Disease severity impacts plerixafor-mobilized stem cell collection in patients with sickle cell disease. Blood Adv 2021;5(9):2403–11.

65. Adler BK, Salzman DE, Carabasi MH, et al. Fatal sickle cell crisis after granulocyte colony-stimulating factor administration. Blood 2001;97(10):3313–4.

66. Fitzhugh CD, Hsieh MM, Bolan CD, et al. Granulocyte colony-stimulating factor (G-CSF) administration in individuals with sickle cell disease: time for a moratorium? Cytotherapy 2009;11(4):464–71.

67. Czechowicz A, Palchaudhuri R, Scheck A, et al. Selective hematopoietic stem cell ablation using CD117-antibody-drug-conjugates enables safe and effective transplantation with immunity preservation. Nat Commun 2019;10(1):617.

68. Chhabra A, Ring AM, Weiskopf K, et al. Hematopoietic stem cell transplantation in immunocompetent hosts without radiation or chemotherapy. Sci Transl Med 2016;8(351):351ra105.

69. Kwon H-S, Logan AC, Chhabra A, et al. Anti-human CD117 antibody-mediated bone marrow niche clearance in nonhuman primates and humanized NSG mice. Blood 2019;133(19):2104–8.

70. Tisdale JF, Donahue RE, Uchida N, et al. A Single Dose of CD117 Antibody Drug Conjugate Enables Autologous Gene-Modified Hematopoietic Stem Cell Transplant (Gene Therapy) in Nonhuman Primates. Blood 2019;134(Supplement_1):610.

71. Uchida N, Stasula U, Hinds M, et al. CD117 Antibody Drug Conjugate-Based Conditioning Allows for Efficient Engraftment of Gene-Modified CD34+ Cells in a Rhesus Gene Therapy Model. Blood 2021;138(Supplement 1):560.

72. Agarwal R, Weinberg KI, Kwon H-S, et al. First Report of Non-Genotoxic Conditioning with JSP191 (anti-CD117) and Hematopoietic Stem Cell Transplantation in a Newly Diagnosed Patient with Severe Combined Immune Deficiency. Blood 2020;136(Supplement 1):10.

73. Agarwal R, Dvorak CC, Kwon H-S, et al. Non-Genotoxic Anti-CD117 Antibody Conditioning Results in Successful Hematopoietic Stem Cell Engraftment in Patients with Severe Combined Immunodeficiency. Blood 2019;134(Supplement_1):800.

74. Fitzhugh CD, Cordes S, Taylor T, et al. At least 20% donor myeloid chimerism is necessary to reverse the sickle phenotype after allogeneic HSCT. Blood 2017; 130(17):1946–8.

75. Li C, Wang H, Georgakopoulou A, et al. In Vivo HSC Gene Therapy Using a Bimodular HDAd5/35++ Vector Cures Sickle Cell Disease in a Mouse Model. Mol Ther 2021;29(2):822–37.

76. Sangamo Announces Transition of SAR445136 Sickle Cell Disease Program From Sanofi to Sangamo [press release]. January 6, 2022 2022.

Hemophilia A/B

Stacy E. Croteau, MD, MMS

KEYWORDS

- Factor VIII • Factor IX • Gene therapy • AAV vector • Hemophilia

KEY POINTS

- A broad, safe range of easily measurable plasma factor protein levels correlating with bleeding phenotype make hemophilia an ideal target for gene therapy.
- Clinically meaningful, intermediate-term FVIII or FIX levels have been observed with several adeno-associated virus (AAV)-based platforms; however, the durability of transgene expression over subsequent years, particularly for FVIII activity, has been variable among programs.
- Hepatocyte cellular responses and immune system responses to AAV-mediated gene transfer require additional investigation to refine vector and transgene engineering.
- Despite generally mild infusion-related reactions in some individuals and asymptomatic ALT elevations, no significant short-term or long-term toxicities attributable to AAV-based gene transfer and no anti-FVIII or FIX antibodies have been observed.
- Next-generation hemophilia gene therapies, including cell-based and gene editing platforms, need to expand the eligible patient population and facilitate improved transgene expression as well as safe, durable FVIII or FIX activity levels.

INTRODUCTION

The landscape of treatments for hemophilia A (factor VIII, FVIII deficiency) and hemophilia B (factor IX, FIX deficiency) has expanded dramatically over the past decade.[1] FVIII and FIX clotting factor concentrates have been the standard of care first for bleed treatment and then bleed prevention (prophylaxis) since the earliest products were licensed in the latter part of the 20th century. As rare, X-linked bleeding disorders, severe FVIII or FIX deficiency affect predominantly men. Around 30,000 individuals are living with hemophilia in the US.[2] The correlation between plasma FVIII or FIX activity levels and bleed phenotype is strong.[3,4] Prophylactic infusion of factor concentrate for individuals with severe disease (<1% activity) or moderate disease (1-<5% activity with a severe bleeding phenotype) starting at an early age (<2–3 years old) is key to hemophilia disease management. The current goal of prophylaxis is to minimize bleeding by maintaining trough factor activity levels of at least 1% to 3%.[5] Access

Boston Children's Hospital, Boston Hemophilia Center, 300 Longwood Avenue, Boston, MA, USA
E-mail address: stacy.croteau@childrens.harvard.edu
Twitter: @croteaumd (S.E.C.)

Hematol Oncol Clin N Am 36 (2022) 797–812
https://doi.org/10.1016/j.hoc.2022.03.009
0889-8588/22/© 2022 Elsevier Inc. All rights reserved.

to and routine infusion of factor concentrate has made a significant impact on mortality, annualized bleed rates (ABRs), hospitalization rate, severity of hemarthropathy, and health-related quality of life (HR-QoL) in the high-resource countries whereby they are available.[3,6]

Innovation in factor concentrates has led from the use of plasma-derived concentrates to expanded design and manufacturing with recombinant clotting factor concentrates, most recently with factor concentrates bioengineered to improve pharmacokinetic characteristics, that is, extended half-life (EHL) products.[7] Despite the substantial advancements in clinical care and outcomes that factor concentrates have afforded individuals with access to these costly therapies,[8] noteworthy unmet medical needs exist and have prompted additional innovation in hemostatic therapeutics, in particular for bleed prevention.[1] Factor concentrates must be administered intravenously as frequently as daily and as infrequently as every 2 weeks depending on the particulars of the type of factor concentrate and the patient's clinical characteristics. This poses a significant administration burden. Patients and caregivers, even with self-infusion skills, often struggle with venous access, in some cases necessitating the placement of central venous catheters, as well as the time and space needed for regular infusions with competing demands of school, work, and life obligations.[9]

The ability to initiate prophylaxis early in life has significantly slowed hemophilic arthropathy both symptomatically and by abnormal MRI findings[3]; however, longitudinal joint health assessments suggest that even with best attempts at prophylaxis, using currently available factor concentrates, children and young adults are still acquiring evidence of abnormal joint findings by MRI by young adulthood.[10] Additionally, FVIII is an immunogenic molecule with about 30% of severe hemophilia A patients developing neutralizing allo-antibodies "inhibitors" to exogenous FVIII concentrates within the first 50 product exposure days necessitating an alternate approach to hemostasis using "bypassing agents" and immune tolerance induction (ITI) in an attempt to eliminate the inhibitors.[11] The incidence of inhibitor development is considerably less ($\sim$5%) among those with severe hemophilia B; however, the associated management challenges are even greater due to low success of ITI and development of FIX antibody-mediated allergic reactions and nephrotic syndrome.[12,13]

Nonfactor replacement therapies (NFTs) including substitution therapy such as emicizumab and rebalancing therapies including the inhibition of antithrombin production (fitusiran) and inhibition of tissue factor pathway inhibitor (TFPI) (concizumab, marstacimab) or activated protein C (serpinPC) provide alternate approaches to bleed prevention for hemophilia A or B (and potentially other coagulation factor deficiencies in the future), **Fig. 1.**[1] Emicizumab, a bispecific antibody mimicking the function of activated FVIII, has been approved for hemophilia A prophylaxis in children and adults by FDA, EMA, and many health authorities across the globe. Features including subcutaneous administration, injection frequency of weekly or less, and less fluctuation in plasma levels compared with factor concentrate, have led to a rapid uptake of emicizumab in clinical practice globally.[8] The rebalancing therapies, although all still investigational, also have the benefit of subcutaneous administration. While a marked improvement in terms of administration ease, the NFTs have drawbacks as well. For example, emicizumab does not normalize hemostasis and interacts with the current, widely available one-stage (PTT-based) clinical coagulation assays artificially normalizing assay results so that they do not accurately reflect *in vivo* hemostasis. There are no available, broadly accepted clinical assays for emicizumab serum levels or "FVIII equivalents." The rebalancing therapies also have the challenge of no clinical assay to quantify improvement in hemostasis and corresponding bleed risk. Most of the

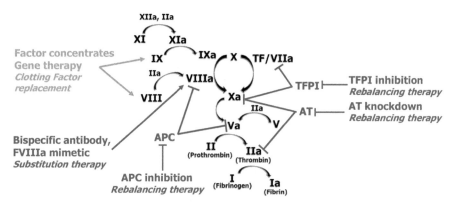

Fig. 1. Overview of clotting cascade (*black*) with anticoagulant proteins (*red*) and location of impact of hemophilia therapies including factor concentrates and FVIII or FIX gene therapy which replace the missing or reduced clotting factor (*green*), and nonfactor replacement therapies (*blue*) including substitution and rebalancing therapies. APC, activated protein C; AT, antithrombin; TFPI, tissue factor pathway inhibitor.

rebalancing therapy clinical trial programs have already encountered issues with thrombotic events requiring the implementation of risk mitigation strategies.[14]

HEMOPHILIA GENE THERAPY, THE EARLY YEARS

Throughout 1990s and 2000s, early attempts at gene transfer for *F8* or *F9* genes were tested including intraperitoneal implantation of dermal fibroblasts transfected with a plasmid containing *F8* sequence,[15] adeno-associated virus (AAV)-mediated gene transfer *F9* into skeletal muscle,[16] and intravenous retrovirus-mediated *F8* gene transfer. These studies demonstrated proof of concept with the detection of transient FVIII or FIX levels in plasma although no durable efficacy of circulating FVIII or FIX proteins in human participants.[17,18] The first liver-directed hemophilia gene transfer was attempted with an AAV2 *F9* construct infused via the hepatic artery.[18] Report of the first successful, sustained hemophilia gene therapy came in 2011.[19] Leveraging an AAV2/8 FIX vector construct, 6 participants received the product intravenously in a dose escalation, 2×10^{11}, 6×10^{11} and 2×10^{12} vg/kg. All had a response ranging from 2% to 11% of normal FIX activity levels. Longitudinally, enduring FIX activity without long-term toxicity, up to 8 years postinfusion, has been reported including 4 additional patients dosed in the highest dose cohort.[20,21] More than a dozen AAV-based hemophilia A or B gene therapy programs have continued to build on this early success.[1] Additionally, both *in vivo* and *ex vivo* platforms leveraging lentiviral (LV)-based gene therapy approaches as well as gene editing technology are also being explored in preclinical and early phase human clinical trials.

ADENO-ASSOCIATED VIRUS GENE TRANSFER

AAV-mediated gene transfer is the leading strategy for hemophilia gene therapy with multiple phase 1 to phase 3 clinical trial programs underway, **Table 1**. Several features make the AAV-based approach desirable for *F8* gene or *F9* gene transfer. AAV is nonpathogenic in humans, and it is administered as a one-time intravenous treatment. Various AAV serotypes have tropism for hepatocytes.[22] Hepatocytes are particularly well suited for protein production and secretion into the circulation where coagulation

Table 1
Current hemophilia A and B AAV gene therapy trials

Investigational Product (Sponsor)	Vector	Transgene	Manufacturing Platform	Dosing	Trial Identifier, Phase
Valoctocogene roxaparvovec (BioMarin)	AAV5	hF8co-SQ	Baculovirus/Sf9 insect cell	6×10^{13} vg/kg	NCT03370913, Phase 3
Giroctocogene fitelparvovec (Pfizer/Sangamo)	AAV2/6	BDD-F8co	Baculovirus/Sf9 insect cell	3×10^{13} vg/kg	NCT04370054, Phase 3
SPK-8011 (Spark Therapeutics)	AAV3-LK03	hF8co-SQ	Plasmid/HEK293 eukaryotic cell	5×10^{11} vg/kg 1×10^{12} vg/kg 2×10^{12} vg/kg	NCT03003533, Phase 1/2
BAY 2599023 (Bayer/Ultragenyx)	AAVhu37	BDD-F8co	Plasmid/HEK293 eukaryotic cell	0.5×10^{13} gc/kg 1×10^{13} gc/kg 2×10^{13} gc/kg 4×10^{13} gc/kg	NCT03588299, Phase 1/2
GO-8 (University College London)	AAV2/8	F8co-V3	Plasmid/HEK293 eukaryotic cell	6×10^{11} vg/kg 2×10^{12} vg/kg 6×10^{12} vg/kg	NCT03001830, Phase 1
TAK-754 (Takeda)	AAV8	BDD-F8	Plasmid/HEK293 eukaryotic cell	2.0×10^{12} cp/kg 6.0×10^{12} cp/kg 1.2×10^{13} cp/kg	NCT03370172, Phase 1
Etranacogene dezaparvovec (UniQure)	AAV5	hF9co-Padua	Baculovirus/Sf9 insect cell	2×10^{13} gc/kg	NCT03569891, Phase 3
Fidanacogene elaparvovec (Pfizer)	Mutant AAV8	hF9co-Padua	Plasmid/HEK293 eukaryotic cell	5×10^{11} vg/kg	NCT03861273, Phase 3
scAAV2/8-LP1-hFIXco (St. Jude Children's Research Hospital)	scAAV2/8	hF9co	Plasmid/HEK293 eukaryotic cell	2×10^{11} vg/kg 6×10^{11} vg/kg 2×10^{12} vg/kg	NCT00979238, Phase 1
Verbrinacogene setparvovec (Freeline Therapeutics)	AAV-S3	hF9co-Padua	proprietary manufacturing platform	7.7×10^{11} vg/kg	NCT05164471, Phase 1/2

proteins are optimally effective and easily measured by standardized coagulation assays. Hepatocytes serve as the normal site of FIX production, while FVIII is synthesized in endothelial cells, predominantly liver sinusoidal endothelial cells. There is a broad normal range, 50% to 150%, of normal FVIII and FIX activity levels and individuals with mild deficiency levels particularly greater than 15% manifest a generally minimal bleeding phenotype in the absence of major injury or surgery.[4] Individuals with moderate and severe disease experience clinically significant reduction in bleeding symptoms even with modest improvement in baseline factor activity levels.

Adeno-Associated Virus Vector Design for Hemophilia

AAV 2/8 and AAV5 are the most common serotypes used for hemophilia gene therapy given their tropism for hepatocytes. Modifications of these and other AAV serotypes have been incorporated across platforms to refine vector design further improving tropism for the human hepatocytes as well as to reduce interaction with preexisting AAV antibodies. AAV neutralizing antibodies (NAbs) are prevalent in the general population due to the frequency of the numerous AAV serotypes in the environment. Several manufacturers have undertaken prevalence studies to better quantify the prevalence of NAbs and their cross-reactivity across various serotypes as well as geographic region.[23,24] AAV2 is reported to have a high NAb rate, 40% to 70% in some populations, whereas NAbs for AAV5 and AAV8 are lower, estimated at 20% to 40%.[25] Early work in the AAV2 trials identified that presence of detectable NAbs interfered with hepatocyte transfection prompting subsequent exclusion of individuals with positive NAb titers to the investigational capsid from the most clinical trials, **Tables 2** and **3**.[26] Interestingly, one of the AAV5-based clinical trial programs [etranacogene dezaparvovec (AMT061)] did not exclude individuals based on this parameter and have not observed a correlation between the presence of NAbs and transgene expression.[27] Assays to detect and quantify NAbs have not been standardized and cannot be compared across clinic trial programs.

Transgene Considerations

The capacity of AAV vector capsids is modest, just 4.7 kb. This is ideal for the incorporation of the $F9$ gene, which is only about 1.5kb; however, poses a challenge for the much larger ($\sim$7 kb) full-length $F8$ gene.[22,28] Although wild-type AAV (wtAAV) variably, but specifically integrates into the AAVS1 site of chromosome 19, removal of the rep gene in the recombinant AAV (rAAV) vectors to make room for the transgene of interest interferes with this integration pattern. Low frequency, random site integration does occur with rAAV; however, the transgene predominately remains episomal reducing the risk of insertional mutagenesis.[29] Specific modifications for the $F8$ transgene include the deletion of the B-domain (BDD), which decreases the $F8$ gene to about 4.4 kb permitting packaging within the small capacity of AAV capsid. The B-domain is cleaved at FVIII activation and does not play a role in coagulation function, though it may have a role in efficient intracellular trafficking. FVIII-BDD has been used in the manufacture of FVIII concentrates to improve production efficiency.[30] Inclusion of a short 14 amino acid linker sequence (rFVIII-SQ) in place of the B-domain provides multiple potential glycosylation sites to improve expression and circulating FVIII levels compared with complete the elimination of the B-domain.[31] A chimeric human/porcine BDD-FVIII (ASC618) is also early in investigation. It is hypothesized that this novel construct may improve protein folding thereby reducing the potential for endoplasmic reticulum (ER) stress response and perhaps overall more reliable and durable transgene expression.[32]

Table 2
Patient population in current hemophilia A AAV gene therapy trials

Investigational Product	Sponsor	Disease Requirement	Sex at Birth	Age	Select Comorbidity Restrictions	Neutralizing AAV-Antibody (NAb) Restrictions
Valoctocogene roxaparvovec (BMN270)	BioMarin	FVIII <1% ≥150 ED	Male	≥18 y	Excluded: HIV, significant liver fibrosis or cirrhosis, chronic or active hepatitis B, active hepatitis C, current/prior FVIII inhibitors	Excluded: detectable antibodies to the AAV5 capsid
Giroctocogene fitelparvovec (SB-525)	Pfizer/Sangamo	FVIII ≤1% ≥150 ED	Male	≥18–64 y	Excluded: significant liver fibrosis or cirrhosis, active hepatitis B or C current/prior FVIII inhibitors; Permitted: HIV CD4+ cell count >200/mm3 and viral load <20 copies/mL	Excluded: AAV6 NAb
SPK-8011	Spark Therapeutics	FVIII ≤2% ≥150 ED	Male	≥18 y	Excluded: significant liver disease, active or on antiviral therapy for hepatitis B or C, current/prior FVIII inhibitors; Permitted: HIV CD4+ cell count >200/mm3 and viral load undetectable	Excluded: AAV-Spark 200 NAb titer ≥1:1
BAY 2599023 (DTX201)	Bayer/Ultragenyx	FVIII <1% ≥150 ED	Male	≥18 y	Excluded: significant liver disease, active or on antiviral therapy for hepatitis B or C, current/prior FVIII inhibitors, BMI > 35 kg/m2; Permitted: HIV CD4+ cell count >200/mm3 and viral load undetectable	Excluded: detectable antibodies reactive with AAVhu37capsid
GO-8	University College, London	FVIII <1% ≥50 ED	Male	≥18 y	Excluded: HIV, significant liver fibrosis or cirrhosis, chronic or active hepatitis B, active hepatitis C, current/prior FVIII inhibitors	Excluded: Detectable AAV8 NAb
TAK-754	Takeda	FVIII <1% >150 ED	Male	≥18–75 y	Excluded: HIV, active hepatitis, chronic hepatitis C, current/prior FVIII inhibitors	Excluded: AAV8 NAb titer ≥1:5

Table 3
Patient population in current hemophilia B AAV gene therapy trials

Investigational Product	Sponsor	Disease Requirement	Sex at Birth	Age	Select Co-morbidity Restrictions	Neutralizing AAV-Antibody (NAb) Restrictions
scAAV2/8-LP1-hFIXco	St. Jude Children's Research Hospital	FIX <1% ≥50 ED	Male	≥18 y	Excluded: significant liver disease, active or on antiviral therapy for hepatitis B or C, current/prior FIX inhibitors Permitted: HIV CD4+ cell count >350 mm3 and viral load <400 copies/mL	Excluded: Detectable antibodies reactive with AAV8
Etranacogene dezaparvovec (AMT061)	UniQure	FIX ≤2%, >150 ED	Male	≥18 y	Excluded: significant liver disease, history of hepatitis B or C exposure, current/prior FIX inhibitors Permitted: HIV controlled on antiviral therapy	none
Fidanacogene elaparvovec (PF-06838435)	Pfizer	FIX ≤2%, ≥50 ED	Male	≥18–65 y	Excluded: significant liver disease, active or on antiviral therapy for hepatitis B or C, current/prior FIX inhibitors Permitted: HIV CD4+ cell count >200/mm3 and viral load undetectable	Excluded: Anti-AAV Spark100 NAb titer ≥ 1:1
Verbrinacogene setparvovec (FLT180a)	Freeline Therapeutics	FIX ≤2%, ≥150 ED	Male	≥18–65 y	Excluded: significant liver disease, active or on antiviral therapy for hepatitis B or C, CMV PCR +, current/prior FIX inhibitors Permitted: controlled HIV with CD4+ cell count >200/mm3	Excluded: Anti-AAV-S3 antibodies > limit of the preestablished clinical cutoff

Although the *F9* gene fits easily within the AAV capsid without significant modification, a naturally occurring *F9* sequence variant FIX-Padua associated with an 8-fold increase in catalytic activity has become the preferred *F9* construct in hemophilia B gene therapy platforms as the circulating functional activity is proportionally higher for a given amount of FIX protein produced and secreted.[33,34] Other emerging *F9* gene variants such as DalcA have been proposed as well.[35] Codon optimization (co) of the selected *F8* or *F9* gene sequence has further enhanced transgene expression several fold.[36] During clinical development, the importance of limiting the number of unmethylated cytosine–guanine dinucleotides (CpGs) motifs was recognized.[37] CpG motifs can be inadvertently introduced during co and enhance a stimulatory CD8[+] T-cell immune response leading to hepatocyte apoptosis.[38]

Administration of Adeno-Associated Virus Gene Transfer for Hemophilia

AAV-based gene therapy has been administered as a single outpatient infusion. Trial participants have generally tolerated infusion of gene therapy products well, although some programs have reported infusion reactions in some individuals including pyrexia, emesis, myalgia within the first 24 hours postinfusion and resolving within a few days.[39–41] Hepatic transfection and transgene expression following gene therapy infusion is relatively swift with the initial rise in FVIII or FIX levels observed as soon as 1 to 2 weeks postinfusion.[19,42–44]

Postinfusion Hepatocyte and Immune System Responses

Although not observed in preclinical mouse or canine studies, early in-human AAV hemophilia studies noted an asymptomatic rise in ALT with a concomitant decline in factor activity seemingly secondary to a cytotoxic T-cell response to vector capsid.[18,19] Participants responded favorably to the initiation of oral corticosteroids with the resolution of the transaminitis and preservation of the transgene expression. ALT rise seemed to be vector dose-responsive and occur about 4 to 12 weeks postinfusion.[45] Subsequent trials observed a similar finding, particularly in the higher dose cohorts prompting some programs to adopt prophylactic initiation of corticosteroids within a few weeks of gene transfer product infusion.[39,40]

The underlying etiology of ALT rise and transgene expression loss/decline in clinical trial participants remains controversial. Inconsistent evidence of a cytotoxic T-cell response with positive interferon-γ enzyme-linked immunospot (ELISPOT) and lack of corticosteroid efficacy in rescuing transgene expression in some participants, led to recognition that the rise in ALT may be attributable to different etiologies among participants and the principal etiology may differ between FVIII and FIX gene therapy platforms.[46] Early innate immune responses that incite transaminitis, cytotoxic T-cell-mediated response against viral capsid peptides, evidence of hepatocyte ER stress due to protein overproduction are among the potential causes.[47] Improved understanding of the complex AAV–host hepatocyte interaction will facilitate improved vector engineering, transgene modifications, and targeted use of immunomodulatory agents (when needed) thus promoting acute and longer term transgene expression. To this end, interest in obtaining strategic liver biopsies, in at least a subset of hemophilia gene therapy clinical trial participants, is growing.[48]

The adverse events reported across gene therapy programs attributable to the use of corticosteroids over several weeks are not inconsequential. Some programs have begun to explore steroid-sparing agents.[40,49] The close laboratory monitoring, twice or thrice weekly, in the early weeks post gene therapy infusion and the potential need for the initiation of corticosteroids or other immunomodulatory agents pose a barrier to successful commercialization. Ensuring consistent and timely patient adherence to laboratory appointments and immunosuppressant therapy when needed over the course of weeks, institutional barriers to rapid, consistent turnaround of clinical laboratories including factor activity levels, and provider expertise to recognize potentially subtle laboratory trends that necessitate the quick implementation of an immunosuppressive agent are important challenges to consider.

Efficacy and Safety Monitoring

Hemophilia population outcome assessments have included laboratory parameters (FVIII or FIX activity by one-stage and chromogenic assays), clinical parameters (ABR and factor concentrate utilization), and patient-reported outcomes. Both FVIII and FIX expression have significant interindividual variability within and among gene therapy programs. The University College London hemophilia B program has the most mature data, with at least 6.7 years of median follow-up reported across all 3 dose cohorts. Mean FIX level in the highest dose cohort [2×10^{12}vg/kg] was 5.1%. There was a 66% decrease in FIX concentrate use and 82% reduction in ABR among all 10 participants. No late toxicities or FIX inhibitors have been reported.[21] The 5 participants in the highest dose cohort [2×10^{13}vg/kg] of the phase 1/2 dose-escalation study (AMT060) achieved a mean FIX activity of 7.1% in the first year which remained stable at 7.4% 4 years postinfusion.[50] The 3 participants that enrolled in the AMT061 phase 2b study which changed to the FIX-Padua variant achieved a mean FIX activity of 44.2% by 2 years postinfusion.[51] The phase 3 etranacogene dezaparvovec (AMT061) trial is ongoing with a mean FIX activity of 36.0% for the 54 participants at least 26 weeks postinfusion.[52] The 15 participants in the fidanacogene elaparvovec phase 1/2a trial have a mean FIX activity of 22.9% at 1 year postinfusion; 12 of 15 experienced zero bleed events.[53]

With regard to FVIII trials, valoctocogene roxaparvovec has completed the enrollment of the phase 3 study with mean FVIII activity 1 year postinfusion of 42.9%. The 7 participants in the highest dose cohort [6×10^{13}vg/kg] of the phase 1/2 trial demonstrated a declining mean chromogenic FVIII activity over the first 3 years of 59%, 36.3%, and 31.3%, respectively. Giroctocogene fitelparvovec reported peak mean chromogenic FVIII activity of 71.7% at week 12 weeks postinfusion among the 5 participants in their highest dose cohort [3×10^{13} vg/kg] with a mean FVIII level of 63.5% at 40 weeks postinfusion. The phase 3 study (NCT04370054) was placed on clinical hold pending review of a proposed protocol amendment in the setting of some participants achieving FVIII levels greater than 150%. The phase 1/2 trial program for SPK-8011 reported an overall mean one-stage FVIII activity of 12.9% over the first 52 weeks and 12% after 52 weeks collectively for the 12 participants who maintained FVIII expression for more than 52 weeks. For the 9 participants in the highest dose cohort [2×10^{12} vg/kg] mean peak chromogenic FVIII activity during the first-year postinfusion was 43.5%. The mean FVIII activity after 52 weeks was 8.14%, for the 7 patients who maintained expression in this subgroup.[40] The phase 1/2 dose-finding study for AAVhu37FVIII (NCT03588299) is ongoing. Of the 6 patients reported so far, 5 have achieved sustained FVIII levels $\geq$5% up to 16 months postinfusion.[54]

Fortunately, no significant long-term safety outcomes attributable to hemophilia gene therapy have been reported for participants to date; however, there are several potential toxicities that continue to require longitudinal assessment. Liver health, particularly given the high prevalence of past HCV and treated HIV infection in this population, mostly attributable to the contaminated blood products in the late 1970s and 1980s, remains an important consideration in individuals with hemophilia. Additionally, concerns for insertional oncogenesis loom although overall integration events are low.[55] One trial participant who received AMT061 was identified to have hepatocellular carcinoma (HCC) just 1 year postgene therapy infusion. This was in the background of both prior HCV and HBV as well as nonalcoholic fatty liver disease. After a detailed investigation, it was determined that this HCC was unlikely related to the gene therapy product.[56]

LENTIVIRAL GENE DELIVERY

Lentiviral (LV) vectors have the capacity to support a larger transgene compared with AAV vectors and also to integrate the transgene into a targeted locus in the host genome potentially supporting more durable expression. This alternate approach for hemophilia gene therapy may broaden the eligible population of hemophilia patients to include individuals with prohibitive AAV NAbs, those with active or prior FVIII or FIX inhibitors, and potentially pediatric patients. Preclinical LV vector approaches in hemophilia are being undertaken both *ex vivo* (transduced autologous hematopoietic stem cells) as well as *in vivo* (hepatocyte-directed).[57–59] In contrast to the *in vivo* approach, *ex vivo* LV gene therapy requires pretreatment with a conditioning regimen (typically alkylating agents with or without additional lymphotoxic medications) to create a niche for hematopoietic stem cells when they are reintroduced following transduction with the either the *F8* or *F9* gene. An actively recruiting phase 1 trial (NCT03818763) is investigating the use of autologous CD34+PBSCs, transduced with an LV vector encoding a BDD-*F8* in adult participants with active FVIII inhibitors following a reduced-intensity conditioning regimen with melphalan and fludarabine.[60] Another LV construct, CD68-ET3-LV, is just entering its first phase 1 trial (NCT04418414) for adult males with severe hemophilia A without inhibitors and will use busulfan and antithymocyte globulin as a conditioning regimen. While *in vivo*, hepatocyte and endothelial cell directed LV vectors have demonstrated promise for both FVIII and FIX constructs in murine and canine models, in-human trials have yet to be announced.[61]

GENE EDITING FOR HEMOPHILIA

Several approaches for gene editing in hemophilia are being explored including the use of zinc finger nucleases (ZFN) and CRISPR-Cas9. Sangamo BioSciences initiated a phase 1 dose-escalation study (NCT02695160) investigating a ZFN-mediated genome editing platform to integrate an *F9* gene construct into the albumin locus of hepatocytes introduced by AAV2/6-derived vectors.[62] Recruitment was difficult and the program was terminated.[63] A similar approach, but leveraging CRISPR-Cas9 to introduce an *F8* or *F9* gene into the hepatocyte albumin locus, is being pursued in hemophilia A and has demonstrated success in murine models for hemophilia B.[32,64]

DISCUSSION

Therapeutic success for hemophilia gene therapy is a moving target. At a time when the goal for the standard of care prophylaxis was to keep factor levels above the severe hemophilia range (trough levels >1%), early gene therapy outcomes achieving factor activity levels sustained in the moderate or low mild hemophilia range were appropriately touted as a major success. For many individuals, consistent factor levels of even a few percent can dramatically improve the bleeding phenotype and reduce the need for factor concentrate infusions. It has been increasingly recognized that the preservation of joint health necessitates factor levels well above 1%. Currently available factor concentrates, particularly for FVIII replacement, make the achievement of trough factor activity of 10% to 15% unrealistic due to the infusion frequency needed and the prohibitive cost. NFTs with alternative mechanisms of action, less frequent and subcutaneous administration, provide an opportunity for less burdensome prophylaxis and potentially improved clinical outcomes. These novel therapies require further investigation of the risk-to-benefit ratio and may be best deployed in specific hemophilia subgroups. Despite the ongoing licensure of multiple new factor concentrates in recent years and the start of approvals for NFTs, the cost of hemophilia therapy continues to rise even for long-established products.

The ultimate goal for gene therapy in hemophilia is to provide a safe, one-time therapy that replaces or corrects the defective *F8* or *F9* gene and renders patients free of their hemophilia. Depending on the age of the individual receiving the gene therapy, hemophilia-related comorbidities, such as hemarthropathy, chronic pain, and for the oldest generations HIV treatment and HCV management and sequelae, may still require long-term monitoring and management. Additionally, if sustained, normal factor levels are not achieved, ongoing hemostasis management in the setting of injury or perioperatively will be needed. Even without the normalization of FVIII or FIX levels, there is significant, clinically meaningful benefit in achieving and sustaining factor levels greater than ~15% of normal. Levels above this threshold, particularly for those without multiple prior hemarthrosis or evidence of joint disease will enable the vast majority of individuals to participate in usual day activities unencumbered by the need for routine intravenous infusions or subcutaneous injections. It is clear that the earlier in life that FVIII or FIX levels are consistently maintained above the severe or moderate hemophilia range, the greater the benefit on joint health and the QoL of both the child and parent. Protection of the more vascular, growing joints of young children is critical for functional preservation into adulthood.

In the US and throughout the globe, networks of hemophilia treatment centers (HTCs), consisting of specialized multi-disciplinary teams, have the expertise to manage mild to complex hemophilia patients, as well as those with other bleeding disorders.[65] HTC teams provide clinical care and education to patients encompassing the breadth of current therapeutic options for bleed treatment and prevention and collaborate with multiple bleeding disorder community groups including strong connections with local, national, and global hemophilia/bleeding disorder patient advocacy, education, and health surveillance groups. The HTCs are optimally poised to help identify individuals well suited to gene therapy as a treatment option and facilitate the informed, joint decision-making process. The HTC team is also well-suited to provide expert safety and efficacy follow-up care for hemophilia gene therapy as well as for the age-related comorbidities associated with hemophilia.

Longitudinal assessment of clinically relevant measures of success is particularly important for hemophilia gene therapy, whereby alternative treatment options exist including factor concentrates and NFTs. While the currently available therapies are associated with low ABRs, at least in clinical trial settings, the additional potential benefits of gene therapy with higher, consistent, and measurable factor levels, the absence of need for routine medication administration, and the impact of these on QoL both in terms of physical function as well as psychological stressors are important to consider.[66]

Vigilance to detect both short-term and longer term safety signals after hemophilia gene therapy remains important. Practitioners should continue to have transparent conversations with patients interested in pursuing gene therapy as a treatment option, about the known challenges as well as the unknown possible side effects inherent in a novel therapeutic modality. The current hemophilia AAV-gene transfer platforms continue to demonstrate at least intermediate-term safety with as yet no specific signals of long-term toxicity. Among and even within gene therapy programs there continues to be substantial variability in initial efficacy and durability and presently redosing is not possible. Increased understanding of capsid architecture, transgene development, and understanding impacts on both the innate and adaptive immune systems is critical. Such understanding will inform needed engineering refinements to the gene therapy products to further improve reliability and predictability of response, and potentially eliminate or at least enable targeted immunosuppressive agents when needed to maximize and sustain transgene expression. Improvements to the current AAV-gene transfer approaches as well as further exploration of LV vectors and gene editing constructs will be needed to safely expand the eligible population with the consideration of important subgroups including female participants with severe disease, pediatric patients, and individuals with FVIII or FIX inhibitors.

DISCLOSURE

S.E. Croteau has served as a consultant for Bayer, BioMarin, CSL-Behring, HEMA Biologics, Pfizer, Sanofi and received institutional research support from Spark Therapeutics.

REFERENCES

1. Croteau SE, Wang M, Wheeler AP. 2021 clinical trials update: Innovations in hemophilia therapy. Am J Hematol 2021;96(1):128–44.
2. Soucie JM, Miller CH, Dupervil B, et al. Occurrence rates of haemophilia among males in the United States based on surveillance conducted in specialized haemophilia treatment centres. Haemophilia 2020;26(3):487–93.
3. Manco-Johnson MJ, Abshire TC, Shapiro AD, et al. Prophylaxis versus episodic treatment to prevent joint disease in boys with severe hemophilia. N Engl J Med 2007;357(6):535–44.
4. Den Uijl IE, Mauser Bunschoten EP, Roosendaal G, et al. Clinical severity of haemophilia A: does the classification of the 1950s still stand? Haemophilia 2011; 17(6):849–53.
5. Srivastava A, Santagostino E, Dougall A, et al. WFH Guidelines for the Management of Hemophilia, 3rd edition. Haemophilia 2020;26(Suppl 6):1–158.
6. Mazepa MA, Monahan PE, Baker JR, et al, Network USHTC. Men with severe hemophilia in the United States: birth cohort analysis of a large national database. Blood 2016;127(24):3073–81.
7. Mannucci PM. Hemophilia therapy: the future has begun. Haematologica 2020; 105(3):545–53.
8. Annual global survey 2020. 2021. Available at: https://www1.wfh.org/publications/files/pdf-2045.pdf. Accessed September 1, 2021.
9. Sun HL, Yang M, Poon MC, et al. The impact of extended half-life factor concentrates on patient reported health outcome measures in persons with hemophilia A and hemophilia B. Res Pract Thromb Haemost 2021;5(7):e12601.
10. Warren BB, Thornhill D, Stein J, et al. Young adult outcomes of childhood prophylaxis for severe hemophilia A: results of the Joint Outcome Continuation Study. Blood Adv 2020;4(11):2451–9.
11. Astermark J. FVIII inhibitors: pathogenesis and avoidance. Blood 2015;125(13): 2045–51.
12. Collins PW, Chalmers E, Hart DP, et al. Diagnosis and treatment of factor VIII and IX inhibitors in congenital haemophilia: (4th edition). UK Haemophilia Centre Doctors Organization. Br J Haematol 2013;160(2):153–70.

13. Astermark J, Holstein K, Abajas YL, et al. The B-Natural study-The outcome of immune tolerance induction therapy in patients with severe haemophilia B. Haemophilia 2021;27(5):802–13.

14. Mahlangu JN. Progress in the development of anti-tissue factor pathway inhibitors for haemophilia management. Front Med (Lausanne) 2021;8:670526.

15. Roth DA, Tawa NE Jr, O'Brien JM, et al. Nonviral transfer of the gene encoding coagulation factor VIII in patients with severe hemophilia A. N Engl J Med 2001;344(23):1735–42.

16. Buchlis G, Podsakoff GM, Radu A, et al. Factor IX expression in skeletal muscle of a severe hemophilia B patient 10 years after AAV-mediated gene transfer. Blood 2012;119(13):3038–41.

17. Powell JS, Ragni MV, White GC 2nd, et al. Phase 1 trial of FVIII gene transfer for severe hemophilia A using a retroviral construct administered by peripheral intravenous infusion. Blood 2003;102(6):2038–45.

18. Manno CS, Pierce GF, Arruda VR, et al. Successful transduction of liver in hemophilia by AAV-Factor IX and limitations imposed by the host immune response. Nat Med 2006;12(3):342–7.

19. Nathwani AC, Tuddenham EG, Rangarajan S, et al. Adenovirus-associated virus vector-mediated gene transfer in hemophilia B. N Engl J Med 2011;365(25): 2357–65.

20. Nathwani AC, Reiss UM, Tuddenham EG, et al. Long-term safety and efficacy of factor IX gene therapy in hemophilia B. N Engl J Med 2014;371(21):1994–2004.

21. Nathwani AC, Reiss U, Tuddenham E, et al. Adeno-associated mediated gene transfer for hemophilia b:8 year follow up and impact of removing "empty viral particles" on safety and efficacy of gene transfer. Blood 2018;132(Supplement 1):491.

22. Wu Z, Asokan A, Samulski RJ. Adeno-associated virus serotypes: vector toolkit for human gene therapy. Mol Ther 2006;14(3):316–27.

23. Kruzik A, Fetahagic D, Hartlieb B, et al. Prevalence of anti-adeno-associated virus immune responses in international cohorts of healthy donors. Mol Ther Methods Clin Dev 2019;14:126–33.

24. Li H, Malani N, Hamilton SR, et al. Assessing the potential for AAV vector genotoxicity in a murine model. Blood 2011;117(12):3311–9.

25. Mingozzi F, High KA. Immune responses to AAV vectors: overcoming barriers to successful gene therapy. Blood 2013;122(1):23–36.

26. High KA. The gene therapy journey for hemophilia: are we there yet? Hematol Am Soc Hematol Educ Program 2012;2012:375–81.

27. Majowicz A, Nijmeijer B, Lampen MH, et al. Therapeutic hFIX Activity Achieved after Single AAV5-hFIX Treatment in Hemophilia B Patients and NHPs with Pre-existing Anti-AAV5 NABs. Mol Ther Methods Clin Dev 2019;14:27–36.

28. Sidonio RF Jr, Pipe SW, Callaghan MU, et al. Discussing investigational AAV gene therapy with hemophilia patients: A guide. Blood Rev 2021;47:100759.

29. Flotte TR, Carter BJ. Adeno-associated virus vectors for gene therapy. Gene Ther 1995;2(6):357–62.

30. Sandberg H, Almstedt A, Brandt J, et al. Structural and functional characterization of B-domain deleted recombinant factor VIII. Semin Hematol 2001;38(2 Suppl 4):4–12.

31. McIntosh J, Lenting PJ, Rosales C, et al. Therapeutic levels of FVIII following a single peripheral vein administration of rAAV vector encoding a novel human factor VIII variant. Blood 2013;121(17):3335–44.

32. Pipe SW, Gonen-Yaacovi G, Segurado OG. Hemophilia A gene therapy: current and next-generation approaches. Expert Opin Biol Ther 2022 Jan;6:1–17. https://doi.org/10.1080/14712598.2022.2002842.

33. Monahan PE, Sun J, Gui T, et al. Employing a gain-of-function factor IX variant R338L to advance the efficacy and safety of hemophilia B human gene therapy: preclinical evaluation supporting an ongoing adeno-associated virus clinical trial. Hum Gene Ther 2015;26(2):69–81.

34. Simioni P, Tormene D, Tognin G, et al. X-linked thrombophilia with a mutant factor IX (factor IX Padua). N Engl J Med 2009;361(17):1671–5.

35. Nair N, De Wolf D, Nguyen PA, et al. Gene therapy for hemophilia B using CB 2679d-GT: a novel factor IX variant with higher potency than factor IX Padua. Blood 2021;137(21):2902–6.

36. Ward NJ, Buckley SM, Waddington SN, et al. Codon optimization of human factor VIII cDNAs leads to high-level expression. Blood 2011;117(3):798–807.

37. Faust SM, Bell P, Cutler BJ, et al. CpG-depleted adeno-associated virus vectors evade immune detection. J Clin Invest 2013;123(7):2994–3001.

38. Konkle BA, Walsh CE, Escobar MA, et al. BAX 335 hemophilia B gene therapy clinical trial results: potential impact of CpG sequences on gene expression. Blood 2021;137(6):763–74.

39. Pasi KJ, Rangarajan S, Mitchell N, et al. Multiyear Follow-up of AAV5-hFVIII-SQ Gene Therapy for Hemophilia A. N Engl J Med 2020;382(1):29–40.

40. George LA, Monahan PE, Eyster ME, et al. Multiyear Factor VIII Expression after AAV Gene Transfer for Hemophilia A. N Engl J Med 2021;385(21):1961–73.

41. Miesbach W, Meijer K, Coppens M, et al. Gene therapy with adeno-associated virus vector 5-human factor IX in adults with hemophilia B. Blood 2018;131(9):1022–31.

42. George LA, Sullivan SK, Giermasz A, et al. Hemophilia B gene therapy with a high-specific-activity factor IX variant. N Engl J Med 2017;377(23):2215–27.

43. Rangarajan S, Walsh L, Lester W, et al. AAV5-Factor VIII Gene Transfer in Severe Hemophilia A. N Engl J Med 2017;377(26):2519–30.

44. Von Drygalski A, Giermasz A, Castaman G, et al. Etranacogene dezaparvovec (AMT-061 phase 2b): normal/near normal FIX activity and bleed cessation in hemophilia B. Blood Adv 2019;3(21):3241–7.

45. Kumar SRP, Hoffman BE, Terhorst C, et al. The Balance between CD8(+) T Cell-Mediated Clearance of AAV-Encoded Antigen in the Liver and Tolerance Is Dependent on the Vector Dose. Mol Ther 2017;25(4):880–91.

46. Zolotukhin I, Markusic DM, Palaschak B, et al. Potential for cellular stress response to hepatic factor VIII expression from AAV vector. Mol Ther Methods Clin Dev 2016;3:16063.

47. Pierce GF, Iorio A. Past, present and future of haemophilia gene therapy: From vectors and transgenes to known and unknown outcomes. Haemophilia 2018;24(Suppl 6):60–7.

48. MASAC Recommendation for Liver Biopsies in Gene Therapy Trials for Hemophilia [press release]. 2019. Available at: https://www.hemophilia.org/healthcare-professionals/guidelines-on-care/masac-documents/masac-document-256-recommendation-for-liver-biopsies-in-gene-therapy-trials-for-hemophilia#:~:text=Takeda%20Shoes-,MASAC%20Document%20256%20%2D%20Recommendation%20for%20Liver%20Biopsies,Gene%20Therapy%20Trials%20for%20Hemophilia&text=Currently%2C%20adeno%2Dassociated%20virus%20(,a%20variety%20of%20monogenic%20diseases.

49. Arruda VR, Favaro P, Finn JD. Strategies to modulate immune responses: a new frontier for gene therapy. Mol Ther 2009;17(9):1492–503.
50. Leebeek FWG, Meijer K, Coppens M, et al. AMT-060 Gene Therapy in Adults with Severe or Moderate-Severe Hemophilia B Confirm Stable FIX Expression and Durable Reductions in Bleeding and Factor IX Consumption for up to 5 Years. Blood 2020;136(Supplement 1):26.
51. Gomez E, Giermasz A, Castaman G, et al. Etranacogene Dezaparvovec (AAV5-Padua hFIX Variant, AMT-061), an Enhanced Vector for Gene Transfer in Adults with Severe or Moderate-severe Hemophilia B: 2.5 Year Data from a Phase 2b Trial [abstract]. Res Pract Thromb Haemost 2021;5(Suppl 2):e12589 p.487. Available at: https://abstracts.isth.org/abstract/etranacogene-dezaparvovec-aav5-padua-hfix-variant-amt-061-an-enhanced-vector-for-gene-transfer-in-adults-with-severe-or-moderate-severe-hemophilia-b-2-5-year-data-from-a-phase-2b-trial/. Accessed September 1, 2021.
52. Pipe SW, Leebeek FW, Recht M, et al. 52 Week Efficacy and Safety of Etranacogene Dezaparvovec in Adults with Severe or Moderate-severe Hemophilia B: Data from the Phase 3 HOPE-B Gene Therapy Trial [abstract]. Res Pract Thromb Haemost 2021;5(Suppl 2):e12591 p.92. Available at: https://abstracts.isth.org/abstract/52-week-efficacy-and-safety-of-etranacogene-dezaparvovec-in-adults-with-severe-or-moderate-severe-hemophilia-b-data-from-the-phase-3-hope-b-gene-therapy-trial/. Accessed September 1, 2021.
53. George LA, Sullivan SK, Rasko JEJ, et al. Efficacy and Safety in 15 Hemophilia B Patients Treated with the AAV Gene Therapy Vector Fidanacogene Elaparvovec and Followed for at Least 1 Year. Blood 2019;134(Supplement_1):3347.
54. Pipe SW, Ferrante F, Reis M, et al. First-in-human gene therapy study of AAVhu37 capsid vector technology in severe hemophilia A - BAY 2599023 has broad patient eligibility and stable and sustained long-term expression of FVIII. Blood 2020;136(Supplement 1):44–5.
55. Colella P, Ronzitti G, Mingozzi F. Emerging issues in AAV-mediated in vivo gene therapy. Mol Ther Methods Clin Dev 2018;8:87–104.
56. Investigation finds hemophilia gene therapy likely did not cause hepatocellular carcinoma. 2021. Available at: https://www.ashclinicalnews.org/online-exclusives/investigation-finds-hemophilia-gene-therapy-likely-not-cause-hepatocellular-carcinoma/.
57. Lytle AM, Brown HC, Paik NY, et al. Effects of FVIII immunity on hepatocyte and hematopoietic stem cell-directed gene therapy of murine hemophilia A. Mol Ther Methods Clin Dev 2016;3:15056.
58. Shi Q. Platelet-targeted gene therapy for hemophilia. Mol Ther Methods Clin Dev 2018;9:100–8.
59. Gong J, Chung TH, Zheng J, et al. Transduction of modified Factor VIII gene improves lentiviral gene therapy efficacy for hemophilia A. J Biol Chem 2021;297(6):101397.
60. Doering CB, Denning G, Shields JE, et al. Preclinical development of a hematopoietic stem and progenitor cell bioengineered factor VIII lentiviral Vector gene therapy for hemophilia A. Hum Gene Ther 2018;29(10):1183–201.
61. Cantore A, Naldini L. WFH State-of-the-art paper 2020: In vivo lentiviral vector gene therapy for haemophilia. Haemophilia 2021;27(S3):122–5.
62. Davidoff AM, Nathwani AC. Genetic targeting of the albumin locus to treat hemophilia. N Engl J Med 2016;374(13):1288–90.
63. Park CY, Lee DR, Sung JJ, et al. Genome-editing technologies for gene correction of hemophilia. Hum Genet 2016;135(9):977–81.

64. Wang Q, Zhong X, Li Q, et al. CRISPR-Cas9-mediated in vivo gene integration at the albumin locus recovers hemostasis in neonatal and adult hemophilia B mice. Mol Ther Methods Clin Dev 2020;18:520–31.
65. Valentino LA, Baker JR, Butler R, et al. Integrated hemophilia patient care via a national network of care centers in the United States: a model for rare coagulation disorders. J Blood Med 2021;12:897–911.
66. Iorio A, Skinner MW, Clearfield E, et al. Core outcome set for gene therapy in haemophilia: Results of the coreHEM multistakeholder project. Haemophilia 2018; 24(4):e167–72.

Gene Therapy for Inborn Errors of Immunity
Severe Combined Immunodeficiencies

Kritika Chetty, MBBS[a], Ben C. Houghton, BSc, PhD[b],
Claire Booth, MBBS, PhD[a,b],*

KEYWORDS

- Lentiviral gene therapy • ADA-SCID • X-SCID • Genome editing

KEY POINTS

- Gene therapy approaches are now in clinical trials for X-SCID, adenosine deaminase (ADA-SCID), Artemis-SCID, and RAG1-SCID.
- Strimvelis, a commercial γ-RV gene therapy product, has EMA approval as a treatment of patients with ADA-SCID.
- Insertional mutagenesis was a significant adverse outcome from initial γ-RV trials; however, self-inactivating lentiviral vectors have demonstrated a significantly improved safety profile.
- Encouraging preclinical gene-editing approaches are approaching clinical translation for X-SCID, RAG1-SCID, and IL7Rα-SCID.

INTRODUCTION

Inborn errors of immunity (IEI) are a diverse group of heterogenous disorders caused by monogenic defects affecting the function of the innate and/or adaptive immune system. Depending on the disease, the prevalence can range between 1 in 8500 to 1 in 100,000.[1] More than 420 mutations have now been identified, with this number expected to increase with further advances in genomic technology.[2]

Severe combined immune deficiency (SCID) is an umbrella term for a group of IEIs characterized by a profound deficiency in the number and function of T lymphocytes, and depending on the defect, variable deficiencies in B and NK cells. Patients present with severe, recurrent opportunistic infections, failure to thrive, and often immune

---

[a] Department of Paediatric Immunology and Gene Therapy, Level 3, Zayed Centre for Research Great Ormond Street Hospital, Great Ormond Street, London, WC1N 3JH, United Kingdom;
[b] UCL Great Ormond Street Institute of Child Health, London, United Kingdom
* Corresponding author. Department of Paediatric Immunology and Gene Therapy, Level 3, Zayed Centre for Research Great Ormond Street Hospital, Great Ormond Street, London, WC1N 3JH, United Kingdom.
E-mail address: c.booth@ucl.ac.uk

Hematol Oncol Clin N Am 36 (2022) 813–827
https://doi.org/10.1016/j.hoc.2022.03.010
0889-8588/22/© 2022 Elsevier Inc. All rights reserved.
hemonc.theclinics.com

dysregulation. Untreated, SCID is fatal within the first 2 years of life. More than 20 different genetic defects have been identified, thought to comprise approximately 90% of the causative defects in SCID.[2,3]

Historically, hematopoeitic stem cell transplant (HSCT) has been the only curative option. Since the first HSCT for SCID in 1968, survival rates have significantly improved, now reaching greater than 90% for some forms due to a combination of earlier disease recognition associated with reduced infectious comorbidities, better transplant protocols, improved graft manipulation techniques including alpha-beta T cell depletion to prevent graft versus host disease (GVHD) and better management of posttransplant complications.[4] HLA-donor type has a major impact on outcome, with matched sibling donors (MSD) leading to the highest survival rates at above 94%.[5–7] Conversely, there is no clear difference in survival between alternative donor types, specifically, matched other related donors, haploidentical donors, and unrelated donors, as evidenced by a retrospective analysis of 662 patients by the Primary Immune Deficiency Treatment Consortium (PIDTC).[7]

A matched sibling donor (MSD) is only available for less than 20% of patients, with survival rates much lower in haploidentical transplants, and immune-related complications remaining a major source of morbidity and mortality, hence the development of gene therapy strategies for these diseases. The use of autologous cells in gene therapy avoids the complication of graft rejection and GVHD traditionally associated with HSCT and permits the use of nonmyeloablative low-dose busulfan conditioning, significantly reducing conditioning-related toxicity.[8] However, the impact of even low exposure busulfan on long-term fertility remains to be seen. Posttransplant immunosuppressive prophylaxis is not required, and the treatment is not dependent on the availability of an allogeneic donor. For both allogeneic HSCT and gene therapy, proceeding early is crucial, with multiple large retrospective studies demonstrating improved survival in infants receiving HSCT at a younger age.[5–7]

SCID was the first genetic disorder successfully treated by gene therapy[9] and today we have gene therapy approaches for four types of SCID in clinical trials: X-SCID, adenosine deaminase-severe combined immune deficiency (ADA-SCID), Artemis, and RAG1-SCID. This review will summarize advances in gene therapy for specific forms of SCID, both in the clinical and preclinical arena, and provide an insight into future directions.

X-SEVERE COMBINED IMMUNE DEFICIENCY
Background

X-SCID is caused by defects in the IL2 Receptor gene (IL2RG), which encodes the common gamma chain protein, a key subunit in the cytokine receptor complex for IL-2, IL-4, IL-7, IL-9, IL-15, and IL-21.[10] Inherited in an x-linked recessive manner, it is the most common form of SCID, accounting for approximately 25% of all cases.[11] It typically presents with absent or significantly reduced T and NK cells and B cells that are present but do not function, due to both a lack of T cell help and an intrinsic defect in B cell signaling (T-B + NK-). Long-term survival from HSCT is greater than 90% if an HLA matched donor is available, however, falls significantly with HLA-mismatch, to a 10-year survival for patients treated after 1995 of 72%.[5,7]

Early Trials in X-Severe Combined Immune Deficiency

X-SCID has proven an excellent target for gene therapy due to the significant survival advantage of gene-corrected cells. Initial proof of principle clinical studies in Paris and London enrolled 20 patients lacking sibling donors.[12–15] CD34+ hematopoeitic stem cells (HSC) were transduced with a Moloney murine leukemia virus-based γ-retroviral (γRV) vector, using the strong promoter/enhancer elements present in the long terminal repeats (LTR) to drive expression of the IL2RG cDNA. After unconditioned infusion of gene-corrected cells, 18/20 patients demonstrated T cell reconstitution with lasting clinical benefit, no opportunistic infections, and normal growth and development.

Vector-Related Adverse Events

6 of the 20 patients developed serious adverse events (SAEs) in the form of clonal T cell ALL, one 15-years postinfusion.[16–19] γRV integration site analysis revealed the vector had inserted into or close to the LMO2 oncogene locus in 5 patients, and the CCND2 oncogene locus in 1 patient, leading to an oncogenic process via transactivation through the LTR enhancer. In most patients, additional pro-oncogenic genetic lesions were found suggesting a "two-hit" theory for the insertional mutagenesis observed. All but one patient survived following ALL-directed chemotherapy. Similar events were also observed in X-linked Chronic Granulomatous Disease (CGD) and Wiskott–Aldrich syndrome (WAS) clinical trials using similar vectors.[20,21]

This significant set-back prompted the community to work toward building safer vectors. Self-inactivating (SIN) vectors were developed via deletion of the 3′LTR U3 domain that was responsible for the long-range promoter/enhancer effect. Transgene expression could then be driven by an internal promoter derived from mammalian housekeeping genes (typically elongation factor 1a-short, or EFS), which was shown to have dramatically reduced transactivation potential.

A trial for X-SCID using a SIN-γRV vector was initiated in Boston, Paris, London, Los Angeles, and Cincinnati.[22] One patient died from overwhelming adenovirus infection before T cell engraftment. No conditioning was used and of the 8 patients surviving, 7 had functional peripheral T-cell reconstitution with the clinical resolution of infections. The kinetics of CD3+ T cell recovery were similar to previous trials with significantly less clustering within proto-oncogenic loci. Follow-up at a median of 8 years revealed none of the patients treated developed myelodysplasia or leukemia (SY Pai 2022, personal communication). However, most patients required ongoing immunoglobulin replacement therapy, suggesting a lack of conditioning was causing incomplete humoral immune recovery. Of note, the last patient treated who received low dose busulfan conditioning secured B cell engraftment, confirming that the inclusion of low dose conditioning in the protocol could improve functional immune recovery.

Recent X-Severe Combined Immune Deficiency Trials

To address this, more recent trials use cytoreduction using low dose busulfan. As an additional safety improvement, SIN lentiviral (SIN-LV) vectors are now preferred due to their more neutral insertion pattern and reduced risk of insertional oncogenesis. 4 older patients with X-SCID with a median age of 16 years received gene therapy as a rescue treatment after unsuccessful haploidentical HSCT.[23] 3-year follow-up for 2 patients demonstrated overall clinical improvement after gene therapy, with multilineage gene marking and reconstitution of humoral immunity. Early results of trials enrolling newly diagnosed infants are promising. Short-term follow-up, with a median duration of 16.4 months, from a study enrolling 8 infants demonstrated the reconstitution of T cell, NK cell, and to a lesser extent B cell function in 7 infants with no clonal insertion events.[24]

ADENOSINE DEAMINASE-SEVERE COMBINED IMMUNE DEFICIENCY
Background

ADA-SCID is an autosomal recessive condition caused by genetic defects in the purine salvage enzyme adenosine deaminase (ADA). The resulting build-up of toxic metabolites inhibits lymphocyte maturation and survival, leading to pan-lymphopenia (T-B-NK-). The estimated incidence is approximately 1 in 500,000, comprising 10% to 20% of all cases of SCID.[11,25] Due to the ubiquitous expression of ADA, the disorder is associated with several nonimmunologic systemic defects including lung abnormalities, skeletal dysplasias, sensorineural deafness, cognitive and behavioral problems, hepatic dysfunction, urogenital defects, and skin abnormalities.[26–33]

ADA enzyme replacement therapy (ERT) allows metabolic detoxification and can promote limited immune recovery. Decreasing T cell numbers and reduced thymic output have been demonstrated over time, and a significant treatment cost prevents it from being a viable long-term option, but its use pre-HSCT and gene therapy is well established.[34]

Unconditioned transplants from matched-related donors have long been the treatment of choice if an appropriate donor is available; however, recent reports of long-term outcomes challenge this paradigm, demonstrating significantly diminished donor engraftment in unconditioned procedures using related or unrelated HLA-matched donors.[35] In those who lack a matched donor, there is significant morbidity and a lower chance of success regardless of whether conditioning is used, with the largest multi-centre series demonstrating only a 43% overall survival with haplo-identical donors.[36]

Clinical Trials in Adenosine Deaminase-Severe Combined Immune Deficiency

Initial trials used unconditioned infusions of transduced lymphocytes or hematopoeitic progenitor cells using a retroviral vector; however, gene marking was extremely low at long-term follow-up and no substantial immunologic improvement was noted.[37,38] Following an improved protocol for γRV transduction of CD34+ cells and the addition of nonmyeloablative conditioning, data from a total of 12 patients treated in Milan were highly encouraging, with the restoration of T cell function in 11 patients and 6 able to cease immunoglobulin replacement therapy.[39,40] This work ultimately led to Strimvelis, a now commercially available γRV gene therapy product for ADA-SCID.[41] The product is a fresh product rather than cryopreserved and due to its short shelf-life, patients must travel to Milan for treatment.

US and London groups used similar protocols involving a fresh γRV product, pausing ERT before infusion, and cytoreductive conditioning.[42–44] 4 of 6 children in the London cohort recovered immune function, and of the 6 subjects in the US cohort who received conditioning, 3 remained well with good gene marking and off ERT up to 5-years postprocedure. Medium-term outcome was reported in 18 patients with a median follow-up of 6.9 years demonstrating long-term engraftment, immune reconstitution, and fewer severe infections in 15 out of 18 patients.[45] Long-term follow-up to 11 years of 10 subjects transduced with an MND-ADA γ-RV vector in the US demonstrated stable multi-lineage gene marking in all 10 patients despite great variability in transduction efficiency between products.[46] Of 10 patients, 9 reconstituted clinically significant immune function to protect against significant infection and were able to cease ERT. 6 patients had evidence of vector integration in proto-oncogenes implicated in insertional oncogenesis; however, none of these patients developed leukemia. Indeed, the safety profile of γ-RV vectors in ADA-SCID is unique in that insertional oncogenesis is extremely rare, with only 1 in at least 50 patients who received the γ-RV product commercially or in clinical trials developing leukemia.[47]

Most recently, a multi-centre trial in the US and UK using a SIN-lentiviral construct has reported very positive results in 50 patients.[48] Overall survival was 100% at 3-years. Persistent gene marking was evident in 48 patients who also had sustained metabolic detoxification and normalization of ADA activity. 90% and 100% of patients were able to discontinue immunoglobulin replacement therapy in the US and UK studies respectively. With the restoration of immunity and no adverse events related to the vector, this outcome data is the most successful to date. The remarkable safety and efficacy outcomes in more than 100 patients with ADA-SCID who received either γ-RV or lentiviral mediated gene therapy led to the consensus that gene therapy is an equivalent first-line option to MSD HSCT.[49] **(Fig. 1)**.

ARTEMIS-SEVERE COMBINED IMMUNE DEFICIENCY
Background

Artemis-SCID is caused by homozygous mutations in the DCLRE1C gene, that en-codes *Artemis*, an exonuclease essential for the repair of DNA double-stranded breaks via nonhomologous end joining.[50,51] Defects lead to a lack of functioning of T and B cells due to impaired VDJ recombination at the T and B cell receptor locus, and increased sensitivity to ionizing radiation and alkylating chemotherapy, with an increased potential for malignant transformation.[52] Like other SCID genotypes, HSCT from MSDs do not need conditioning, however, differ in that these patients never achieve full T cell immunity and rarely have B cell reconstitution.[8,53,54] As most patients do not have MSDs available, conditioning is required to reduce risks associated with graft rejection and optimize immune restoration. With alkylating chemotherapeutic agents poorly tolerated and an increased risk of late complications after HSCT in these patients, *Artemis*-SCID remains one of the most difficult SCID ge-notypes to transplant.[53,54]

Artemis GT Clinical Trials

Early results of a phase I/II clinical trial in 5 newly diagnosed infants with *Artemis*-SCID show multilineage gene marking and reconstitution of T cell immunity in all 3 evaluable patients. The protocol uses a novel self-inactivating lentiviral vector expressing DCLRE1C driven by the human endogenous *Artemis* promoter (AProArt), and conditioning with targeted low dose busulfan conditioning.[55,56] A trial is anticipated to open in Paris with patients planned to receive autologous CD34+ cells transduced with the G2ARTE lentiviral vector expressing the DCLRE1C cDNA (NCT05071222).[57,58]

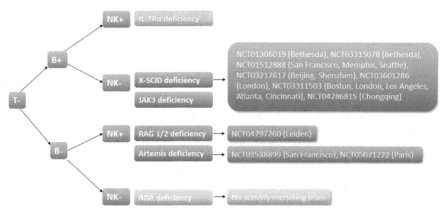

Fig. 1. SCID immunophenotypes with corresponding current gene therapy clinical trials by ClinicalTrials.gov Identifier.

RAG1-SEVERE COMBINED IMMUNE DEFICIENCY
Background and Preclinical Work

Similar to *Artemis*, defects in RAG1 and RAG2 proteins lead to a T-B-NK + phenotype due to the inability to initiate VDJ recombination.[59] Gene therapy poses unique difficulties in *RAG1*-SCID as ectopic expression of *RAG1* may be harmful, and too few corrected cells may lead to immune dysregulation. Several preclinical efforts to correct *RAG1* deficiency have produced variable results, with cases of clonal proliferation and phenotypes resembling human Omenn syndrome in different studies based on varying promoters and differing levels of gene expression.[60–62]

Favorable preclinical safety and efficacy data using a lentiviral codon-optimized human *RAG1* SIN vector have led to the development of a clinical program for gene therapy for RAG1-SCID, now underway in Leiden and soon to open to recruitment in London (NCT04797260).[63] Children up to 24 months of age lacking an HLA-matched donor will be infused with autologous CD34+ cells transduced with a SIN-LV-RAG1 vector after conditioning.

Omenn syndrome, mostly due to hypomorphic variants in *RAG1* or *RAG2*, describes a clinical- and immune-phenotype characterized by failure to thrive, opportunistic infections, erythrodermatous rash, organomegaly, autologous oligoclonal autoreactive T cells, high IgE and hypereosinophilia. Residual *RAG* function partially permits T cell development leading to immune dysregulation. The efficacy of lentiviral-mediated gene therapy was tested in a murine model of Omenn syndrome.[64] There was significant amelioration of immunodeficiency in treated mice, with the normalization of immunoglobulin levels and T-cell repertoire, good response to in vivo challenges, and dramatic improvement of autoimmune manifestations. *RAG2* preclinical models have also proved encouraging, with both γ-RV and lentiviral vectors demonstrating effective correction of immunodeficiency without vector-related complications.[65,66]

IL-7 RECEPTOR (IL-7R) DEFICIENCY SEVERE COMBINED IMMUNE DEFICIENCY

IL-7R deficiency causes approximately 10% of SCID and is caused by biallelic defects of the *IL-7R* alpha chain gene that forms a complete receptor in complex with IL2RG. IL-7 signaling is required for T cell receptor rearrangement and T cell maintenance, and deficiencies lead to a T-B + NK + SCID. In contrast, mice lacking IL7R (*Il7r*) lacks both T and B cells. A γRV vector-based approach was tested in the *Il7r* knockout mouse model, which restored T cells and variably restored B cells, but was associated with, significant myeloproliferation, neutrophilia, and splenomegaly.[67] Recent data evaluating a lentiviral vector using the human *IL7R* gene demonstrated improved outcomes, with further evaluation underway.[68]

JAK-3 SEVERE COMBINED IMMUNE DEFICIENCY

JAK-3 belongs to a family of nonreceptor protein tyrosine kinases involved in intracellular signal transduction. JAK-3 specifically plays a crucial role in cytokine signaling through interaction with the common gamma chain (γc), and therefore mutations affecting JAK-3 function produce an autosomal recessive form of inherited immunodeficiency resembling X-SCID (T-B + NK-). A gene therapy approach was investigated by using a retroviral vector containing the normal JAK-3 cDNA to reconstitute the expression of JAK-3 protein in B cell lines from patients with JAK-3 SCID.[69] JAK-3 expression was restored, and transduced cells were able to proliferate normally in response to IL-2, indicating efficient in vitro correction. A clinical gene therapy approach was attempted using a JAK3-gRV vector and no conditioning regimen for a 2 and half-year-old boy, after 2 previous unsuccessful allogeneic HSCTs using his mother as a donor.[70] Adequate vector gene transfer and expression were noted at 7-month follow-up; however, no immune reconstitution was evident.

In Vivo Approaches

In vivo delivery approaches may offer advantages to a conventional ex vivo HSC procedure by removing the need to culture HSC ex vivo, a process that can be associated with reduced "stemness." Furthermore, an in vivo approach could reduce the intensity of chemotherapeutic conditioning of the patient and allow a faster route to patient treatment postdiagnosis, without the need for specialized manufacture of cells. However, the efficacy of VSV-G pseudotyped lentiviral vectors is limited in the human setting due to serum inactivation, indicating the need for alternative vector technologies.[71] Foamy viral vectors, and cocal-pseudotyped lentiviral vectors are resistant to serum inactivation, and both have been trialed as gene delivery platforms in a canine model of X-SCID.

Foamy viruses can effectively transduce HSC and, as an integrating retrovirus, exhibit an attractive integration profile.[72] X-SCID canines receiving a G-CSF and AMD3100 mobilization regimen before PGK-IL2RG FV infusion showed increased thymic output and broad TCR diversity, although B cell and myeloid gene marking remained low.[73] No genotoxicity was observed in longer follow-up studies, but further studies will be required before the full safety profile of this approach can be determined.[74,75] (**Table 1**).

Gene Editing in Severe Combined Immune Deficiency

Precision gene correction is becoming a promising future therapeutic approach for immune deficiencies with a number of platforms now available to perform targeted gene correction; zinc finger nucleases (ZFNs), transcription activator-like effector nucleases (TALENs), and the increasingly popular CRISPR/Cas system. Correcting a target gene in situ should allow for the expression of that gene from endogenous regulatory elements, thereby achieving a more physiologic expression profile than with conventional additive gene therapy strategies. This is a particularly attractive technique for conditions whereby partial expression or aberrant expression could be detrimental, for example, as seen in CD40 ligand deficiency whereby unregulated transgene expression leads to lymphoproliferation.[76] Gene-editing platforms combine site-specific sequences (targeted to the loci of interest) and endonucleases capable of initiating a double-stranded break (DSB) in the DNA at that precise location. The DSB can then be repaired by nonhomologous end-joining (NHEJ), useful for gene knockout, or through homology-directed repair (HDR) which allows accurate correction from a donor template.

X-SCID was an early disease target to demonstrate this technology could potentially offer therapeutic benefits as corrected cells show a strong survival advantage. Using ZFNs targeting the first intron of the IL2R gene and providing HDR template in the form of integration deficient lentivirus (IDLV), Genovese and colleagues[77] showed functional correction of gene-edited X-SCID CD34+ cells in an NSG mouse model. Building on this work, Schiroli and colleagues[78] then provided proof of efficacy for this approach in a humanized X-SCID mouse model alongside demonstrating that functional reconstitution could be achieved with less than 10% correction of hematopoeitic progenitors. They also improved editing efficiency in human CD34+ cells by using AAV6 to deliver corrective DNA sequences. This approach was both highly translatable and transferable to other monogenic disorders.

Table 1
Current gene therapy trials for SCID

Disease	Trial Number	Recruitment	Vector	Transgene	Promoter	Start Date	Age	Conditioning	Location	Sponsorship	Estimated Enrollment	Reference
X-SCID	NCT01129544	Active, not recruiting	SIN-γRV	IL2RG	EFS	2010	Not specified	Busulfan	Boston, Los Angeles, Cincinnati	Academic	9*	Hacein-Bey-Abina et al,[14] 2010
	NCT01306019	Recruiting	Lentivirus	IL2RG	EF1 α with 400-bp insulator fragment from the chicken beta-globin locus	2012	2–40 y	Busulfan	Bethesda	Academic	30	Mamcarz et al,[24] 2019
	NCT03315078	Recruiting	Lentivirus	IL2RG	As above	2012	2–40 y	Busulfan	Bethesda	Academic	13	Mamcarz et al,[24] 2019
	NCT01512888	Recruiting	Lentivirus	IL2RG	As above	2016	< 2 y	Busulfan	San Francisco, Memphis, Seattle	Academic	28	Kwan et al,[25] 2014
	NCT03217617	Recruiting	Lentivirus	IL2RG	Not available	2017	1 m–10 y	Not available	Beijing, Shenzhen	Academic	10	
	NCT03601286	Recruiting	Lentivirus	IL2RG	EFS	2018	2 m–5 y	Busulfan	London	Academic	5	
	NCT03311503	Recruiting	Lentivirus	IL2RG	EFS	2018	< 5 y	Busulfan	Boston, London, Los Angeles, Atlanta, Cincinnati	Academic	10	
	NCT04286815	Recruiting	Lentivirus	IL2RG	Not available	2020	< 18 y	Not available	Chongqing	Academic	10	
ADA-SCID	NCT03765632	Active, not recruiting	Lentivirus	ADA	EFS	2018	< 17 y	Busulfan	London	Academic	13	
RAG1-SCID	NCT04797260	Recruiting	Lentivirus	RAG	MND	2021	2 m–2 y	Busulfan and Fludarabine	Leiden	Academic	10	
Artemis-SCID	NCT03538899	Recruiting	Lentivirus	DCLERE1C	AProArt	2018	< 2 m	Busulfan	San Francisco	Academic	25	Punwani et al,[56] 2017
	NCT05071222	Not yet recruiting	Lentivirus	DCLERE1C	AProArt	2021	< 1 y	Busulfan	Paris	Academic	5	

*Actual enrollment 8 patients

Subsequently, the CRISPR/Cas system has been used together with an AAV6 donor targeting integration of the AAV6 delivered cDNA to the endogenous start codon of the IL2R gene. Pavel-Dinu achieved up to 20% targeted integration in long-term HSCs with a median targeting efficiency of 45% in CD34+ cells from 6 patients with X-SCID.[79] Xenotransplant experiments using those patient corrected cells demonstrated rescue of lymphoid defects both in vitro and in vivo. No abnormalities of hematopoiesis were identified and there was no evidence of off-target events.

Currently, there are no clinical trials of gene-editing underway for any form of SCID, but several groups are working to translate encouraging preclinical studies to the clinic for X-SCID, RAG-SCID, and IL7Rα deficient SCID. Achieving clinically relevant levels of HDR-mediated correction remains a significant challenge for the field although a great deal of effort is focused on improving this and undoubtedly, we will see early phase clinical trials reaching the clinic in the coming years.

Future Directions/Challenges

While significant progress has been made in bringing gene therapy and precision gene editing to the clinic for various types of SCID, several advances are occurring to optimize patient outcomes beyond the direct improvements in transduction protocols and vector technology. Newborn screening of SCID has reduced patient morbidity by earlier disease diagnosis and therefore earlier definitive treatment before infections.[80] Vast improvements in genetic technologies are allowing for precise identification of pathogenic variants, assisting in earlier diagnosis and definitive therapy. Despite the advantage of needing lower dose conditioning agents, acute and long-term toxicity still occur, albeit at lower rates than in HSCT. A move toward safe and effective cytoreduction without chemotherapy would further reduce the risk of toxicity in both HSCT and gene therapy, and work in this field is underway with the development of monoclonal antibodies, c-kit antibodies, and antibodies against CD45+ and other stem cell markers.[81,82]

Advances in molecular diagnostics and fetal surgical techniques, in allowing for earlier disease identification and safer delivery of gene therapy vectors within the fetus are paving the way for in utero gene therapy. Preemptive definitive therapy seeks to transform patient outcomes, not only with respect to potential improved success rates but also in preventing irreversible damage that can occur during fetal development in certain forms of SCID. A sterile maternal womb would facilitate immune reconstitution before pathogen exposure, and a smaller fetus would necessitate a reduced cell dose. In-utero treatment has the potential to significantly optimize patient outcomes; however, the procedure is still in its infancy and several challenges remain, including the ability to develop appropriate animal models.

Despite these significant advances, challenges remain in the gene therapy development pipeline. Notwithstanding the complexities of the products, strict requirements by oversight entities with associated personnel, facilities, quality assurance, and regulatory requirements all contribute to the substantial costs in bringing these medicines to the market. Furthermore, additional work is needed in certain forms of SCID in establishing functional levels of protein expression, and without the results of any gene-editing clinical trials, it remains to be seen if gene editing is more beneficial than additive gene therapy.

CLINICS CARE POINTS

- Gene therapy approaches are now in clinical trials for X-SCID, ADA-SCID, Artemis-SCID, and RAG1-SCID.

- Strimvelis, a commercial γ-RV gene therapy product, has EMA approval as a treatment of patients with ADA-SCID.
- Insertional mutagenesis was a significant adverse outcome from initial X-SCID trials using a γ-RV product; however, self-inactivating vectors have demonstrated a significantly improved safety profile.
- Encouraging preclinical gene-editing approaches are being translated to the clinic for X-SCID, RAG1-SCID, and IL7Rα-SCID.

SUMMARY

SCID has been the exemplar condition for successful cellular therapies, from the first reported HSCT in an X-SCID patient in 1968 to the first clinical gene therapy trial in ADA-SCID in 1990. Conversely, SCID has also been the forerunner condition in demonstrating genotoxicity from first-generation gene therapy vectors. Despite these initial setbacks, developments in the field are now accelerating, with the first commercial gene therapy product approved in 2016 in Europe, the establishment of more clinical trials for rarer forms of SCID, and expansion of both ex vivo and in vivo gene-editing technologies. Challenges remain in overcoming potentially prohibitive costs in bringing these complex medicines to market, however, with the advent of newborn screening, safer cytoreductive techniques and in utero treatments, improved outcomes for patients with SCID are likely to continue.

FUNDING

Research at Great Ormond Street Hospital is supported by the GOSH NIHR BRC.

REFERENCES

1. Kobrynski L, Powell RW, Bowen S. Prevalence and morbidity of primary immunodeficiency diseases, United States 2001-2007. J Clin Immunol 2014;34(8):954–61.
2. Bousfiha A, Jeddane L, Picard C, et al. Human Inborn Errors of Immunity: 2019 Update of the IUIS Phenotypical Classification. J Clin Immunol 2020;40(1):66–81.
3. Gaspar BH, Qasim W, Davies GE, et al. How i treat severe combined immunodeficiency. Blood 2013;122(23):3749–58.
4. Slatter MA, Gennery AR. Hematopoietic cell transplantation in primary immunodeficiency – conventional and emerging indications. Expert Rev Clin Immunol 2018;14(2):103–14.
5. Pai SY, Logan BR, Griffith LM, et al. Transplantation Outcomes for Severe Combined Immunodeficiency, 2000–2009. N Engl J Med 2014;371(5):434–46.
6. Heimall J, Logan BR, Cowan MJ, et al. Immune reconstitution and survival of 100 SCID patients post–hematopoietic cell transplant: a PIDTC natural history study. Blood 2017;130(25):2718–27.
7. Haddad E, Logan BR, Griffith LM, et al. SCID genotype and 6-month posttransplant CD4 count predict survival and immune recovery. Blood 2018;132(17):1737–49.
8. O'Marcaigh AS, DeSantes K, Hu D, et al. Bone marrow transplantation for T-B- severe combined immunodeficiency disease in Athabascan-speaking native Americans. Bone Marrow Transplant 2001;27(7):703–9.

9. Bordignon C, Notarangelo LD, Nobili N, et al. Gene therapy in peripheral blood lymphocytes and bone marrow for ADA- immunodeficient patients. Science 1995;270(5235):470–5.

10. Noguchi M, Yi H, Rosenblatt HM, et al. Interleukin-2 receptor γ chain mutation results in X-linked severe combined immunodeficiency in humans. Cell 1993;73(1):147–57.

11. Dvorak CC, Haddad E, Buckley RH, et al. The genetic landscape of severe combined immunodeficiency in the United States and Canada in the current era (2010-2018). J Allergy Clin Immunol 2019;143(1):405–7.

12. Cavazzana-Calvo M, Hacein-Bey S, De Saint Basile G, et al. Gene therapy of human severe combined immunodeficiency (SCID)-X1 disease. Science 2000;288(5466):669–72.

13. Hacein-Bey-Abina S, Le Deist F, Carlier F, et al. Sustained correction of X-linked severe combined immunodeficiency by ex vivo gene therapy. N Engl J Med 2002;346(16):1185–93.

14. Hacein-Bey-Abina S, Hauer J, Lim A, et al. Efficacy of Gene Therapy for X-Linked Severe Combined Immunodeficiency. N Engl J Med 2010;363(4):355–64.

15. Gaspar HB, Parsley KL, Howe S, et al. Gene therapy of X-linked severe combined immunodeficiency by use of a pseudotyped gammaretroviral vector. Lancet 2004;364(9452):2181–7.

16. Hacein-Bey-Abina S, Garrigue A, Wang GP, et al. Insertional oncogenesis in 4 patients after retrovirus-mediated gene therapy of SCID-X1. J Clin Invest 2008;118(9):3132–42.

17. Howe SJ, Mansour MR, Schwarzwaelder K, et al. Insertional mutagenesis combined with acquired somatic mutations causes leukemogenesis following gene therapy of SCID-X1 patients. J Clin Invest 2008;118(9):3143.

18. Fischer A, Hacein-Bey-Abina S. Gene therapy for severe combined immunodeficiencies and beyond. J Exp Med 2020;217(2):e20190607.

19. Six E, Gandemer V, Magnani A, et al. LMO2 associated clonal T cell proliferation 15 years after gamma-retrovirus mediated gene therapy for SCIDX1. Mol Ther 2017;25(5):347–8.

20. Stein S, Ott MG, Schultze-Strasser S, et al. Genomic instability and myelodysplasia with monosomy 7 consequent to EVI1 activation after gene therapy for chronic granulomatous disease. Nat Med 2010;16(2):198–204.

21. Braun CJ, Boztug K, Paruzynski A, et al. Gene therapy for Wiskott-Aldrich syndrome-long-term efficacy and genotoxicity. Sci Translational Med 2014;6(227):227ra33.

22. Hacein-Bey-Abina S, Pai SY, Gaspar HB, et al. A modified γ-retrovirus vector for X-linked severe combined immunodeficiency. N Engl J Med 2014;371(15):1407–17.

23. de Ravin SS, Wu X, Moir S, et al. Lentiviral hematopoietic stem cell gene therapy for X-linked severe combined immunodeficiency. Sci Translational Med 2016;8(335):335ra57.

24. Mamcarz E, Zhou S, Lockey T, et al. Lentiviral Gene Therapy Combined with Low-Dose Busulfan in Infants with SCID-X1. N Engl J Med 2019;380(16):1525–34.

25. Kwan A, Abraham RS, Currier R, et al. Newborn Screening for Severe Combined Immunodeficiency in 11 Screening Programs in the United States. JAMA 2014;312(7):729.

26. Cederbaum SD, Kaitila I, Rimoin DL, et al. The chondro-osseous dysplasia of adenosine deaminase deficiency with severe combined immunodeficiency. J Pediatr 1976;89(5):737–42.

27. Albuquerque W, Gaspar HB. Bilateral sensorineural deafness in adenosine deaminase-deficient severe combined immunodeficiency. J Pediatr 2004; 144(2):278–80.
28. Bollinger ME, Arredondo-Vega FX, Santisteban I, et al. Hepatic Dysfunction as a Complication of Adenosine Deaminase Deficiency. N Engl J Med 1996;334(21): 1367–72.
29. Keightley RG, Lawton AR, Cooper MD, et al. Successful fetal transplantation in a child with severe combined immunodeficiency. Lancet 1975;306(7940):850–3.
30. Rogers MH, Lwin R, Fairbanks L, et al. Cognitive and behavioral abnormalities in adenosine deaminase deficient severe combined immunodeficiency. J Pediatr 2001;139(1):44–50.
31. Grunebaum E, Cutz E, Roifman CM. Pulmonary alveolar proteinosis in patients with adenosine deaminase deficiency. J Allergy Clin Immunol 2012;129(6): 1588–93.
32. Kesserwan C, Sokolic R, Cowen EW, et al. Multicentric dermatofibrosarcoma protuberans in patients with adenosine deaminase–deficient severe combined immune deficiency. J Allergy Clin Immunol 2012;129(3):762–9.e1.
33. Pajno R, Pacillo L, Recupero S, et al. Urogenital abnormalities in adenosine deaminase deficiency. J Clin Immunol 2020;40(4):610–8.
34. Chan B, Wara D, Bastian J, et al. Long-term efficacy of enzyme replacement therapy for Adenosine deaminase (ADA)-deficient Severe Combined Immunodeficiency (SCID). Clin Immunol 2005;117(2):133–43.
35. Kreins AY, Velasco HF, Cheong KN, et al. Long-Term Immune Recovery After Hematopoietic Stem Cell Transplantation for ADA Deficiency: a Single-Center Experience. J Clin Immunol 2021. https://doi.org/10.1007/s10875-021-01145-w.
36. Hassan A, Booth C, Brightwell A, et al. Outcome of hematopoietic stem cell transplantation for adenosine deaminase-deficient severe combined immunodeficiency. Blood 2012;120(17):3615–24.
37. Muul LM, Tuschong LM, Soenen SL, et al. Persistence and expression of the adenosine deaminase gene for 12 years and immune reaction to gene transfer components: long-term results of the first clinical gene therapy trial. Blood 2003;101(7):2563–9.
38. Aiuti A, Vai S, Mortellaro A, et al. Immune reconstitution in ADA-SCID after PBL gene therapy and discontinuation of enzyme replacement. Nat Med 2002;8(5): 423–5.
39. Aiuti A, Slavin S, Aker M, et al. Correction of ADA-SCID by Stem Cell Gene Therapy Combined with Nonmyeloablative Conditioning. Science 2002;296(5577): 2410–3.
40. Aiuti A, Cattaneo F, Galimberti S, et al. Gene therapy for immunodeficiency due to adenosine deaminase deficiency. N Engl J Med 2009;360(5):447–58.
41. Aiuti A, Roncarolo MG, Naldini L. Gene therapy for ADA-SCID, the first marketing approval of an ex vivo gene therapy in Europe: paving the road for the next generation of advanced therapy medicinal products. EMBO Mol Med 2017;9(6): 737–40.
42. Gaspar HB, Bjorkegren E, Parsley K, et al. Successful Reconstitution of Immunity in ADA-SCID by Stem Cell Gene Therapy Following Cessation of PEG-ADA and Use of Mild Preconditioning. Mol Ther 2006;14(4):505–13.
43. Gaspar HB, Cooray S, Gilmour KC, et al. Immunodeficiency: Hematopoietic stem cell gene therapy for adenosine deaminase-deficient severe combined immunodeficiency leads to long-term immunological recovery and metabolic correction. Sci Translational Med 2011;3(97):97ra80.

44. Candotti F, Shaw KL, Muul L, et al. Gene therapy for adenosine deaminase-deficient severe combined immune deficiency: clinical comparison of retroviral vectors and treatment plans. Blood 2012;120(18):3635–46.

45. Cicalese MP, Ferrua F, Castagnaro L, et al. Update on the safety and efficacy of retroviral gene therapy for immunodeficiency due to adenosine deaminase deficiency. Blood 2016;128(1):45–54.

46. Reinhardt B, Habib O, Shaw KL, et al. Long-term outcomes after gene therapy for adenosine deaminase severe combined immune deficiency. Blood 2021;138(15): 1304–16.

47. Orchard Therapeutics. Press Releases Orchard Statement on Strimvelis®, a Gammaretroviral Vector-Based Gene Therapy for ADA-SCID.; 2020.

48. Kohn DB, Booth C, Shaw KL, et al. Autologous Ex Vivo lentiviral gene therapy for adenosine deaminase deficiency. N Engl J Med 2021;384(21):2002–13.

49. Kohn DB, Hershfield MS, Puck JM, et al. Consensus approach for the management of severe combined immune deficiency caused by adenosine deaminase deficiency. J Allergy Clin Immunol 2019;143(3):852–63.

50. Moshous D, Li L, de Chasseval R, et al. A new gene involved in DNA double-strand break repair and V(D)J recombination is located on human chromosome 10p. Hum Mol Genet 2000;9(4):583–8.

51. Moshous D, Callebaut I, de Chasseval R, et al. Artemis, a novel DNA double-strand break repair/V(D)J recombination protein, is mutated in human severe combined immune deficiency. Cell 2001;105(2):177–86.

52. de Miranda NFCC, Björkman A, Pan-Hammarström Q. DNA repair: the link between primary immunodeficiency and cancer. Ann N Y Acad Sci 2011;1246(1): 50–63.

53. Neven B, Leroy S, Decaluwe H, et al. Long-term outcome after hematopoietic stem cell transplantation of a single-center cohort of 90 patients with severe combined immunodeficiency. Blood 2009;113(17):4114–24.

54. Schuetz C, Neven B, Dvorak CC, et al. SCID patients with ARTEMIS vs RAG deficiencies following HCT: increased risk of late toxicity in ARTEMIS-deficient SCID. Blood 2014;123(2):281–9.

55. Cowan MJ, Yu J, Facchino J, et al. Early Outcome of a Phase I/II Clinical Trial (NCT03538899) of Gene-Corrected Autologous CD34+ Hematopoietic Cells and Low-Exposure Busulfan in Newly Diagnosed Patients with Artemis-Deficient Severe Combined Immunodeficiency (ART-SCID). Biol Blood Marrow Transplant 2020;26(3):S88–9.

56. Punwani D, Kawahara M, Yu J, et al. Lentivirus Mediated Correction of Artemis-Deficient Severe Combined Immunodeficiency. Hum Gene Ther 2017;28(1): 112–24.

57. Benjelloun F, Garrigue A, Demerens-de Chappedelaine C, et al. Stable and functional lymphoid reconstitution in artemis-deficient mice following lentiviral artemis gene transfer into hematopoietic stem cells. Mol Ther 2008;16(8):1490–9.

58. Charrier S, Lagresle-Peyrou C, Poletti V, et al. Biosafety Studies of a Clinically Applicable Lentiviral Vector for the Gene Therapy of Artemis-SCID. Mol Ther Methods Clin Dev 2019;15:232–45. https://doi.org/10.1016/j.omtm.2019.08.014.

59. Alt FW, Rathbun G, Oltz E, et al. Function and Control of Recombination-Activating Gene Activity. Ann New York Acad Sci 1992;651(1):277–94.

60. Lagresle-Peyrou C, Yates F, Malassis-Séris M, et al. Long-term immune reconstitution in RAG-1-deficient mice treated by retroviral gene therapy: a balance between efficiency and toxicity. Blood 2006;107(1):63–72.

61. Pike-Overzet K, Rodijk M, Ng YY, et al. Correction of murine Rag1 deficiency by self-inactivating lentiviral vector-mediated gene transfer. Leukemia 2011;25(9): 1471–83.

62. van Til NP, Sarwari R, Visser TP, et al. Recombination-activating gene 1 (Rag1)–deficient mice with severe combined immunodeficiency treated with lentiviral gene therapy demonstrate autoimmune Omenn-like syndrome. J Allergy Clin Immunol 2014;133(4):1116–23.

63. Garcia-Perez L, van Eggermond M, van Roon L, et al. Successful Preclinical Development of Gene Therapy for Recombinase-Activating Gene-1-Deficient SCID. Mol Ther Methods Clin Dev 2020;17:666–82.

64. Capo V, Castiello MC, Fontana E, et al. Efficacy of lentivirus-mediated gene therapy in an Omenn syndrome recombination-activating gene 2 mouse model is not hindered by inflammation and immune dysregulation. J Allergy Clin Immunol 2018;142(3):928–41.e8.

65. Yates F, Malassis-Séris M, Stockholm D, et al. Gene therapy of RAG-2−/− mice: sustained correction of the immunodeficiency. Blood 2002;100(12):3942–9.

66. van Til NP, de Boer H, Mashamba N, et al. Correction of murine Rag2 severe combined immunodeficiency by lentiviral gene therapy using a codon-optimized RAG2 therapeutic transgene. Mol Ther 2012;20(10):1968–80.

67. Jiang Q, Li WQ, Aiello FB, et al. Retroviral transduction of IL-7Rα into IL-7Rα−/− bone marrow progenitors: correction of lymphoid deficiency and induction of neutrophilia. Gene Ther 2005;12(24):1761–8.

68. Triebwasser M, Jarocha DJ, Breda L, et al. Rescue of Murine IL-7 receptor deficiency with human IL-7 receptor gene therapy. Blood 2021;138:3131. https://doi.org/10.1182/blood-2021-151040.

69. Candotti F, Oakes SA, Johnston JA, et al. In vitro correction of JAK3-deficient severe combined immunodeficiency by retroviral-mediated gene transduction. J Exp Med 1996;183(6):2687–92.

70. Sorrentino BP, Lu T, James I, et al. 1164. A clinical attempt to treat JAK3-deficient SCID using retroviral-mediated gene transfer to bone marrow CD34+ Cells. Mol Ther 2003;7(5):S449.

71. DePolo NJ, Reed JD, Sheridan PL, et al. VSV-G Pseudotyped lentiviral vector particles produced in human cells are inactivated by human serum. Mol Ther 2000; 2(3):218–22.

72. Simantirakis E, Tsironis I, Vassilopoulos G. FV vectors as alternative gene vehicles for gene transfer in HSCs. Viruses 2020;12(3):332.

73. Humbert O, Chan F, Rajawat YS, et al. Rapid immune reconstitution of SCID-X1 canines after G-CSF/AMD3100 mobilization and in vivo gene therapy. Blood Adv 2018;2(9):987–99.

74. Trobridge GD, Wu RA, Hansen M, et al. Cocal-pseudotyped lentiviral vectors resist inactivation by human serum and efficiently transduce primate hematopoietic repopulating cells. Mol Ther 2010;18(4):725–33.

75. Rajawat YS, Humbert O, Cook SM, et al. In Vivo Gene Therapy for Canine SCID-X1 Using Cocal-Pseudotyped Lentiviral Vector. Hum Gene Ther 2020;32(1–2): 113–27.

76. Sacco MG, Ungari M, Catò EM, et al. Lymphoid abnormalities in CD40 ligand transgenic mice suggest the need for tight regulation in gene therapy approaches to hyper immunoglobulin M (IgM) syndrome. Cancer Gene Ther 2000;7(10):1299–306.

77. Genovese P, Schiroli G, Escobar G, et al. Targeted genome editing in human repopulating haematopoietic stem cells. Nature 2014;510(7504):235–40.

78. Schiroli G, Ferrari S, Conway A, et al. Preclinical modeling highlights the thera-peutic potential of hematopoietic stem cell gene editing for correction of SCID-X1. Sci Translational Med 2017;9(411):eaan0820.
79. Pavel-Dinu M, Wiebking V, Dejene BT, et al. Gene correction for SCID-X1 in long-term hematopoietic stem cells. Nat Commun 2019;10(1):1–15.
80. Dorsey MJ, Puck JM. Newborn Screening for Severe Combined Immunodefi-ciency in the United States: Lessons Learned. Immunol Allergy Clin 2019; 39(1):1–11.
81. Kwon HS, Logan AC, Chhabra A, et al. Anti-human CD117 antibody-mediated bone marrow niche clearance in nonhuman primates and humanized NSG mice. Blood 2019;133(19):2104–8.
82. Palchaudhuri R, Saez B, Hoggatt J, et al. Non-genotoxic conditioning for hemato-poietic stem cell transplantation using a hematopoietic-cell-specific internalizing immunotoxin. Nat Biotechnol 2016;34(7):738–45.

Genes as Medicine

The Development of Gene Therapies for Inborn Errors of Immunity

Joseph D. Long, MS[a], Edward C. Trope, MS[a], Jennifer Yang, BS[b],
Kristen Rector, MS[c], Caroline Y. Kuo, MD[a],*

KEYWORDS

- Gene modification • Viral vector gene therapy • Gene editing
- Inborn errors of immunity • Primary immunodeficiency

KEY POINTS

- Genome modification approaches can be broadly categorized into viral vector-mediated gene therapy, site-specific gene editing, and gene silencing.
- Viral vector-mediated gene addition has progressed the farthest with several clinical trials for IEI.
- Certain genes need more tightly regulated expression profiles and require either gene editing or improved vector design.
- Both on- and off-target activity of gene editing platforms need to be fully characterized before translation to the clinic.
- The field of gene modification holds great promise for the development of new and improved therapies for IEI.

The field of gene therapy has experienced tremendous growth in the last decade ranging from improvements in the design of viral vectors for gene addition of therapeutic gene cassettes to the discovery of site-specific nucleases targeting transgenes to desired locations in the genome. Such advancements have not only enabled the development of disease models but also created opportunities for the development of tailored therapeutic approaches. There are 3 main methods of gene modification that can be used for the prevention or treatment of disease. This includes viral vector-mediated gene therapy to supply or bypass a missing/defective gene, gene editing enabled by programmable nucleases to create sequence-specific alterations

[a] Division of Allergy & Immunology, Department of Pediatrics, David Geffen School of Medicine at the University of California, Los Angeles, 10833 Le Conte, MDCC 12-430, Los Angeles, CA 90095, USA; [b] Department of Psychology, University of California, Los Angeles, 1285 Psychology Building, Box 951563, Los Angeles, CA 90095, USA; [c] No affiliation
* Corresponding author.
E-mail address: ckuo@mednet.ucla.edu

Hematol Oncol Clin N Am 36 (2022) 829–851
https://doi.org/10.1016/j.hoc.2022.03.011
0889-8588/22/© 2022 Elsevier Inc. All rights reserved.

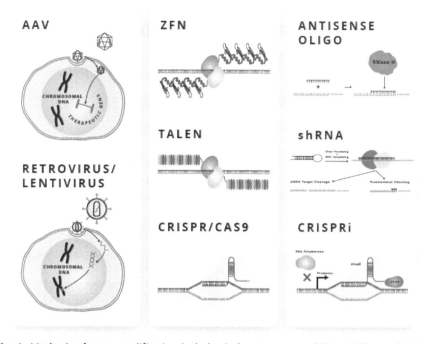

Fig. 1. Methods of gene modification include viral vector gene addition (*left panel*), site-specific gene editing (*middle panel*), and gene silencing (*right panel*).

in the genome, and gene silencing to reduce the expression of a gene or genes (**Fig. 1**). These gene-modification platforms can be delivered either *in vivo*, for which the therapy is injected directed into a patient's body, or *ex vivo*, in which cells are harvested from a patient and modified in a laboratory setting, and then returned to the patient (**Fig. 2**).

The development of genome modification as a therapeutic has been particularly prolific for diseases classified as inborn errors of immunity (IEI). This includes more than 400 known monogenic germline mutations resulting in increased susceptibility to a range of infectious diseases with associated comorbidities such as autoimmunity, inflammation, atopy, and malignancy.[1] To encourage a deeper understanding of the gene modification approaches and portray the current landscape of gene therapies for primary immune deficiencies, this review focuses on a selection of non-severe combined immunodeficiency (SCID) IEI as examples of (1) when viral vector gene therapy may be the most beneficial approach, (2) when gene editing is essential, and (3) diseases in which extensive preclinical and clinical experience with viral vector gene therapy has been successful but has also highlighted the need for either improved vector designs or a more targeted approach.

VIRAL VECTOR GENE THERAPY

Retroviral vectors efficiently deliver transgenes owing to their high transduction ability and long evolved mechanisms for innate immune avoidance. Following the infection of a host cell, reverse transcriptase converts viral RNA into a DNA copy, which then stably integrates into the host genome. Two subtypes of retroviruses, gamma-

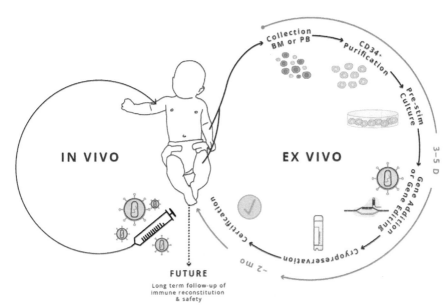

Fig. 2. *In vivo* and *ex vivo* delivery methods for gene therapy. The *ex vivo* diagram depicts the process commonly used for treating diseases of the hematopoietic system such as inborn errors of immunity. HSCT can be collected from the peripheral blood or bone marrow, purified for the more primitive CD34+ fraction which is then placed in culture for gene addition or editing. Following gene modification, cells are cryopreserved and then undergo full certification before being returned to the patient as an autologous transplant.

retroviruses and lentiviruses, have been used extensively for research and clinical gene therapy purposes.[2]

Gamma-retroviral vectors (gRVs), a simple retrovirus, are characterized by high titers as well as high transduction efficiency, but cannot shuttle their cargo across the nuclear membrane. Instead, gRVs wait until the breakdown of the nuclear membrane during mitosis, limiting their use to actively dividing cells. Early clinical studies using these vectors noted concerning insertional mutagenesis following integration near a proto-oncogene and transactivation by strong retroviral enhancers. On the other hand, lentiviral vectors (LVs) based on human immunodeficiency virus-1 (HIV-1) are more versatile as they can be used to infect both dividing and nondividing cell types. Moreover, the LV is highly optimized and there are now 2nd generation and 3rd generation systems that differ in terms of accessory proteins, number of packaging plasmids, and the promoter driving the expression of the viral RNA. The 3rd generation further improves on the safety profile of the 2nd generation with more replication-incompetent features and a self-inactivating (SIN) design by the elimination of the promoter in the U3 region of 3′LTR of the provirus. Due to the improved safety profile as well as the ability to transduce nondividing cell types, the use of LVs for gene therapy has become more common than yRVs.[3,4] A summary of clinical trials of gene therapy for non-SCID IEI is shown in **Table 1** while approaches in development are shown in **Table 2**.

Fanconi Anemia is an IEI for which viral vector gene therapy may be the most beneficial gene modification approach. FANCA is one of the largest genes in the Fanconi complementation group and accounts for Fanconi Anemia in >60% of cases. FANCA

Table 1
Clinical trials of gene therapy for non-SCID inborn errors of immunity

Disease	Approach	HSPC Source	NCT#	Outcomes	Reference
Fanconi Anemia	γRV: G1FASVNa FANCC	PBSC	NCT00001399	• G-CSF mobilization alone provided poor mobilization in 2/3 patients • No correction in engrafted LT-HSCs but transient improvement noted	Liu et al,[8]1999
	γRV: MSCV-FANCA	PBSC	NCT00271089 NCT00272857	• Significant depletion of CD34 compartment before pancytopenia • Extended mobilization and multiple collections may be necessary	Croop et al,[79]2001; Kelly et al,[7]2007
	LV: PGK-FANCA-WPRE	PBSC	NCT01331018	• Highlighted need for more robust CD34 enrichment strategies • Gene marking noted only in primitive populations	Tolar et al,[80]2011
		PBSC	NCT02931071 NCT02678533 FANCOLEN-I	• 55% of total PB and BM cells gene corrected in patients without conditioning (at 30 mo posttreatment)	www.Eurofancolen.eu
	LV: PGK-FANCA-WPRE	PBSC	NCT03157804	• 43.5% of BM CD34 gene marked at 24 mo posttreatment	Rio et al,[5]2019

Disease	Vector			Details	Reference
Chronic Granulomatous Disease	γRV: MFGS-p47	PBSC	-	• 5 patients treated • Peak short-term correction of 0.004%–0.05% of total peripheral blood granulocytes • No conditioning administered	Malech et al,[23] 1997
	γRV: MFGS-gp91^{phox}	PBSC	-	• 6 patients treated • Only short-term gene marking in neutrophils • No conditioning administered	Malech et al,[81] 2004, E. M. Kang et al,[24] 2010a
	γRV: SFFV-gp91phox	PBSC	00,927,134	• 2 patients treated • Activating insertions in MDS1-EVI1, PRDM16 or SETBP1	Ott et al,[25] 2006
	γRV: MFGS-gp91^{phox}	PBSC	-	• 3 patients treated • Long-term marking in 1.1% and 0.03% of neutrophils in 2 patients • No clonal dominance	E. M. Kang et al,[24] 2010
	γRV: MT-gp91	PBSC	-	• 2 patients treated • Gene-marked cells ranged from 0.08% to 0.5% after 3 y (0.05%–0.21% NADPH oxidase activity) • No abnormal cell expansion, but vector integration sites observed near proto-oncogenes (MDS1-EVI1, PRDM16, and CCND2)	H. J. Kang et al,[82] 2011
	LV: pCCLchimGP91WPRE (G1XCGD)	PBSC	01,855,685 02,234,934	• 13 patients treated (analysis available for 9)	Kohn, Booth, et al,[84] 2020

(continued on next page)

Table 1
(continued)

Disease	Approach	HSPC Source	NCT#	Outcomes	Reference
				• 2 died of preexisting disease • 6 of 7 surviving patients with stable VCN and oxidase-positive neutrophils • 3 newly treated pediatric patients had initially high neutrophil recovery but poor engraftment of gene-marked cells	
Leukocyte Adhesion Deficiency Type I	γRV: MLV-CD18	BM	-	• 2 patients treated • No significant engraftment • No conditioning administered	Bauer & Hickstein,[83]2000
	LV: Chim-CD18-WPRE	PBSC	03,812,263	• 9 patients treated • No drug-related SAEs • All with sustained CD18 restoration	Kohn, Rao, et al[84]2020
Wiskott-Aldrich Syndrome	γRV: SFFV-WAS	PBSC	-	• 10 patients treated, 9 with gene marking • 7 (and possibly up to 9) had myelodysplasia related to insertional oncogenesis	Braun et al,[36]2014
	LV: w1.6_hWASP_WPRE (LV-w1.6 W)	BM or PBSC	01,515,462	• 3 patients treated • Reduced-intensity conditioning • Stable engraftment of WASP-expression cells	Aiuti et al,[38]2013

Vector	Cell source	Identifier	Outcomes	Reference
LV: w1.6_hWASP_WPRE (LV-w1.6 W)	BM or PBSC	02,333,760 01,347,346 01,347,242	• 9 patients treated • Myeloablative conditioning • 8 of 9 living with stable engraftment of gene-marked cells and no vector-related toxicity	Hacein-Bey Abina et al,[85]2015 Magnani et al,[86]2022
LV: w1.6_hWASP_WPRE (LV-w1.6 W)	PBSC and/or BM	01,410,825	• 5 patients treated • Stable multilineage vector gene marking • No clonal expansion • Myeloablative conditioning	Labrosse et al,[41]2019

Table 2
Gene modification approaches in development for non-SCID inborn errors of immunity

Disease	Approach	Corrective Donor	Reference
Ataxia telangiectasia	LV	EF1α-ATM-WPRE	Carranza et al,[87]2018
CARD9 deficiency	LV	CARD9[a]	Kreitzer et al,[88]2020
IL10RB deficiency	LV or Editing (TALEN)	LV: CBX3-EFS-IL10RB-WPRE[b] Editing: AAV6 cDNA[b]	Hoffman et al,2021
IFNγR1	LV	SFFV.Ifnγr1, miR223. Ifnγr1, or MSP.Ifnγr1	Hetzel et al,[89]2018
	LV	SFFV.IFNγR1.iGFP	Hahn et al,[90]2020
MUNC13 (HLH)	γRV	EFS-LNGFR-P2A-MUNC13D-WPRE[1]	Dettmer et al,[91]2019
	LV	MND-UNC13D[b] EFS-UNC13D[b]	Takushi et al,[92]2020
Perforin (HLH)	LV	PGK/PRF-Perforin1[a]	Tiwari et al,[93]2015
	γRV	PGK-PRF	Ghosh et al,[94]2018
IPEX	LV	EF1α-FOXP3	Passerini et al,[64]2013
	LV	EF1α-FOXP3	Santoni De Sio et al,[66]2017
		PGK-FOXP3	
	LV	CNS123p-FOXP3	Masiuk et al,[67]2019
	LV	EF1α-FOXP3	Sato et al,[65]2020
	LV or Editing (CRISPR/Cas9)	LV: EF1a-FOXP3[1] Editing: AAV6 cDNA[1]	Goodwin et al,[95]2020
Severe Congenital Neutropenia	Editing (CRISPR/Cas9)	N/A (frameshift mutations)	Rao et al,[96]2019
	Editing (CRISPR/Cas9)	AAV6 Exons 1–3[b] or AAV6 Exons 4–5[b]	Ritter et al,[97]2019
	Editing (CRISPR/Cas9)	AAV6 Exon 4[b]	Tran et al,[98]2020
STAT3 Hyper IgE Syndrome	Editing (Adenine Base Editing)	N/A	Eberherr et al,[99]2021

Disease	Approach	Construct	Reference
X-linked Agammaglobulinemia	γRV	MSCV-huBTK-SAR	Yu et al,[47]2004
	LV	EμB29-Btk-WPRE	Kerns et al,[100]2010
	LV	EFS-coBtk-WPRE[b]	Ng et al,[101]2010
		CD19-coBtk-WPRE[b]	
	LV	UCOE-BTKp-CoBTK[b]	Seymour et al,[53]2021
	Editing (CRISPR/Cas9)	AAV6 cDNA[b]	Gray et al,[55]2021
X-linked Chronic Granulomatous Disease	Editing (ZFN targeting AAVS1)	AAV6 cDNA	De Ravin et al,[30]2016; Merling et al,[29]2015, Zou et al,[31]2011
	Editing (TALEN or CRISPR/Cas9)	ssODN targeting CYBB C676 T mutation	De Ravin et al,[102]2017
	Editing (CRISPR/Cas9)	ssODN targeting CYBB C676 T mutation	De Ravin et al,[34]2021
X-linked Hyper-IgM Syndrome	Editing (TALEN)	AAV6 cDNA[b]	Hubbard et al,[16]2016
	Editing (TALEN or CRISPR/Cas9)	AAV6 cDNA[b]	Kuo et al,[17]2018
	Gene Editing (CRISPR/Cas9)	AAV6 cDNA[b]	Vavassori et al,[18]2021
X-linked Lymphoproliferative disease	LV	EFS-SAP-WPRE[b]	Rivat et al,[103]2013
	γRV or LV	EFS-SAP-WPRE[b]	Panchal et al,[104]2018
XMEN	Editing (CRISPR/Cas9)	AAV6 cDNA[b]	Brault et al,[105]2021
WAS	Editing (TALEN or CRISPR/Cas9)	AAV6 cDNA[a]	Khan et al,[106]2016
	Editing (CRISPR/Cas9)	AAV6 cDNA[b]	Rai et al,[43]2020
	Editing (CRISPR/Cas9 nanoblades)	AAV6 SFFV-GFP	Gutierrez-Guerrero et al,[107]2021

[a] Indicates promoter and/or codon-optimization not reported.
[b] Indicates use of codon-optimized/codon-divergent donor sequence.

spans 79 kilobases (kb) on chromosome 16 with a cDNA length of 5452 bp and 1455 amino acids (AA) in the protein. FANCA plays an important role in DNA repair and shows a preference for single-stranded DNA (ssDNA) over double-stranded DNA (dsDNA). FANCA is also thought to participate in hematopoiesis during the development of the embryo as mutations in the gene lead to severe defects in hematopoiesis during the first decade of life with 70% to 80% of patients experiencing bone marrow failure.[5] The high rates of marrow failure create the need for early-treatment of the disease and make patients with Fanconi Anemia excellent candidates for gene therapy.

Current clinical translation focuses on gRV as well as LV therapies and will likely remain this way for some time. When combined with homology arms, the longest transcript far exceeds the 4.7 kb packaging capacity of adeno-associated virus (AAV) used in gene-editing approaches. LVs lacks stringent size cutoffs for transgenes, and the reduction in titer and transduction efficiency common for large cargos[6] can be overcome to some degree with transduction enhancers.

Hematopoietic stem cells (HSC) from a patient affected by Fanconi Anemia are highly sensitive to oxygen and TNF-a levels. The sensitivity of Fanconi Anemia HSCs places restrictions on the culture conditions and may restrict gene therapy approaches to lentiviral mediated therapies. Numerous efforts in the clinic, as well as xenogeneic transplant models, failed to achieve detectable numbers of engraftable cells and transduction protocols were revised to tailor to the unique properties of these cells.[7,8] Río and colleagues demonstrated that shortening *ex vivo* culture time to 24 hours (as opposed to 48), culturing patient cells in hypoxic conditions, and adding the antioxidant N-acetylcysteine to cultures could lead to human cell engraftment in a mouse model.[5] The viability of the cells remained more than 88% and resulted in a final average VCN of about 0.4 copies/cell using their highly modified protocol. Interestingly, the group also confirmed the long hypothesized increased fitness of corrected cells with a 6.4-fold increase in progenitors after 4 weeks *in vivo* compared with *in vitro* results. Investigators then translated these preclinical results into the first clinical study to achieve engraftment of gene-corrected cells in patients. The response in patients was highly variable, with final VCNs in bone marrow CD34s ranging from 0.05 to 0.4. It should be noted that inclusion criteria for patients were evidence of bone marrow failure and earlier treatment following further clinical validation could lead to more consistent results due to improved stem cell health and numbers at collection (but potentially less selective advantage). Nevertheless, robust competition was noted with patients reaching gene marking in 55% of peripheral blood leukocytes.

Site-Specific Gene Editing

Viral vectors pose 3 major safety concerns: the possibility of replication-competent virus production, oncogenesis from random insertion, and deleterious effects due to dysregulated expression of the therapeutic transgene. To avoid these complications, targeted gene editing has gained popularity in the field. Gene insertion is mediated by site-specific programmable nucleases, most commonly zinc finger nucleases (ZFN), transcription activator-like effector nucleases (TALEN), and CRISPR/Cas9. Nuclease-mediated cleavage of the genomic target may then be resolved by nonhomologous end joining (NHEJ), homology-directed repair (HDR), or, in the case of base editing, the base excision repair pathway (**Fig. 3**A).

Following the creation of double-stranded breaks (DSB) by any of the nuclease platforms, either NHEJ or HDR may occur to repair the breakage. For the NHEJ-mediated DSB repair pathway, the broken ends recruit the Ku70/Ku80 heterodimer, which binds DNA-PK and DNA lig-IV to help join the compatible ends together. As a result, NHEJ commonly results in small insertions or deletions (indels) that cause loss-of-function

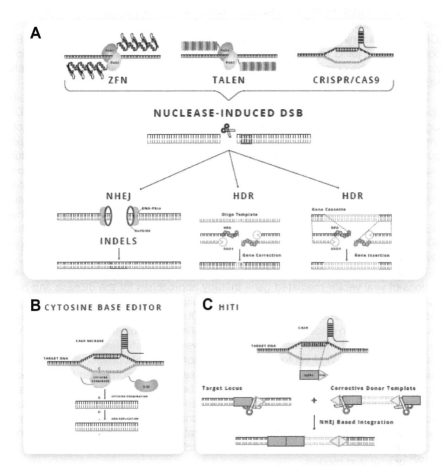

Fig. 3. (*A*) DNA repair pathways following nuclease-mediated DSBs can result in NHEJ-mediated indels or HDR events using homologous donors delivered as single-stranded oligo-deoxynucleotides or larger gene cassettes. (*B*) Schematic of a cytosine base editor. (*C*) Homology Independent Targeted Integration (HITI), an NHEJ-based gene-editing approach. NHEJ is an error-prone process and can occur during any phase of the cell cycle. HDR requires a homologous template and is generally restricted to the S/G2 phases of the cell cycle. Both base editors and HITI would not be affected by the cell cycle state.

mutations of the targeted gene. To achieve more precise editing such as single nucleotide changes or insertions of larger DNA cassettes, HDR-mediated DSB repair pathway using a homologous donor template is required. For therapeutic correction of mutations, the donor template is typically either single-stranded oligos (ssODN) or an AAV delivered HDR template. As opposed to NHEJ, which occurs throughout all cell cycles, HDR is restricted to the S and G_2 phases of the cell cycle. For this reason, researchers have attempted to improve integration efficiency by exploiting the NHEJ pathway through Homology Independent Targeted Integration (HITI), in which flanking guide RNA target sites excise the donor cassette to facilitate end-trapping at the genomic locus.

Lastly, to overcome the limitations of HDR, base editors (BEs) were developed to install small substitutions.[9] There are currently 2 types of BEs—cytosine base editors (CBEs) and adenine base editors (ABEs) (**Fig. 3**B). Without making DSBs, CBEs convert C to T (or G to A on the complementary strand), and ABEs convert A to G (or T to C on the complementary strand). For genomic targeting, newer generation BEs use Cas9 nickase bound to a cytidine or adenine deaminase.

X-Linked Hyper IgM Syndrome is the classic example of an IEI that requires site-specific gene modification approaches. The disease results from defects in CD40 Ligand (CD40L), a transmembrane protein transiently expressed on the surface of T lymphocytes during immune activation that binds to CD40 on B cells to the signal production of class-switched immunoglobulin. Affected individuals are unable to produce class-switched antibodies and are therefore susceptible to a range of infections, including recurrent upper and lower respiratory tract infections, opportunistic infections, and gastrointestinal infections with hepatobiliary disease and a predisposition to develop autoimmune/autoinflammatory complications and malignancy. Allogeneic HSCT can be curative with posttransplant survival rates ranging from 60 to more than 80%. However, up to 40% of patients have been reported to develop significant acute GvHD, veno-occlusive disease, worsening or infections, and death.[10–12]

The tightly regulated nature of CD40L expression was emphasized in early investigations of viral vector-mediated gene therapy approaches for the disease and highlights this as one in which targeted gene editing is essential. Using the murine model of disease, gene addition of murine CD40L cDNA through gRVs resulted in immune reconstitution evidenced by immunoglobulin production and immune responses to vaccination and infectious challenges. However, constitutive expression of the transgene from the viral vector resulted in abnormal lymphoproliferation with many mice progressing to frank lymphomas.[13,14] These results emphasized that the modification of very tightly regulated genes needs to be accomplished in a more regulated manner, making this an ideal candidate for gene-editing approaches. Subsequent work investigating LVs that delivered CD40L under control of a 1.3kb fragment of the endogenous proximal promoter demonstrated near-physiologic expression in T cells on immune stimulation,[15] but this approach has not been evaluated in primary HSPC or in *in vivo* models.

Gene editing in primary T cells was first reported for XHIM using TALEN mRNA targeting the 5′UTR of the gene codelivered with an AAV6 carrying a codon-divergent CD40L cDNA followed by the endogenous 3′UTR or the WPRE sequence.[16] Gene-editing rates of ~35% and ~45% were achieved using each of the homologous donor constructs, with normal protein expression and binding to CD40 as measured by flow cytometry. In addition, edited XHIM-patient CD4 T cells possessed a broad TCR repertoire and were able to induce naïve B-cell class switching *in vitro*. Following this initial report, TALENs and CRISPRs were compared for their editing ability at the CD40L gene in XHIM patient T cells as well as healthy donor-derived HPSC.[17] Both nuclease platforms achieved efficient gene integration in primary T lymphocytes with physiologically restored protein expression and function. In addition, healthy donor-derived HPSC achieved average editing rates of 21% with TALENS and 15% with CRISPR/Cas9 *in vitro*. The addition of adenoviral helper proteins (E4Orf6 and E1B55K H354 mutant), which were previously reported to enhance CRISPR-mediated gene disruption and augment AAV transduction of certain cells, increased integration rates by about 1.5-fold *in vitro*. Similar to other studies of gene editing of human hematopoietic stem cells, levels of gene editing decreased *in vivo* when transplanted into immunodeficient NSG mice. On average, integration rates in the bone marrow of transplanted mice ranged from 0.3% to 22% and averaged 4.4% across treatment groups. CRISPR/Cas9 gene editing for XHIM has been additionally demonstrated by other groups focusing on the translation of T cell editing for early-stage clinical trials.[18]

Lessons Learned from Current Clinical Trials of Gene Therapy for IEI

There are several IEI for which gene therapy has been tested extensively in preclinical work and in clinical trials. The following diseases are primary immune deficiency diseases for which vector gene therapy has shown great promise, and even life-saving for many individuals, but also highlight that improvement in vector design or a more targeted approach may be needed.

Chronic granulomatous disease (CGD) encompasses a group of defects in the nicotinamide adenine dinucleotide phosphate (NADPH) oxidase complex in phagocytes that result in the inability of neutrophils, macrophages, and monocytes to eliminate bacterial and fungal pathogens. Patients are prone to developing granulomas of various organs, particularly the gastrointestinal and genitourinary tracts. The most common form of CGD is X-linked due to mutations in the CYBB gene that encodes gp91phox, a member of the 5-protein complex that makes up NADPH. On diagnosis, patients are started on antibacterial and antifungal prophylaxis with close monitoring of and aggressive treatment of infectious complications. Allogeneic HSCT can be curative for the disease, and while there are generally better outcomes in younger patients, there have also been promising outcomes with reduced-intensity conditioning regimens in older patients with CGD-related infections and inflammatory issues.[19]

The utility of gene therapy for the treatment of X-linked chronic granulomatous disease (XCGD) was initially demonstrated in the 1990s using gRV gene transfer.[20,21] Even relatively low levels of oxidase activity was predicted to result in clinical benefit as female carriers with skewed lyonization for the mutated allele but with at least 10% neutrophil activity were reported to lack infectious complications.[22] Early phase clinical trials achieved very low levels of gene marking, particularly without Busulfan conditioning.[23,24] Additional patients enrolled in Europe and Asia using gRVs combined with reduced-intensity conditioning experienced clinical benefit from the treatment, but 3 developed myelodysplasia due to vector insertions near growth promoting genes, particularly MDS1/EVI1 and PRDM16, followed by transactivation by the spleen focus-forming virus (SFFV) LTR.[25,26] To improve on the safety of the vector, current clinical trials for XCGD use LVs containing a chimeric internal promoter designed to drive gp91phox expression in phagocytes.[27] In ongoing parallel clinical trials in the United States, United Kingdom, and a compassionate-use program, additional patients with severe XCGD have been treated with significant clinical benefit in surviving patients and no evidence of clonal dysregulation thus far.[28]

While viral-mediated gene therapy for XCGD has evolved significantly in the last 30 years and has been life-saving for many patients, there remains the risk of insertional oncogenesis as well as lower levels of protein production compared with cells from unaffected individuals.[28] Multiple strategies for site-specific gene insertion at the CYBB locus, beginning with ZFN-mediated integration of a gp91phox cassette at the AAVS1 "safe harbor" locus within intron 1 of the PPP1R12C gene, have been investigated.[29–31]

To evaluate targeted gene transfer at the endogenous CYBB locus, TALENs and Cas9 were also designed to target either replacement of a single exon or an exon 1 to 13 minigene at exon 1.[32] In patient-derived iPSC, site-specific replacement of exon 5 restored gp91phox expression and ROS production but the insertion of a larger minigene only restored gp91phox and ROS activity when leaving exon/intron1 and replacing only exons 2 to 13. These results highlighted that for certain genes, retention of intronic sequences may be needed for expression when using the endogenous promoter. In addition to evaluating single exon replacement, single-stranded oligo-deoxynucleotides (ssODN) were also used to repair a frequent C676 substitution in exon 7 of the *CYBB* gene.[33] Rates of gene editing in patient-derived X-CGD HSPC ranged from 12% to 31% *in vitro,* and when transplanted into NSG mice, about 16% of human myeloid cells present in the peripheral blood of mice expressed gp91phox and possessed NADPH oxidase activity as measured by DHR. Transient inhibition of p53-binding protein 1 (53BP1), a protein that favors nonhomologous end-joining, though i53 mRNA doubled rates of gene integration when using a ssODN donor but not with AAV6 to deliver larger gene cassettes.[34]

Wiskott-Aldrich Syndrome (WAS) Between 2006 and 2009, 10 patients were enrolled in the first clinical trial of gene therapy for severe WAS, a disease classically characterized by bleeding episodes due to small platelets, eczema, and recurrent infections with a predisposition for autoimmunity and lymphoid malignancies. Patients were conditioned with reduced-intensity Busulfan condition and received autologous HSPC transduced with a gRV expressing the WAS protein (WASp). 9 of 10 patients reconstituted with gene marked cells, and while there was initial improvement in the laboratory and clinical indices, at least 7 (and possibly up to 9) have been reported to have myelodysplasia or leukemia, many of which were related to *LMO2* and *MDS-EVI1* insertional oncogenesis.[35,36] This initial clinical trial highlighted the need for improved gene therapy approaches, particularly as allogeneic HSCT outcomes have significantly improved in recent years. For instance, in a recent report of 129 patients with WAS who were transplanted between 2005 and 2015 throughout various centers in the US and Canada, the 5-year overall survival was 91% regardless of stem cell source.[37]

Subsequently, LV-based clinical trials opened in Europe and the US; while the same vector design using a 1.6kb fragment of the endogenous WAS promoter to regulate WASp expression was used at 4 clinical trial sites, different degrees of myelo-/immunosuppression were implemented. As reviewed by Ferrua and colleagues, at least 34 patients have been treated with 31 currently living.[38–42] Patients experienced clinical benefits including improved immune function, decreased need for antimicrobials or IVIG, and overall decreased incidence of severe bleeding episodes. However, because WASp expression was suboptimal, some patients continued to have bleeding events and required intermittent platelet transfusions.

To achieve more physiologic expression of WASp, a CRISPR/Cas9 editing approach at the endogenous gene locus has been demonstrated to be effective in primary HPSC.[43] Co-delivery of Cas9 with an AAV6 containing a promoterless WAS cDNA achieved an average of 46% or 25% targeted integration depending on the donor construct used (BGH polyA signal or WAS 3'UTR, respectively). In addition, the percentage of cells that expressed WASp by flow cytometry correlated almost exactly with the percentage of gene integration, in contrast to cells transduced with the clinical WAS LV in which a VCN of 1 restored WASp expression in only about 34% of cells. Gene-modified patient-derived HSPC gave rise to functional macrophages and mature platelets with normal WASp expression in *in vitro* differentiation protocols. In addition, gene-editing WAS HSPC retained repopulating ability in murine models with WASp expression of 37% in primary and 16% in secondary transplants in the bone marrow. This work is currently in the translational stage of development moving toward an early phase clinical trial.

X-linked agammaglobulinemia (XLA) is an immune deficiency caused by loss-of-function mutations in the Bruton's Tyrosine Kinase (*BTK*) gene. The disease is characterized by a block in early B cell development, which results in a lack of mature B cells and antibody production. Without functional antibodies, patients with XLA suffer from multiple infectious complications including respiratory and skin infections, gastroenteritis, and invasive infections such as sepsis and meningitis.[44,45] While allogeneic HSCT can be curative for XLA,[46] life-long antibody supplementation remains the preferable treatment option given the potential risks that accompany transplant.

Over the last decade, multiple groups have explored *ex vivo* gene addition strategies through the use of gRVs or LVs. Earlier work showed that a gRV expressing human BTK successfully rescued BTK-dependent B cell development and function in the XLA analogous Btk$^{-/-}$Tec$^{-/-}$ mouse model. This work established the feasibility of gene therapy for the treatment of XLA and provided evidence for the selective advantage of cells that carry a functional copy of *BTK*.[47–50] Following reports of insertional oncogenesis related to gRV, there was a shift to the exploration of LVs as a safer alternative for gene addition in the treatment of XLA.

The first LV-based gene transfer for XLA also showed Btk-dependent B cell reconstitution in the XLA mouse model, as well as improved T-independent immune response and proliferation in response to B-cell mitogens. The viral construct contained the Eμ immunoglobulin heavy chain enhancer and B29 minimal promoter elements to help drive B-lineage specific expression. While largely successful, there was evidence of epigenetic silencing of the promoter/enhancer elements in secondary transplants. In addition, restoration of BTK expression was limited to the B-cell lineage and was absent in myeloid cells, which are known to express BTK.[51] Inclusion of the ubiquitous chromatin opening elements (UCOEs)[52] to address epigenetic silencing and an endogenous BTK minimal promoter element facilitated BTK expression in both B- and myeloid cells.[53]

An important point raised in the above studies was the relative expression of BTK from a transgene compared with endogenous BTK expression. While lower expression may limit therapeutic potential, aiming to achieve the highest possible BTK expression is unlikely a viable strategy. There is concern that overexpression of BTK relative to normal physiologic levels may be correlated with certain B lymphoid leukemias.[54] Because of the tight regulation of endogenous BTK expression, a targeted editing strategy may represent a safer alternative. Recent work exploring this gene-editing approach in cell lines showed that sgRNA targeting intron 1 of *BTK* in combination with a cDNA donor template resulted in BTK protein expression close to WT levels. Up to 20% targeted integration was achieved in healthy donor PBSCs.[55]

While this level of targeted integration is seemingly enough to result in therapeutic levels of BTK expression, multiple groups have shown low engraftment and/or reduction in the editing of HDR-based edited HSPCs when transitioning to *in vivo* models.[56,57] This phenomenon is in part due to the quiescent nature of the most primitive HSC that exist mostly in G$_0$/G$_1$ and are less likely to undergo HDR which preferentially occurs during S/G$_2$.[58,59] To address this issue, BTK cDNA corrective donor templates that use non–HDR-based DNA repair mechanisms such as NHEJ and MMEJ have also been explored. Most of the editing events were found to occur in the more differentiated progenitor cells while there were comparable levels of targeted integration in the immunophenotypic HSC fraction (CD34+, CD38-, CD45RA-, CD90+) with NHEJ, MMEJ, and HDR-based repair approaches.[60]

Immune dysregulation, polyendocrinopathy, enteropathy, X-linked (IPEX) syndrome is a severe monogenic, immune disorder caused by mutations in the *FOXP3* gene. It is an early-onset multiorgan disease with autoimmune-related manifestations such as eczema, enteropathy, and type 1 diabetes, with deaths typically in infancy or early childhood.[61] FOXP3 is known as the master transcription factor in T$_{reg}$ cells, playing a critical in their regulatory function. Treatment of IPEX is currently limited to symptom management through immunosuppression or replacement therapies, with HSCT as the only available curative option.[62,63]

Gene addition-based approaches to overexpress normal FOXP3 in IPEX CD4+ T cells have been demonstrated using LVs. Treated CD4^{FOXP3} T cells acquired T_{reg} like characteristics and function *in vitro* and *in vivo*.[64,65] However, the long-term efficacy and survivability of T_{reg} cells *in vivo* remains unknown, and there are known adverse effects of FOXP3 overexpression on HSPC proliferation and differentiation.[66] Therefore, any FOXP3 gene therapy hoping to use long-term HSPCs likely needs to be under more regulated FOXP3 control, which has been accomplished through the inclusion of endogenous FOXP3 regulatory elements.[67]

Recent work exploring targeted gene editing for IPEX used a Cas9 targeting exon 1 of FOXP3 along with a FOXP3 cDNA donor template as AAV6. ~30% gene integration of the FOXP3 donor construct was detected in human CD34$^+$ HSPCs, which were able to engraft and differentiate *in vivo*. FOXP3 edited primary T_{eff} also had similar FOXP3 protein expression levels, cytokine production levels, and proliferation rates to WT unmodified T cells. However, while edited T_{regs} showed similar T_{reg} marker expression profiles (CD25, CTLA-4, HELIOS) to WT unmodified T_{regs}, the overall suppressive capacity was diminished in comparison. It was noted that this was likely due to the lower overall FOXP3 protein expression in the edited T_{regs}. Importantly, after transplant of edited HSPCs in neonatal NSG-SGM3 mice, FOXP3$^+$ T_{regs} isolated from the spleen were found to have a similar suppressive capacity compared with their WT counterpart.[66] Overall, this work is an important step forward toward realizing targeted gene editing as a viable therapeutic strategy for IPEX.

Challenges in Gene Editing

Nuclease specificity

One of the major challenges for any of the gene-editing platforms is genotoxicity. Identification of the optimal locus for on-target editing while minimizing off-target activity is a critical aspect of their use and can be aided by *in silico* design tools available that account for not only the DNA sequence but also more complex factors such as G/C content, chromatin state, and exon position.[56] There have also been improvements in nuclease and sgRNA technology and production such as more specific high fidelity Cas9 proteins, chemically synthesized/modified sgRNAs, as well as obligate heterodimeric Fok1 nuclease in the case of ZFNs or TALENs.[68–71] Despite these advances, off-target activity remains a real concern and the use of any targeted nuclease must be accompanied by multiple detection methods of unintended genome modification. GUIDE-seq, CIRCLE-seq, DIGENOME-seq, and DISCOVER-seq are only some of the techniques available to identify these off-target sites or chromosomal aberrations and help establish an overall greater safety profile of targeted nucleases.

Adeno-Associated Virus Packaging/Donor Template Limitations

A significant challenge specific to the targeted gene integration strategy is in the introduction of the homologous donor template and more specifically the delivery of large transgenes. Currently, the use of an adeno-associated virus is the most efficient method for introducing the donor template molecule, but they are limited by their 4.5kb cargo capacity. While 4.5kb is sufficient for some IEI, many others such as DOCK8 deficiency require a much larger capacity. Potential solutions for large transgene delivery include division of the donor template into several sections or the use of alternative viral vectors with larger packaging capacities such as Integrase-defective lentivirus (IDLV).[72–74] However, the therapeutic potential of the multi-AAV or IDLV approach in the context of PIDs remains to be explored.

Homology-Directed Repair and Maintaining Hematopoietic Stem Cell Repopulating Capacity

Reaching the highest levels of HDR while maintaining the self-renewing and engrafting characteristics of HSC is likely the biggest challenge facing HDR-based editing. HSPCs naturally exist in a quiescent G_0/G_1 state, making NHEJ the preferred DNA repair pathway. To circumvent this cell cycle limitation, groups have implemented modifications to reduce Cas9 activity in G_1 while maintaining editing capacity in S/G_2,[75] while others have implemented the use of small molecules to either inhibit NHEJ or increase rates of HDR.[76,77] In addition, the use of transient i53 expression to inhibit the NHEJ promoting repair protein 53BP1 has been reported to achieve higher HDR rates in HSPCs *in vitro*.[32] While maximizing HDR rates is an important factor, maintaining the long-term engraftment potential of edited HSPCs is also critical. Several groups have reported substantial loss or lack of persistence of HDR-based edited HSPCs *in vivo*. To overcome this issue, there has been a significant investigation into optimizing HSC culture conditions, fine-tuning editing protocols, and inclusion of small molecules such as StemRegenin 1, dmPGE2, and UM171.[10,72,78] This will be a critical element to allow gene-editing approaches to continue to advance to the clinic.

SUMMARY

In all, the field of gene therapy possesses great potential to change the way many monogenic diseases, particularly of the immune system, are treated. As improvements in genome modification approaches are developed along with improvements in early diagnosis of disease, medical management, and bone marrow conditioning, it is hoped that there can be even better outcomes for those with rare and once fatal diseases.

CLINICS CARE POINTS

- Clinical trials of viral vector gene therapy is available for several IEI including Fanconi Anemia, Chronic Granulomatous Disease, Leukocyte Adhesion Deficiency Type I, and Wiskott-Aldrich Syndrome.

- Early gene therapy trials have demonstrated that some degree of bone marrow conditioning is required to create room in the marrow niche for gene modified cells to engraft.

DISCLOSURE

The authors have nothing to disclose.

REFERENCES

1. Tangye SG, Al-Herz Waleed, Bousfiha Aziz, et al. Human Inborn Errors of Immunity: 2019 Update on the Classification from the International Union of Immunological Societies Expert Committee. J Clin Immunol 2020;40:24–64.
2. Thomas CE, Ehrhardt A, Kay MA. Progress and problems with the use of viral vectors for gene therapy. Nat Rev Genet 2003;4:346–58.
3. Milone MC, O'Doherty U. Clinical use of lentiviral vectors. Leukemia 2018;32:1529–41.

4. Bulcha JT, Wang Y, Ma H, et al. Viral vector platforms within the gene therapy landscape. Signal Transduct Target Ther 2021;6.

5. Río P, Navarro S, Wang W, et al. Successful engraftment of gene-corrected hematopoietic stem cells in non-conditioned patients with Fanconi anemia. Nat Med 2019;25:1396–401.

6. Han J, Tam K, Ma F, et al. β-Globin Lentiviral Vectors Have Reduced Titers due to Incomplete Vector RNA Genomes and Lowered Virion Production. Stem Cell Rep 2021;16:198–211.

7. Kelly PF, Radtke S, von Kalle C, et al. Stem cell collection and gene transfer in fanconi anemia. Mol Ther 2007;15:211–9.

8. Liu JM, Kim S, Read EJ, et al. Engraftment of hematopoietic progenitor cells transduced with the Fanconi anemia group C gene (FANCC). Hum Gene Ther 1999;10:2337–46.

9. Gaudelli NM, Komor AC, Rees HA, et al. Programmable base editing of T to G C in genomic DNA without DNA cleavage. Nature 2017;551:464–71.

10. Genovese P, Schiroli G, Escobar G, et al. Targeted genome editing in human repopulating haematopoietic stem cells. Nature 2014;510:235–40.

11. Mitsui-Sekinaka K, Imai K, Sato H, et al. Clinical features and hematopoietic stem cell transplantations for CD40 ligand deficiency in Japan. J Allergy Clin Immunol 2015;1–7. https://doi.org/10.1016/j.jaci.2015.02.020.

12. de la Morena MT, Leonard D, Torgerson TR, et al. Long-term outcomes of 176 patients with X-linked hyper-IgM syndrome treated with or without hematopoietic cell transplantation. J Allergy Clin Immunol 2017;139:1282–92.

13. Sacco MG, Ungari M, Cato EM, et al. Suggest the need for tight regulation in gene therapy approaches to hyper immunoglobulin M (IgM) syndrome. Cancer Gene Ther 2000;7:1299–306.

14. Brown MP, Topham DJ, Sangster MY, et al. Thymic lymphoproliferative disease after successful correction of CD40 ligand deficiency by gene transfer in mice. Nat Med 1998;4:1253–60.

15. Romero Z, Torres S, Cobo M, et al. A tissue-specific, activation-inducible, lentiviral vector regulated by human CD40L proximal promoter sequences. Gene Ther 2011;18:364–71.

16. Hubbard N, Hagin D, Sommer K, et al. Targeted gene editing restores regulated CD40L expression and function in X-HIGM T cells. Blood 2016. https://doi.org/10.1182/blood-2015-11-683235.

17. Kuo CY, Long JD, Campo-Fernandez B, et al. Site-Specific Gene Editing of Human Hematopoietic Stem Cells for X-Linked Hyper-IgM Syndrome. Cell Rep 2018;23:2606–16.

18. Vavassori V, Mercuri E, Marcovecchio GE, et al. Modeling, optimization, and comparable efficacy of T cell and hematopoietic stem cell gene editing for treating hyper-IgM syndrome. EMBO Mol Med 2021;1–25. https://doi.org/10.15252/emmm.202013545.

19. Güngör T, Teira P, Slatter M, et al. Reduced-intensity conditioning and HLA-matched haemopoietic stem-cell transplantation in patients with chronic granulomatous disease: A prospective multicentre study. Lancet 2014;383:436–48.

20. Porter C, Parkar M, Levinsky R, et al. X-linked chronic granulomatous disease: correction of NADPH oxidase defect by retrovirus-mediated expression of gp91-phox. Blood 1993;82:2196–202.

21. Dinauer MC, Li LL, Bjo H, et al. Long-term correction of phagocyte NADPH oxidase activity. Blood 1999;94:914–22.

22. Marciano BE, Zerbe CS, Falcone EL, et al. X-linked carriers of chronic granulomatous disease: Illness, lyonization, and stability. J Allergy Clin Immunol 2018; 141:365–71.
23. Malech HL, Maples PB, Whiting-Theobald N, et al. Prolonged production of NADPH oxidase-corrected granulocytes after gene therapy of chronic granulomatous disease. Proc Natl Acad Sci USA 1997;94:12133–8.
24. Kang EM, Choi U, Theobald N, et al. Retrovirus gene therapy for X-linked chronic granulomatous disease can achieve stable long-term correction of oxidase activity in peripheral blood neutrophils. Blood 2010;115:783–91.
25. Ott MG, Schmidt M, Schwarzwaelder K, et al. Correction of X-linked chronic granulomatous disease by gene therapy, augmented by insertional activation of MDS1-EVI1, PRDM16 or SETBP1. Nat Med 2006;12:401–9.
26. Stein S, Ott MG, Schultze-Strasser S, et al. Genomic instability and myelodysplasia with monosomy 7 consequent to EVI1 activation after gene therapy for chronic granulomatous disease. Nat Med 2010;16:198–204.
27. Santilli G, Almarza E, Brendel C, et al. Biochemical correction of X-CGD by a novel chimeric promoter regulating high levels of transgene expression in myeloid cells. Mol Ther 2011;19:122–32.
28. Kohn DB, Booth C, Kang EM, et al. Lentiviral gene therapy for X-linked chronic granulomatous disease. Nat Med 2020;26:200–6.
29. Merling RK, Sweeney CL, Chu J, et al. An AAVS1-targeted minigene platform for correction of iPSCs from all five types of chronic granulomatous disease. Mol Ther 2015;23:147–57.
30. De Ravin SS, Reik A, Liu PQ, et al. Targeted gene addition in human CD34 + hematopoietic cells for correction of X-linked chronic granulomatous disease. Nat Biotechnol 2016;34:424–9.
31. Zou J, Sweeney CL, Chou BK, et al. Oxidase-deficient neutrophils from X-linked chronic granulomatous disease iPS cells: functional correction by zinc finger nuclease-mediated safe harbor targeting. Blood 2011;117:5561–72.
32. Sweeney CL, Zou J, Choi U, et al. Targeted repair of CYBB in X-CGD iPSCs requires retention of intronic sequences for expression and functional correction. Mol Ther 2017;25:321–30.
33. De Ravin SS, Li L, Wu X, et al. CRISPR-Cas9 gene repair of hematopoietic stem cells from patients with X-linked chronic granulomatous disease. Sci Transl Med 2017;1.
34. De Ravin SS, Brault J, Meis RJ, et al. Enhanced homology-directed repair for highly efficient gene editing in hematopoietic stem/progenitor cells. Blood 2021;137:2598–608.
35. Cavazzana M, Bushman FD, Miccio A, et al. Gene therapy targeting haematopoietic stem cells for inherited diseases: progress and challenges. Nat Rev Drug Discov 2019;18:447–62.
36. Braun CJ, Boztug K, Paruzynski A, et al. Gene therapy for wiskott-Aldrich syndrome–long-term efficacy and genotoxicity. Sci Transl Med 2014;6:227ra33.
37. Burroughs LM, Petrovic A, Brazauskas R, et al. Excellent outcomes following hematopoietic cell transplantation for Wiskott-Aldrich syndrome: a PIDTC report. Blood 2020;135:2094–105.
38. Aiuti A, Biasco L, Scaramuzza S, et al. Lentiviral hematopoietic stem cell gene therapy in patients with wiskott-aldrich syndrome. Science 2013;80:341.
39. Ferrua F, Cicalese MP, Galimberti S, et al. Lentiviral haemopoietic stem/progenitor cell gene therapy for treatment of Wiskott-Aldrich syndrome: interim results

of a non-randomised, open-label, phase 1/2 clinical study. Lancet Haematol 2019;6:e239–53.

40. Sereni L, Castiello MC, Di Silverstre D, et al. Lentiviral gene therapy corrects platelet phenotype and function in patients with Wiskott-Aldrich syndrome. J Allergy Clin Immunol 2019;144:825–38.

41. Labrosse R, Chu J, Armant M, et al. Development of hematopoietic stem cell gene therapy for Wiskott-Aldrich syndrome. Blood 2019;1:4629.

42. Ferrua F, Marangoni F, Aiuti A, et al. Gene therapy for Wiskott-Aldrich syndrome: History, new vectors, future directions. J Allergy Clin Immunol 2020;146:262–5.

43. Rai R, Romito M, Rivers E, et al. Targeted gene correction of human hematopoietic stem cells for the treatment of Wiskott - Aldrich Syndrome. Nat Commun 2020;11.

44. Vetrie D, Vorechovsky I, Sideras P, et al. The gene involved in X-linked agammaglobulinaemia is a member of the src family of protein-tyrosine kinases. Nature 1993;361:226–33.

45. Lougaris V, Soresina A, Baronio M, et al. Long-term follow-up of 168 patients with X-linked agammaglobulinemia reveals increased morbidity and mortality. J Allergy Clin Immunol 2020;146:429–37.

46. Ikegame K, Imai K, Yamashita M, et al. Allogeneic stem cell transplantation for X-linked agammaglobulinemia using reduced intensity conditioning as a model of the reconstitution of humoral immunity. J Hematol Oncol 2016;9:9.

47. Yu PW, Tabuchi RS, Kato RM, et al. Sustained correction of B-cell development and function in a murine model of X-linked agammaglobulinemia (XLA) using retroviral-mediated gene transfer. Blood 2004;104:1281–90.

48. Nomura K, Kanegane H, Karasuyama H, et al. Genetic defect in human X-linked agammaglobulinemia impedes a maturational evolution of pro-B cells into a later stage of pre-B cells in the B-cell differentiation pathway. Blood 2000;96:610–7.

49. Rohrer J, Conley ME. Correction of X-linked immunodeficient mice by competitive reconstitution with limiting numbers of normal bone marrow cells. Blood 1999;94:3358–65.

50. Hendriks RW, Bruijn M F De, Maas A, et al. Inactivation of Btk by insertion of lacZ reveals defects in B cell development ony past the pre-B cell stage. EMBO J 1996;15:4862–72.

51. Kerns HM, Ryu BY, Stirling BV, et al. B cell-specific lentiviral gene therapy leads to sustained B-cell functional recovery in a murine model of X-linked agammaglobulinemia. Blood 2010;115:2146–55.

52. Neville JJ, Orlando J, Mann K, et al. Ubiquitous chromatin-opening elements (UCOEs): applications in biomanufacturing and gene therapy. Biotechnol Adv 2017;35:557–64.

53. Seymour BJ, Singh S, Certo HM, et al. Effective, safe, and sustained correction of murine XLA using a UCOE-BTK promoter-based lentiviral vector. Mol.Ther.-Methods Clin.Dev 2021;20:635–51.

54. Kokabee L, Wang X, Sevinsky CJ, et al. Bruton's tyrosine kinase is a potential therapeutic target in prostate cancer. Cancer Biol Ther 2015;16:1604–15.

55. Gray DH, Villegas I, Long J, et al. Optimizing Integration and Expression of Transgenic Bruton's Tyrosine Kinase for CRISPR-Cas9-Mediated Gene Editing of X-Linked Agammaglobulinemia. CRISPR J 2021;4:191–206.

56. Zhang ZY, Thrasher AJ, Zhang F. Gene therapy and genome editing for primary immunodeficiency diseases. Genes Dis 2020;7:38–51.

57. Yu K-R, Natanson H, Dunbar CE. Gene Editing of Human Hematopoietic Stem and Progenitor Cells: Promise and Potential Hurdles. Hum Gene Ther 2016; 27:729–40.

58. Branzei D, Foiani M. Regulation of DNA repair throughout the cell cycle. Nat.Rev.Mol Cell Biol 2008;9:297–308.

59. Pietras EM, Warr MR, Passegué E. Cell cycle regulation in hematopoietic stem cells. J Cell Biol 2011;195:709–20.

60. Gray DH, Santos J, Keir AG, et al. A comparison of DNA repair pathways to achieve a site-specific gene modification of the Bruton's tyrosine kinase gene. Mol.Ther Nucleic Acids 2022;27:505–16.

61. Barzaghi F, Amaya Hernandez LC, Neven B, et al. Long-term follow-up of IPEX syndrome patients after different therapeutic strategies: an international multicenter retrospective study. J.Allergy Clin.Immunol 2018;141:1036–49, e5.

62. d'Hennezel E, Dhuban K Bin, Torgerson T, et al. The immunogenetics of immune dysregulation, polyendocrinopathy, enteropathy, X linked (IPEX) syndrome. J.Med.Genet 2012;49:291–302.

63. Bacchetta R, Barzaghi F, Roncarolo MG. From IPEX syndrome to FOXP3 mutation: a lesson on immune dysregulation. Ann N Y Acad Sci 2016;1417:5–22.

64. Passerini L, Mel ER, Sartirana C, et al. CD4+ T cells from IPEX patients convert into functional and stable regulatory T cells by FOXP3 gene transfer. Sci.-Transl.Med 2013;5:1–11.

65. Sato Y, Passerini L, Piening BD, et al. Human-engineered Treg-like cells suppress FOXP3-deficient T cells but preserve adaptive immune responses in vivo. Clin Transl Immunol 2020;9.

66. Santoni De Sio FR, Passerini L, Valente MM, et al. Ectopic FOXP3 Expression Preserves Primitive Features of Human Hematopoietic Stem Cells while Impairing Functional T Cell Differentiation. Sci Rep 2017;7:1–10.

67. Masiuk KE, Laborada J, Roncarolo MG, et al. Lentiviral gene therapy in HSCs restores lineage-specific Foxp3 expression and suppresses autoimmunity in a mouse model of IPEX syndrome. Cell Stem Cell 2019;24:309–17, e7.

68. Vakulskas CA, Dever DP, Rettig GR, et al. A high-fidelity Cas9 mutant delivered as a ribonucleoprotein complex enables efficient gene editing in human hematopoietic stem and progenitor cells. Nat Med 2018;24:1216–24.

69. Guilinger JP, Pattanayak V, Reyon D, et al. Broad specificity profiling of TALENs results in engineered nucleases with improved DNA-cleavage specificity. Nat Methods 2014;11:429–35.

70. Doyon Y, Vo TD, Mendel MC, et al. Enhancing zinc-finger-nuclease activity with improved obligate heterodimeric architectures. Nat Methods 2011;8:74–9.

71. Hendel A, Bak RO, Clark JT, et al. Chemically modified gRNAs enhance CRISPR/Cas editing in human cells. Nat Biotechnol 2015;33:985–9.

72. Bak RO, Dever DP, Porteus MH. CRISPR/Cas9 genome editing in human hematopoietic stem cells. Nat Protoc 2018;13:358–76.

73. Hoban MD, Lumaquin D, Kuo CY, et al. CRISPR/Cas9-mediated correction of the sickle mutation in human CD34+ cells. Mol Ther 2016;1–9. https://doi.org/10.1038/mt.2016.148.

74. Petrillo C, Thorne LG, Unali G, et al. Cyclosporine H overcomes innate immune restrictions to improve lentiviral transduction and gene editing in human hematopoietic stem cells. Cell Stem Cell 2018;23:820–32, e9.

75. Lomova A, Clark DN, Romero Z, et al. Improving Gene Editing in Human Hematopoietic Stem Cells by Temporal Control of DNA Repair. Mol Ther 2018; 26:87.

76. Maruyama T, Dougan SK, Truttmann M, et al. Inhibition of non-homologous end joining increases the efficiency of CRISPR/Cas9-mediated precise [TM: inserted] genome editing. Nature 2015;33:538–42.

77. Song J, Yang D, Xu J, et al. RS-1 enhances CRISPR/Cas9- and TALEN-mediated knock-in efficiency. Nat Commun 2016;7.

78. Pavel-Dinu M, Wiebking V, Dejene BT, et al. Gene correction for SCID-X1 in long-term hematopoietic stem cells. Nat Commun 2019;10.

79. Croop JM, Cooper R, Fernandez C, et al. Mobilization and collection of peripheral blood CD34 + cells from patients with Fanconi anemia. Blood 2001;98: 2917–21.

80. Tolar J, Adair JE, Antoniou M, et al. Stem cell gene therapy for fanconi anemia: report from the 1st international fanconi anemia gene therapy working group meeting. Mol Ther 2011;19:1193–8.

81. Malech HL, Choi U, Brenner S. Progress toward effective gene therapy for chronic granulomatous disease. Jpn.J.Infect.Dis 2004;57:27–8.

82. Kang HJ, Bartholomae CC, Paruzynski A, et al. Retroviral gene therapy for X-linked chronic granulomatous disease: results from phase I/II trial. Mol.Ther 2011;19:2092–101.

83. Bauer TR, Schwartz BR, Liles WC, et al. Retroviral-mediated gene transfer of the leukocyte integrin CD18 into peripheral blood CD34+ cells derived from a patient with leukocyte adhesion deficiency type 1. Blood 1998;91:1520–6.

84. Kohn DB, Rao GR, Almarza E, et al. A phase 1/2 study of lentiviral-mediated ex-vivo gene therapy for pediatric patients with severe leukocyte adhesion deficiency-I (LAD-I): results from phase 1. Blood 2020;136:15.

85. Hacein-Bey Abina S, Gaspar HB, Blondeau J, et al. Outcomes following gene therapy in patients with severe wiskott-aldrich syndrome. JAMA 2015;313:1550.

86. Magnani A, Semeraro M, Adam F, et al. Long-term safety and efficacy of lentiviral hematopoietic stem/progenitor cell gene therapy for Wiskott–Aldrich syndrome. Nat Med 2022;28:71–80.

87. Carranza D, Torres-Rusillo S, Ceballos-Perez G, et al. Reconstitution of the ataxia-telangiectasia cellular phenotype with lentiviral vectors. Front.Immunol 2018;9:1–10.

88. Kreitzer CR, Choi U, Swamydas M, et al. Development of a Lentiviral Gene Therapy Vector for Treatment of CARD9 Deficiency. Mol Ther 2020;28:168.

89. Hetzel M, Mucci A, Blank P, et al. Hematopoietic stem cell gene therapy for IFNγR1 deficiency protects mice from mycobacterial infections. Blood 2018; 131:533–45.

90. Hahn K, Pollmann L, Nowak J, et al. Human lentiviral gene therapy restores the cellular phenotype of autosomal recessive complete IFN-γR1 deficiency. Mol.Ther Methods Clin Dev 2020;17:785–95.

91. Dettmer V, Bloom K, Gross M, et al. Retroviral UNC13D gene transfer restores cytotoxic activity of t cells derived from familial hemophagocytic lymphohistiocytosis type 3 patients in vitro. Hum.Gene Ther 2019;30:975–84.

92. Takushi SE, Paik NY, Fedanov A, et al. Lentiviral gene therapy for familial hemophagocytic lymphohistiocytosis type 3, caused by UNC13D Genetic defects. Hum.Gene Ther 2020;31:626–38.

93. Tiwari S, Hontz A, Terrell C, et al. Genetic therapy for perforin deficiency associated hemophagocytic lymphohistiocytosis requires high level expression of the perforin gene for adequate correction. Mol.Ther 2015;23:S93.

94. Ghosh S, Carmo M, Calero-Garcia M, et al. T-cell gene therapy for perforin deficiency corrects cytotoxicity defects and prevents hemophagocytic lymphohistiocytosis manifestations. J.Allergy Clin.Immunol 2018;142:904–13, e3.

95. Goodwin M, Lee E, Lakshmanan U, et al. CRISPR-based gene editing enables FOXP3 gene repair in IPEX patient cells. Sci.Adv 2020;6.

96. Rao S, Brito-Frazao J, Serbin AV, et al. Gene editing ELANE in human hematopoietic stem and progenitor cells reveals disease mechanisms and therapeutic strategies for severe congenital neutropenia. Blood 2019;134:3.

97. Ritter MU, Secker B, Klimiankou M, et al. Efficient correction of ELANE mutations in primary HSPCs of severe congenital neutropenia patients using CRISPR/Cas9 and rAVV6 HDR repair templates. Blood 2019;134:1036.

98. Tran NT, Graf R, Wulf-Goldenberg A, et al. CRISPR-Cas9-mediated ELANE mutation correction in hematopoietic stem and progenitor cells to treat severe congenital neutropenia. Mol Ther 2020;28:2621–34.

99. Eberherr AC, Maaske A, Wolf C, et al. Rescue of STAT3 function in hyper-IgE syndrome using adenine base editing. Cris J 2021;4:178–90.

100. Kerns HM, Ryu BY, Stirling BD, et al. B cell – specific lentiviral gene therapy leads to sustained B-cell functional recovery in a murine model of X-linked agammaglobulinemia. Gene Ther 2010;115:2146–55.

101. Ng YY, Baert MRM, Pike-Overzet K, et al. Correction of B-cell development in Btk-deficient mice using lentiviral vectors with codon-optimized human BTK. Leuk.Off J.Leuk Soc.Am.Leuk.Res.Fund U.K 2010;24:1617–30.

102. De Ravin SS, Li L, Wu X, et al. CRISPR-Cas9 gene repair of hematopoietic stem cells from patients with X-linked chronic granulomatous disease. Sci Transl Med 2017;9.

103. Rivat C, Booth c>, Alonso-Ferrero M, et al. SAP gene transfer restores cellular and humoral immune function in a murine model of X-linked lymphoproliferative disease. Blood 2013;121:1073–6.

104. Panchal N, Houghton B, Diez B, et al. Transfer of gene-corrected T cells corrects humoral and cytotoxic defects in patients with X-linked lymphoproliferative disease. J Allergy Clin Immunol 2018;142:235–45, e6.

105. Brault J, Liu T, Bello E, et al. CRISPR-targeted MAGT1 insertion restores XMEN patient hematopoietic stem cells and lymphocytes. Blood 2021;138:2768–80.

106. Khan IF, Wang Y, Clough C, et al. Precision editing of the WAS locus via homologous recombination in primary human hematopoietic cells mediated by either TALEN or CRISPR/Cas nucleases. Mol.Ther 2016;24:S227.

107. Gutierrez-Guerrero A, Abrey Recalde MJ, Mangeot PE, et al. Baboon envelope pseudotyped "Nanoblades" carrying Cas9/gRNA complexes allow efficient genome editing in human T, B, and CD34+ cells and knock-in of AAV6-encoded donor DNA in CD34+ cells. Front Genome Ed 2021;3.

Gene Therapy for Pediatric Neurologic Disease

Lauren Jimenez-Kurlander, MD[a,b], Christine N. Duncan, MD[a,b],*

KEYWORDS

- Neurologic disorders • Gene therapy • Ex vivo • In vivo
- Lysosomal storage disorders • Peroxisomal storage disorders • Leukodystrophies
- Motor neuron disease

KEY POINTS

- Lysosomal and peroxisomal storage disorders, leukodystrophies, and motor neuron diseases include diverse groups of monogenic disorders with a spectrum of neurologic manifestations that affect the pediatric population with limited definitive treatment options currently.
- Gene therapy allows for the transduction of target cells with functional gene; the selection of a promoter of sufficient activity, combined in some cases with a codon-optimized transgene, results in supraphysiologic functional enzyme production that has the potential to treat nearby unmodified impaired cells via cross-correction in several pediatric neurologic conditions.
- Ex vivo gene therapies systemically distribute functional enzyme, which allows for the targeting of multi-organ systems, including the central and peripheral nervous systems.
- In vivo delivery of functional gene is ideal for targeting select organ systems with lower cell turnover, including the brain.
- Future directions are focused on enhancing gene therapy methods, including minimizing the likelihood of insertional oncogenesis, improving the penetration of the blood–brain barrier, and optimizing tissue uptake.

INTRODUCTION
Gene Therapy Definitions and Rationale

Gene therapy refers to several modalities of nucleic acid delivery that aim to correct impaired cellular function due to a dysfunctional gene or genes in some cases. The use of recombinant laboratory-designed viral vectors to deliver functional genes has been trialed over the past several decades for a variety of diseases and disorders, specifically through genome integration in actively dividing cells or episomal retention

---

[a] Department of Pediatric Hematology and Oncology, Boston Children's Hospital, Boston, MA 02115, USA; [b] Department of Pediatric Oncology, Dana-Farber Cancer Institute, Boston, MA 02215, USA
* Corresponding author. 450 Brookline Avenue, Boston, MA 02115.
E-mail address: Christine_Duncan@dfci.harvard.edu

Hematol Oncol Clin N Am 36 (2022) 853–864
https://doi.org/10.1016/j.hoc.2022.05.003
0889-8588/22/© 2022 Elsevier Inc. All rights reserved.
hemonc.theclinics.com

in nondividing cells.[1] This effort largely aims to cure diseases without definitive treatment or those for which the only available cell-based therapy is allogeneic hematopoietic stem cell transplantation (allo-HCT), which carries significant limitations, such as difficulty identifying immunocompatible donors, and transplant-related toxicities, including the potential development of graft versus host disease (GVHD). For those diseases and disorders that impact the nervous system, curative therapies are frequently unattainable due to historically limited treatment options for neuronal degeneration and difficulty in penetrating the blood–brain barrier (BBB). This makes gene therapy an attractive potential solution as the luminal surface of the BBB includes molecules that can interact with some viral ligands used in gene therapy efforts.[2,3] Monogenic neurologic disorders are primed as optimal gene therapy candidates as target cells can be transduced by viral vectors, allowing for the production of therapeutic protein.[4,5] This makes the neuropathic subset of lysosomal storage and peroxisomal disorders, leukodystrophies, and motor neuron diseases ideal candidates for gene therapy (**Fig. 1**). The current standard of care for some of these diseases is enzyme replacement therapy (ERT) whereby enzyme is purified ex vivo and then infused into the patient. However, ERT is suboptimal therapy given the potential to develop an immune response against the exogenous enzyme over time, inability of most to cross the BBB, as well as the financial and social complications of repeated lifetime therapy. Comparatively, gene therapy has the potential to treat patients without the need for repeated administration throughout a lifetime.[1] Target cells can either be modified in vivo or modified ex vivo and subsequently autotransplanted.[5] Their respective mechanisms of action are described in-depth later in this review.

One of the earliest viral vectors trialed clinically was the nonintegrating adenovirus, whose pitfalls included significant immunogenicity and short-lived transgene expression. An alternative vector, adeno-associated virus (AAV), has been used more recently given its decreased immunogenicity, broader tropism, and long-term expression in nondividing cells. As a result, AAVs may serve as optimal vectors for in vivo delivery to select organ systems with lower cell turnover, including the brain.[1] With respect to ex vivo delivery, many early trials for immunodeficiencies used the gamma-retrovirus (γ-RV), which clinically revealed a risk of oncogene transactivation following insertional mutagenesis. The need for self-inactivating vectors has since led

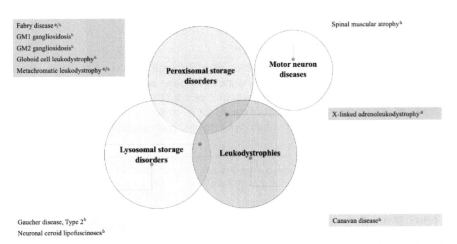

Fabry disease [a/b]
GM1 gangliosidosis [b]
GM2 gangliosidosis [b]
Globoid cell leukodystrophy [b]
Metachromatic leukodystrophy [a/b]

Spinal muscular atrophy [b]

Peroxisomal storage disorders

Motor neuron diseases

X-linked adrenoleukodystrophy [a]

Lysosomal storage disorders

Leukodystrophies

Gaucher disease, Type 2 [b]
Neuronal ceroid lipofuscinoses [b]

Canavan disease [b]

Fig. 1. Pediatric neurologic disorders being targeted by gene therapy currently. [a]ex vivo trials, [b]in vivo trials.

to the extensive use of the HIV-1-derived lentivirus (LV).[1,5–7] These lentiviral vectors have treated more than 200 patients with 10 hematologic disorders (including metabolic disorders, primary immunodeficiencies, and hemoglobinopathies).[5]

Background of Storage Disorders and Leukodystrophies

Storage disorders are a heterogeneous group of inherited disorders that arise from monogenic defects of enzyme or transporter production, specifically those critical to peroxisomal or lysosomal function.[8] Peroxisomal storage disorders (PSDs) refer to the subset of storage disorders with impaired enzymes or transporters that typically reside in peroxisomes, the intracellular organelles responsible for lipid metabolism, including b-oxidation of very long-chain fatty acids (VLCFAs) and cholesterol synthesis.[9] PSDs include disorders of peroxisome biogenesis, which are caused by PEX gene defects; single peroxisomal enzyme deficiencies; and a contiguous gene deletion syndrome.[10] Due to the accumulation of VLCFAs in neuronal membranes, PSDs have a wide spectrum of neurologic manifestations as a result of demyelination and neuronal death. In the pediatric population, gene therapy has been trialed as the treatment for one of the single peroxisomal enzyme deficiencies, X-linked cerebral adrenoleukodystrophy (X-ALD).

Lysosomal storage disorders (LSDs) refer to the subset of storage disorders with impaired enzymes or transporters that typically reside in lysosomes, the intracellular organelles responsible for the degradation and recycling of intra-and extracellular waste. Without adequate enzymatic function, substrates such as lipids and/or polysaccharides accumulate and secondarily cause the accumulation of other macromolecules, organelle dysfunction, and oxidative stress that impacts end-organ function.[1] The specific substrate determines the clinical manifestation of disease, which may include the central and/or peripheral nervous systems. Central nervous system (CNS) effects include microglial activation, neuroinflammation, and axonal degeneration, ultimately resulting in neuronal death and/or demyelination, contributing to poor clinical prognoses for patients and limiting effective treatment options.[1,9]

More than 60 LSDs have been identified with an overall incidence of 1 in 5000 to 7000 people.[11] Of those, about two-thirds have neurologic manifestations including: Fabry disease, type 2 Gaucher disease, GM1 and GM2 gangliosidoses, neuronal ceroid lipofuscinoses, globoid cell leukodystrophy (GLD), and metachromatic leukodystrophy (MLD).[4] Lysosomal enzymes are synthesized in the endoplasmic reticulum and trafficked to lysosomes by their specific substrate marker mannose-6-phosphate (M6P) via vesicular transport. While some lysosomal enzymes bind to intracellular M6P receptor (M6PR), they can also be secreted into the extracellular space. The M6PR is expressed on the surface of many cell types, which helps to scavenge extracellular enzyme back to the lysosome.[12] Using cell-based therapy, this process can be exploited in a phenomenon known as cross-correction whereby cellular modification to overexpress enzyme allows for neighboring unmodified cellular enzyme uptake.[1,4]

Alternatively, degenerative neurologic disease can also be classified by neuropathological findings. Leukodystrophies are a subset of neurologic disease defined by pathologic abnormalities of the CNS glial cells.[13] As glial cells form the membranous myelin sheath, clinical effects vary depending on the part of the myelin sheath affected in each specific leukodystrophy. Some LSDs and PSDs are also classified as leukodystrophies, including X-ALD, Fabry Disease, GM1 and GM2 gangliosidoses, GLD, and MLD (**Fig. 1**). Another leukodystrophy, Canavan disease, is also targetable by gene therapy given its monogenic etiology and lack of alternative effective treatment.[14] An additional class of degenerative neurologic disease is motor neuron disease (MND), which is characterized by progressive motor neuron destruction, with clinical manifestations dependent on the involvement of upper and/or lower motor neurons.[15] One type of MND, spinal muscular atrophy (SMA), is caused by monogenic defects of the *SMN1* gene, which makes it an attractive target for gene therapies.[15,16]

This review outlines the pediatric neurologic disorders that have been targeted by clinical gene therapies at this time, highlights the relevant recent or ongoing clinical trials, and identifies complications and future directions of gene therapy efforts.

EX VIVO DELIVERY
Mechanism of Action

As introduced above, ex vivo delivery of the corrected gene of interest builds on the established techniques of HCT. As in autologous HCT, hematopoietic stem and progenitor cells (HSPCs) are either harvested from the patient's bone marrow or mobilized into the peripheral blood circulation; samples are collected by leukapheresis and enriched in culture for CD34+ cells.[7] Meanwhile, an integrating retroviral (either a gammaretroviral or lentiviral) vector is selected that can accommodate the gene of interest, relying on viral and/or cellular gene promoters, which act to drive the transgene.[17] Potential clinical benefit is optimized through the use of ubiquitous promoters that lead to supraphysiologic levels of gene expression, which is distinct from many other disease entities that require cell-type-specific or regulated expression.[1] Some approaches incorporate codon optimization of the transgene to heighten protein expression by up to >1000-fold.[18] The retroviral vector of choice can also be modified to minimize genotoxicity. For example, self-inactivation is one such modification that involves controlling therapeutic gene expression by removing strong viral enhancers from the 3′ long-terminal repeat (LTR). An exogenous promoter is placed in the internal position instead of the LTR in these cases to drive the transgene. This process effectively removes the original viral genes and regulatory elements.[5,9] Another common modification is the deletion of promoter viral sequences in the LTRs.[7] Lentiviral vectors preferentially integrate into gene bodies over promoters, which reduce the risk for aberrant transcriptional activation.[7] Using lentiviral vectors, up to 8 kb of transgene are able to be delivered to the HSPCs; this allows stable genomic integration of the vector with permanent transgene expression of all progeny cells.[5] The HSPCs are transduced with the retroviral vectors that carry the cDNA (which may be codon optimized) of the disease-causing gene.[8] The patient receives either a submyeloablative or myeloablative chemotherapeutic conditioning regimen before the reinfusion of the modified HSPCs, optimizing successful engraftment by creating space in the marrow niche.[7] Preclinical studies suggest that myeloablative regimens with CNS penetration using agents such as busulfan are critical to allow for myeloid engraftment in the brain.[9] The reinfused modified HSPCs secrete extracellular vesicles containing both plasmid DNA and protein and, in many cases, can be taken up by neighboring cells via cross-correction.[4] As a result, the overexpression of the corrective enzyme throughout the body, including in the CNS, results in the detoxification of neurons and glial cells, clinically reversing neurodegenerative metabolic disease.[5,7,9]

Diseases

Cerebral X-linked adrenoleukodystrophy
X-linked adrenoleukodystrophy background. The most common PSD is X-linked adrenoleukodystrophy (X-ALD), a single gene peroxisomal enzyme deficiency caused by a defect in the gene *ABCD1* (ATP-binding cassette, subfamily D, member 1) and subsequent deficiency of the peroxisomal ABC half-transporter ALD protein.[19] As a result, there is VLCFA accumulation that predominantly affects adrenal and nervous

system tissues. When VLCFA accumulation occurs in oligodendrocytes, the cholesterol metabolic pathway is unable to produce adequate myelin.[9] This can lead to demyelination and neurodegeneration, a hallmark of the phenotype known as cerebral ALD.[9,19] Cerebral ALD (cALD) manifests in approximately 35% of patients with ALD typically at age less than 12 years old, while older individuals are less likely to develop the cerebral phenotype.[19] Cognitive and behavioral impairment often manifests clinically between ages 3 and 15 years; this is followed by rapid neurologic deterioration with most patients dying within a decade after diagnosis if they do not receive a successful allo-HCT, the only effective available therapy currently.[20]

In 1990, Aubourg and colleagues published the first report of a therapeutic allo-HCT in a boy with early-stage cALD.[21] Since that time, allo-HCT has been used as therapy with optimal success when performed in early-stage cerebral disease whereby there is minimal demyelination. As the peroxisomal ABC half-transporter ALD protein is a structural protein, the likely mechanism of allo-HCT is cell-mediated as opposed to through cross-correction. Amelioration of disease is dependent on the replacement of the host's abnormally functioning microglia by donor-derived cells over time. Typically, demyelination continues for about 12 to 18 months after cellular therapy before arresting.[9] As a result, early diagnosis and rapid donor identification are critical for effective treatment. Of note, neither allo-HCT nor gene insertion is expected to effectively treat the phenotypes of adrenomyeloneuropathy or adrenal insufficiency in cALD.[19]

Cerebral X-adrenoleukodystrophy ex vivo gene therapy data. Preclinical studies on nonobese diabetic/severe combined immunodeficiency (SCID) mice set the foundation for successful lentiviral transduction of human CD34+ cells expressing the ALD protein. These studies demonstrated that xenotransplant in the mice resulted in successful cellular migration to the mice's brains with subsequent differentiation into perivascular myeloid cells expressing the ALD protein.[22]

Cartier and colleagues subsequently developed a lentivirus that coded for the wild-type *ABCD1* cDNA (CG1711hALD-LV) under the expression of the MND (myeloproliferative sarcoma virus enhancer, negative control region deleted, dl587rev primer binding site substituted) promoter. Using this vector, they used the first ex vivo gene therapy clinical trial for 4 boys with cerebral ALD in 2009.[23] Autologous HSPCs were transduced with the therapeutic lentivirus and auto-transplanted following conditioning with busulfan.[24] For the 2 patients whose results have been reported, polyclonal reconstitution was confirmed after 24 to 30 months of follow-up with 9% to 14% of granulocytes, monocytes, and T and B lymphocytes expressing the ALD protein. Clinically, the patients' progressive cerebral demyelination stopped 14 to 16 months after infusion, which is a comparable timeline to outcomes following allo-HCT in this population.[23,24]

Since that time, a 2013 large multicenter phase II/III clinical trial has reported results for 17 boys with early-stage cerebral ALD who received elivaldogene tavalentivec (Lenti-D) gene therapy following conditioning with busulfan and cyclophosphamide **(Table 1)**.[19] Similar to the CG1711hALD-LV, Lenti-D is a lentiviral vector that codes for *ABCD1* cDNA using an MNDU3 an internal promoter. Preliminary results showed measurable ALD protein in all patients. At a median follow-up of 29.4 months, 88% of patients had minimal clinical symptoms. Two patients in the study were unable to achieve the stabilization of disease; the first died of rapid neurologic progression before the time required for cerebral myeloid reconstitution, and the second opted to withdraw from the study in favor of allo-HCT and later died from transplantation associated complications.[19] The American Food and Drug Administration (FDA)

Table 1
Recent or ongoing ex vivo LV-mediated gene therapy studies for pediatric neurologic disorders

Disease	Trial Phase	Conditioning	No. pts	Age (y)	Start - End Date	Sponsor	Site(s)	Status	Trial ID
Fabry disease	I/II	Not specified	12	16–50	2/21/18–11/21	AVROBIO	New Jersey, Australia, Canada	Recruiting	NCT03454893
MLD	I/II	Not specified	20	Up to 7	4/9/10 – e4/23	Orchard Therapeutics	Italy	Active, not recruiting	NCT01560182
MLD	II	Bu	10	Up to 6	1/25/18 – e8/2028	Orchard Therapeutics	Italy	Active, not recruiting	NCT03392987
MLD	III	Bu	6	Up to 17	12/31/20 - e1/32	Orchard Therapeutics	Italy	Recruiting	NCT04283227
MLD and X-ALD	I/II	Not specified	50	2–45	1/15 – e10/25	Shenzhen Second People's Hospital	China	Recruiting	NCT02559830
Cerebral X-ALD	II/III	Bu/Cy	32	Up to 17	1/21/13–3/21	Bluebird bio	California, Massachusetts, Minnesota, Argentina, Australia, France, Germany, England	Completed	NCT01896102
Cerebral X-ALD	III	Bu/Flu	35	Up to 17	1/24/19 – e2/24	Bluebird bio	California, Massachusetts, Minnesota, France, Germany, Italy, Netherlands, England	Active, not recruiting	NCT03852498

Abbreviations: Bu, busulfan; Cy, cyclophosphamide; e, estimated; Flu, fludarabine; LV, lentiviral; MLD, metachromatic leukodystrophy; no., number; pts, patients; VSV-G, vesicular stomatitis virus glycoprotein G; X-ALD, X-linked adrenoleukodystrophy; y, years
Data collected from a search performed on December 10, 2021 at https://www.clinicaltrials.gov.

designated Lenti-D as a breakthrough therapy following this report.[9] In October 2020 The European Medicines Agency accepted bluebird bio's marketing authorization application for Lenti-D gene therapy for the treatment of patients with cALD. A phase III multicenter clinical trial was opened in January 2019 with plans to enroll 35 pediatric patients with cerebral ALD by 2024 for therapeutic Lenti-D administration following conditioning with busulfan and fludarabine (**Table 1**). The clinical trial was placed on hold by the FDA in August 2021 following the development of myelodysplastic syndrome (MDS), likely mediated by lentiviral vector, in a study participant.[25] MDS was subsequently reported in two additional children. The investigation into these events is ongoing.

Fabry disease

Fabry disease background. Fabry disease is an LSD that occurs due to mutations in the X-linked *GLA* gene and subsequent deficiency of lysosomal α-galactosidase A. Without adequate α-galactosidase A, there is impaired degradation of the membrane glycosphingolipid ceramide trihexoside (GL-3), which accumulates in the vascular epithelium and other cells, predominantly impacting the kidneys, heart, and brain.[26] Clinically, symptoms present in childhood and adolescence, most commonly between 6 years old and sexual maturity with neuropathic pain and gastrointestinal problems.[26,27] Symptoms are typically mild and well-controlled in the childhood years.[1] As a result, mortality is rare in the pediatric population with anticipated life expectancies around the fifth to sixth decades, but there have been reports of significant morbidity including cerebral vascular accidents (CVAs) in children.[28] Given the relatively lower cerebral involvement in Fabry disease as compared with other LSDs, gene therapy efforts may be able to use less intensive conditioning regimens as effective treatment may be achieved even without brain remodeling by the transduced myeloid cells.[1]

Fabry disease ex vivo gene therapy data. Preclinical studies using a murine Fabry disease model used a lentiviral vector to transduce HSPCs with a functional *GLA* gene using the mammalian elongation factor 1 α (EF-1 α) promoter. They used codon optimization and demonstrated stable engraftment with supraphysiologic α-galactosidase A activity with corresponding reduction in GL-3 substrate accumulation 12 weeks after xenotransplantation.[29] Following these results, in 2018, a single-arm phase I trial conducted in Canada used an LV vector to administer corrected *GLA* gene to 5 adult males following nonmyeloablative conditioning with melphalan, and α-galactosidase A activity was produced to near-normal levels within 1 week in all patients. Clinical evaluations are ongoing with the first patient now 3-years posttreatment.[30] The same LV-modified HSPC method is now being used in another phase I/II trial (NCT03454893) with sites in New Jersey, Canada, and Australia, recruiting adolescents at least 16 years old as well as adults (**Table 1**).

Metachromatic leukodystrophy

Metachromatic leukodystrophy background. Metachromatic leukodystrophy (MLD) is an LSD characterized by the deficiency of the lysosomal enzyme arylsulfatase A (ARSA), caused by variants in the *ARSA* gene or, rarely, the *PSAP* gene.[31] Without sufficient ARSA, there is an accumulation of sulfatides that particularly impacts oligodendrocytes, resulting in severe demyelination. Clinically, this manifests as one of the 3 subtypes: late infantile, juvenile, or adult.[9] Subtypes are characterized by age of symptom onset as well as severity. About 40% to 60% of affected patients have late infantile MLD whereby disease onset occurs before 4 years old, typically manifesting as difficulty ambulating, and clinical symptoms are severe with progression typically resulting in immobility and death within 5 years of diagnosis. The juvenile form affects

20% to 30% of patients with MLD and involves symptom onset between 4 years old and sexual maturity, often manifesting initially as school difficulty or behavioral problems but occasionally presents with motor impairments.[26] Late infantile MLD has no currently available treatment as allo-HCT is ineffective, even in cases of presymptomatic disease. Comparatively, juvenile MLD can benefit from allo-HCT, which effectively halts or slows cerebral demyelination. However, allo-HCT is unable to slow disease progression in the peripheral nervous system, resulting in severe peripheral neuropathy-related motor deficits years after transplantation.[32]

Metachromatic leukodystrophy ex vivo gene therapy data. Using a murine MLD model, Biffi and colleagues demonstrated successful CNS microglial reconstitution following LV-mediated transduction of HSPCs with the corrected *ARSA* gene using the phosphoglycerate kinase (PGK) promoter.[33,34] Interestingly, mice demonstrated better clinical and neuropathological outcomes as compared with those who received wild-type HSPC transplantation, suggesting a therapeutic benefit to the supraphysiologic enzyme expression attainable with gene therapy.[33] Following these results, a single-arm phase I/II clinical trial in Milan was initiated in 2010 using the infusion of LV-mediated *ARSA* transduced HSPCs, controlled by the PGK promoter, following conditioning with busulfan in children with presymptomatic MLD (**Table 1**).[35] Vector copy numbers of greater than 2 diploid genomes/cell were targeted to achieve supraphysiologic expression. Preliminary results of the first 9 of 20 patients after 18 to 54 months of follow-up showed stable engraftment of gene-corrected cells and recovery of ARSA activity in all HSPC lineages as well as the cerebral spinal fluid (CSF) as early as 6 months after gene therapy administration. The ongoing phase II trial (**Table 1**) is assessing outcomes using cryopreserved cells instead of fresh cell products in children up to 6 years old (NCT03392987).

COMPLICATIONS AND CONCERNS

Challenges related to gene therapy administration and potential late effects remain. Patients' inflammatory states can impair effective reconstitution, autotransplanted HSPCs can be altered by the disease environment, and myeloablative conditioning regimens carry potential late effects that must be monitored lifelong.[5] For successful, long-term therapeutic success, treatment must achieve durable, high levels of gene-corrected cell chimerism in the CNS that maintains appropriate levels of functional enzyme.[9] Insufficient enzyme will result in incompletely treated disease, while excessive enzyme can result in cytotoxicity.[1,9] Delivering sufficient corrected gene copies to the appropriately targeted cells remains a challenge, and optimization of LV vector promoters should help to regulate therapeutic gene expression appropriately.

The potential for insertional oncogenesis remains a paramount concern. Since the first lentiviral clinical trial over a decade ago, large amounts of transduced HSPCs (ie, 5–20 million per kg body weight) have been administered to more than 200 patients.[5] Clonal expansions and leukemias were first identified after the integration of unmodified gammaretroviral vectors within cancer-related genes for other diseases. For example, leukemias were reported following the activation of the *LMO2* oncogene in the first gene therapy trial for X-linked severe combined immunodeficiency type 1 (SCID-X1).[6] These concerns were largely but not fully mitigated by the shift in the field to the use of LV vectors. Recently, a multicenter phase III gene therapy trial using a self-inactivating LV vector for sickle cell disease (NCT04293185) was suspended because of the development of acute myeloid leukemia (AML) in 2 patients and myelodysplastic syndrome (MDS) in a second patient. Both cases of AML were determined to be unrelated to vector insertion, while the case of MDS was determined to be related to the patient's conditioning regimen (see Chapter 8). The significant clonal expansions that have resulted from LV vector integration within cancer-related genes suggest there is potential to promote cellular growth with unclear clinical implications. Cellular growth seems less aggressive than those resulting from the earlier gammaretroviral vectors, which had intact, potent enhancers in the LTR region, but nonetheless warrants close ongoing monitoring.[5] At this time, 3 serious adverse events (SAEs) of myelodysplastic syndrome (MDS) have been reported in patients who received the Lenti-D vector as part of the phase III trial ALD-104 (NCT03852498, **Table 1**). Data suggest that the initial patient's MDS was likely mediated by Lenti-D vector insertion and occurred over a year after treatment. Analyses of the etiology of the latter 2 patients' cases are ongoing.

FUTURE DIRECTIONS

To enhance efficacy and minimize risks, especially with respect to insertional oncogenesis, efforts to optimize gene therapy mechanisms are underway, particularly with gene-editing techniques. Site-specific editing of the human genome can act to correct a dysfunctional gene or add a copy of the therapeutic gene to its physiologic location. One example of an emerging gene-editing system uses the clustered regularly interspaced short palindromic repeats-associated protein-9 nuclease (CRISPR/Cas9), which delivers a Cas9 nuclease and short guide RNA (sgRNA) to the target cells.[36] The Cas9 nuclease then creates a double-stranded DNA break at the target site as guided by the sgRNA, and homologous recombination can then be used to incorporate the corrected gene. By inserting the gene at its physiologic locus, it is downstream of its endogenous promoter.[36] However, it is unclear at this time whether this will result in sufficient quantities of enzyme production as supraphysiologic levels may be necessary to achieve the cross-correction of nearby cells.[9] At this time, a preclinical effort using CRISPR/Cas9 methodology has been trialed for GLD, specifically using human fetal brain-derived neural stem cells (NSCs) to express galactosylceramidase in a murine disease model.[37]

Furthermore, treatment of neurologic disorders requires traversing the BBB; optimization of LV vectors moving forward can help to ensure adequate CNS delivery. For example, LV vectors can be built to express fusion enzymes known to physiologically cross the BBB such as apolipoprotein E or B-derived domains.[1] There is often a challenge in achieving sufficient enzyme levels across multiple organ systems, as these neurologic disorders can have clinical manifestations of other organ systems. Future efforts may incorporate multiple delivery modalities simultaneously. For example, preclinical trials by Rafi and colleagues used a murine model of GLD and delivered AAVrh10/GALC via intracerebroventricular, intracerebellar, and intravenous routes with subsequent high brain GALC activity and moderate to high spinal cord and peripheral GALC activity.[38] The use of multiple injection sites can help to overcome the difficulty of site-specific delivery and potential need for repeat administration to maintain enzyme levels.

SUMMARY

Lysosomal and peroxisomal storage disorders, leukodystrophies, and motor neuron diseases include diverse groups of monogenic disorders that have a spectrum of devastating neurologic manifestations that affect the pediatric population. Currently, many of these disorders and diseases lack any definitive treatment despite efforts over the past several decades to exploit cross-correction through ERT and allo-HCT. Gene therapy is a cell-based method to administer corrected gene to patients, which allows for the secretion of functional enzymes. Appropriate conditioning regimens enable cerebral myeloid remodeling for the potential arrest or reversal of cerebral disease. In many cases, there is also the potential to treat nearby unmodified impaired cells via cross-correction.

Ex vivo gene therapies systemically distribute functional enzyme, which allows for the targeting of multi-organ systems, including the central and peripheral nervous systems. This is being trialed for many disorders, including X-ALD, Fabry disease, and MLD with promising preliminary results. By transducing autologous HSPCs with corrected gene using LV vectors, the patient's body recognizes the foreign gene product as self, alleviating concerns of immunogenicity.[39] In vivo delivery of functional gene is ideal for targeting select organ systems with relatively lower cell turnover, including the brain. In vivo efforts are currently being trialed for many disorders as well, including Canavan disease, Fabry disease, GD2, GLD, GM1 and GM2 gangliosidoses, neuronal ceroid lipofuscinoses, and SMA. Potential complications and concerns related to these therapeutic methods include the risks associated with conditioning regimens as well as the potential for insertional oncogenesis. Future directions are focused on enhancing gene therapy methods, including minimizing the likelihood of insertional oncogenesis, improving the penetration of the BBB, and optimizing tissue uptake.

CLINICS CARE POINTS

- Pediatric patients with neurologic disease from select underlying lysosomal and peroxisomal storage disorders, leukodystrophies, or motor neuron diseases may be candidates for gene therapy under ongoing clinical trials.
- Early diagnosis is critical for the effective treatment of pediatric neurologic disorders as superior outcomes exist for patients who are presymptomatic or have the early disease.
- Supraphysiologic enzyme levels may be required to sustain the clinical arrest of neurodegeneration following gene therapy for pediatric neurologic disorders.
- Patients who have received gene therapy may be at increased risk of secondary malignancy related to insertional oncogenesis or to the conditioning regimen.

DISCLOSURE

Dr C.N. Duncan is a consultant for bluebird bio, Omeros, and Novartis.

REFERENCES

1. Nagree MS, Scalia S, McKillop WM, et al. An update on gene therapy for lysosomal storage disorders. Expert Opin Biol Ther 2019;19(7):655–70.
2. Piguet F, Alves S, Cartier N. Clinical Gene Therapy for Neurodegenerative Diseases: Past, Present, and Future. Hum Gene Ther 2017;28(11):988–1003.
3. Ndemazie NB, Inkoom A, Morfaw EF, et al. Multi-disciplinary Approach for Drug and Gene Delivery Systems to the Brain. AAPS PharmSciTech 2021;23(1):11.
4. Graceffa V. Clinical Development of Cell Therapies to Halt Lysosomal Storage Diseases: Results and Lessons Learned. Curr Gene Ther 2022;22(3):191–213.
5. Cavazzana M, Bushman FD, Miccio A, et al. Gene therapy targeting haematopoietic stem cells for inherited diseases: progress and challenges. Nat Rev Drug Discov 2019;18(6):447–62.
6. von Kalle C, Fehse B, Layh-Schmitt G, et al. Stem cell clonality and genotoxicity in hematopoietic cells: gene activation side effects should be avoidable. Semin Hematol 2004;41(4):303–18.

7. Ferrari G, Thrasher AJ, Aiuti A. Gene therapy using haematopoietic stem and progenitor cells. Nat Rev Genet 2021;22(4):216–34.

8. Biffi A. Gene therapy for lysosomal storage disorders: a good start. Hum Mol Genet 2016;25(R1):R65–75.

9. Poletti V, Biffi A. Gene-Based Approaches to Inherited Neurometabolic Diseases. Hum Gene Ther 2019;30(10):1222–35.

10. Shimozawa N. Molecular and clinical aspects of peroxisomal diseases. J Inherit Metab Dis 2007;30(2):193–7.

11. Fuller M, Meikle PJ, Hopwood JJ. Epidemiology of lysosomal storage diseases: an overview. In: Mehta A, Beck M, Sunder-Plassmann G, editors. Fabry disease: Perspectives from 5 Years of FOS. Oxford: Oxford PharmaGenesis Copyright © 2006, Oxford PharmaGenesis™; 2006.

12. Neufeld EF. The uptake of enzymes into lysosomes: an overview. Birth Defects Orig Artic Ser 1980;16(1):77–84.

13. Maegawa GHB. Lysosomal Leukodystrophies Lysosomal Storage Diseases Associated With White Matter Abnormalities. J Child Neurol 2019;34(6):339–58.

14. Lotun A, Gessler DJ, Gao G. Canavan Disease as a Model for Gene Therapy-Mediated Myelin Repair. Front Cell Neurosci 2021;15:661928.

15. Miccio A, Antoniou P, Ciura S, et al. Novel genome-editing-based approaches to treat motor neuron diseases: Promises and challenges. Mol Ther 2022;30(1):47–53.

16. Goemans N. Gene therapy for spinal muscular atrophy: hope and caution. Lancet Neurol 2021;20(4):251–2.

17. Kurian KM, Watson CJ, Wyllie AH. Retroviral vectors. Mol Pathol 2000;53(4):173–6.

18. Mauro VP. Codon Optimization in the Production of Recombinant Biotherapeutics: Potential Risks and Considerations. BioDrugs 2018;32(1):69–81.

19. Eichler F, Duncan C, Musolino PL, et al. Hematopoietic Stem-Cell Gene Therapy for Cerebral Adrenoleukodystrophy. N Engl J Med 2017;377(17):1630–8.

20. Mahmood A, Raymond GV, Dubey P, et al. Survival analysis of haematopoietic cell transplantation for childhood cerebral X-linked adrenoleukodystrophy: a comparison study. Lancet Neurol 2007;6(8):687–92.

21. Aubourg P, Blanche S, Jambaqué I, et al. Reversal of early neurologic and neuroradiologic manifestations of X-linked adrenoleukodystrophy by bone marrow transplantation. N Engl J Med 1990;322(26):1860–6.

22. Asheuer M, Pflumio F, Benhamida S, et al. Human CD34$^+$ cells differentiate into microglia and express recombinant therapeutic protein. Proc Natl Acad Sci U S A 2004;101(10):3557–62.

23. Cartier N, Hacein-Bey-Abina S, Bartholomae CC, et al. Hematopoietic stem cell gene therapy with a lentiviral vector in X-linked adrenoleukodystrophy. Science 2009;326(5954):818–23.

24. Cartier N, Hacein-Bey-Abina S, Bartholomae CC, et al. Lentiviral hematopoietic cell gene therapy for X-linked adrenoleukodystrophy. Methods Enzymol 2012;507:187–98.

25. Bluebird bio Announces FDA Priority review of Biologics License application for eli-cel gene therapy for cerebral adrenoleukodystrophy (CALD) in patients without a Matched Sibling donor. Available at: https://www.businesswire.com/news/home/20211217005659/en/bluebird-bio-Announces-FDA-Priority-Review-of-Biologics-License-Application-for-eli-cel-Gene-Therapy-for-Cerebral-Adreno leukodystrophy-CALD-in-Patients-Without-a-Matched-Sibling-Donor. Accessed March 6, 2022.

26. Wang RY, Bodamer OA, Watson MS, et al. Lysosomal storage diseases: diagnostic confirmation and management of presymptomatic individuals. Genet Med 2011;13(5):457–84.

27. Ries M, Gupta S, Moore DF, et al. Pediatric Fabry disease. Pediatrics 2005;115(3):e344-355.

28. Pintos-Morell G, Beck M. Fabry disease in children and the effects of enzyme replacement treatment. Eur J Pediatr 2009;168(11):1355–63.

29. Huang J, Khan A, Au BC, et al. Lentivector Iterations and Pre-Clinical Scale-Up/Toxicity Testing: Targeting Mobilized CD34(+) Cells for Correction of Fabry Disease. Mol Ther Methods Clin Dev 2017;5:241–58.

30. Khan A, Barber DL, Huang J, et al. Lentivirus-mediated gene therapy for Fabry disease. Nat Commun 2021;12(1):1178.

31. Cesani M, Lorioli L, Grossi S, et al. Mutation Update of ARSA and PSAP Genes Causing Metachromatic Leukodystrophy. Hum Mutat 2016;37(1):16–27.

32. Sevin C, Aubourg P, Cartier N. Enzyme, cell and gene-based therapies for metachromatic leukodystrophy. J Inherit Metab Dis 2007;30(2):175–83.

33. Biffi A, De Palma M, Quattrini A, et al. Correction of metachromatic leukodystrophy in the mouse model by transplantation of genetically modified hematopoietic stem cells. J Clin Invest 2004;113(8):1118–29.

34. Biffi A, Capotondo A, Fasano S, et al. Gene therapy of metachromatic leukodystrophy reverses neurological damage and deficits in mice. J Clin Invest 2006;116(11):3070–82.

35. Sessa M, Lorioli L, Fumagalli F, et al. Lentiviral haemopoietic stem-cell gene therapy in early-onset metachromatic leukodystrophy: an ad-hoc analysis of a non-randomised, open-label, phase 1/2 trial. Lancet 2016;388(10043):476–87.

36. Gaj T, Gersbach CA, Barbas CF 3rd. ZFN, TALEN, and CRISPR/Cas-based methods for genome engineering. Trends Biotechnol 2013;31(7):397–405.

37. Dever DP, Scharenberg SG, Camarena J, et al. CRISPR/Cas9 Genome Engineering in Engraftable Human Brain-Derived Neural Stem Cells. iScience 2019;15:524–35.

38. Rafi MA, Rao HZ, Luzi P, et al. Extended normal life after AAVrh10-mediated gene therapy in the mouse model of Krabbe disease. Mol Ther 2012;20(11):2031–42.

39. Sack BK, Herzog RW, Terhorst C, et al. Development of Gene Transfer for Induction of Antigen-specific Tolerance. Mol Ther Methods Clin Dev 2014;1:14013.

Ex Vivo and In Vivo Gene Therapy for Mucopolysaccharidoses: State of the Art

Giulia Consiglieri, MD[a,b,c], Maria Ester Bernardo, MD, PhD[a,b,d], Nicola Brunetti-Pierri, MD[e,f,g,1], Alessandro Aiuti, MD, PhD[a,b,d,1,*]

KEYWORDS

- Mucopolysaccharidoses • Invivo gene therapy • Exvivo gene therapy
- Enzyme replacement therapy • Hematopoietic stem cell transplantation

KEY POINTS

- Current treatments, enzyme replacement therapy (ERT) and hematopoietic stem cell transplantation (HSCT), for mucopolysaccharidoses (MPSs) have limitations including lack of efficacy on brain and skeletal manifestations, high costs, and safety issues.
- Gene therapy (GT) in MPSs aims at obtaining high levels of the therapeutic enzyme in multiple tissues either by engrafted gene-modified hematopoietic stem progenitor cells or by direct infusion in-vivo of the viral vector.
- Preliminary results of ex-vivo GT clinical trials in MPS type I, Hurler variant, and mucopolysaccharidosis type IIIA patients have shown a good safety profile together with encouraging biochemical and early clinical outcomes.
- In-vivo GT by local brain delivery or systemic intravenous injections of viral vectors resulted in biochemical and clinical improvements in preclinical models and early clinical trials of various MPSs.

[a] Pediatric Immunohematology and Bone Marrow Transplantation Unit, IRCCS San Raffaele Scientific Institute, Milan, Italy; [b] San Raffaele Telethon Institute for Gene Therapy (SR-Tiget), IRCSS San Raffaele Scientific Institute, Milan, Italy; [c] Department of Biomedicine and Prevention, University of Rome Tor Vergata, Rome, Italy; [d] Vita-Salute San Raffaele University, Milan, Italy; [e] Department of Translational Medicine, Federico II University, Naples, Italy; [f] Telethon Institute of Genetics and Medicine, Pozzuoli, Naples, Italy; [g] Scuola Superiore Meridionale, School for Advanced Studies, Naples, Italy
[1] Equal contribution.
* Corresponding author. Pediatric Immunohematology and Bone Marrow Transplantation Unit, IRCCS San Raffaele Scientific Institute, Milan, Italy.
E-mail address: aiuti.alessandro@hsr.it

Hematol Oncol Clin N Am 36 (2022) 865–878
https://doi.org/10.1016/j.hoc.2022.03.012
0889-8588/22/© 2022 Elsevier Inc. All rights reserved.

hemonc.theclinics.com

INTRODUCTION

Mucopolysaccharidoses (MPSs) comprise a group of rare inherited lysosomal storage disorders (LSDs) with an overall incidence of 1:25,000 live births,[1] caused by deficiency of enzymes involved in degradation of glycosaminoglycans (GAGs).

Clinical manifestations depend on accumulation of undegraded GAGs in the lysosomes of several cell types, and thus, they are multisystemic and characterized by the involvement of both the central nervous system (CNS) and visceral organs with hepatosplenomegaly, cardiac valve disease, respiratory disease, and skeletal abnormalities.

Primary CNS involvement is present in the severe forms of mucopolysaccharidosis (MPS) type I and II, all type III subtypes, and type VII.[2,3] Although the biochemical abnormalities can be detected at birth, MPS patients are rarely recognized clinically before they show coarse facial features and cognitive impairment. Mortality is high in the first 2 to 3 decades of life, largely due to respiratory infections, heart disease, and/or severe neurodegeneration.

Besides supportive treatments, enzyme replacement therapy (ERT) and allogeneic hematopoietic stem cell transplantation (HSCT), aiming at delivering the deficient enzyme and reducing GAG accumulation, are standard treatments for several MPSs.[4–6] ERT is currently available for MPS type I, II, IVA, VI, and VII and is based on repeated intravenous (iv) administrations of the recombinant enzyme. The efficacy of ERT is based on the uptake by diseased cells of circulating lysosomal enzymes via the mannose-6-phosphate receptor, followed by enzyme internalization, and targeting to lysosomes.

Although clinical benefits have been observed for visceral organs, several tissues remain refractory to ERT, such as the CNS due to the inability of the enzyme to cross the blood-brain barrier (BBB) and to penetrate the skeleton, and the eye. Moreover, ERT is often associated with immunologic responses, potentially compromising its efficacy.[5,6] For delivering the recombinant enzyme to the brain, intrathecal ERT has been investigated in clinical trials for MPS type I, II, and IIIA. Unfortunately, severe adverse events and malfunction of the intrathecal drug delivery device are major challenges, and data on the efficacy of ERT by this route of administration are still inconclusive.[7–9]

Despite the potential of treating neurologic manifestations by providing a permanent source of the missing enzyme at the CNS level, HSCT is associated with transplant-related mortality (TRM) and residual disease burden particularly at skeletal and CNS levels.[10–12] Therefore, there is an unmet need for a safe and more effective treatment resulting in enzyme delivery to the affected tissues, especially the skeleton and the brain.

GT approaches aiming at correction of the genetic defect have been extensively investigated over the last years and represent an attractive and potentially more effective alternative strategy to overcome the limitations of conventional treatments.[13–15] Gene transfer can be achieved by either in-vivo or ex-vivo procedures (**Fig. 1**). Ex-vivo GT requires the harvest from patients of hematopoietic stem progenitor cells (HSPC), which are genetically modified in-vitro with a viral vector to express the therapeutic gene at normal or supranormal concentrations. Subsequently, the gene-corrected cells are infused after chemotherapy into the patient where they engraft and differentiate into multiple hematopoietic lineages expressing the functional enzyme. Efficacy in the CNS is based on HSPC migrating into the brain and differentiating into microglial cells, which provide a source of enzyme for cross-correction of neighboring cells. Conversely, in-vivo GT consists of the direct injection of viral vectors expressing the therapeutic gene into the patient, by different routes of administration including systemic iv injection or local CNS delivery (eg, intracerebral [IC], intracerebroventricular [ICV], and intracisternal injections) in order to obtain specific organ targeting.

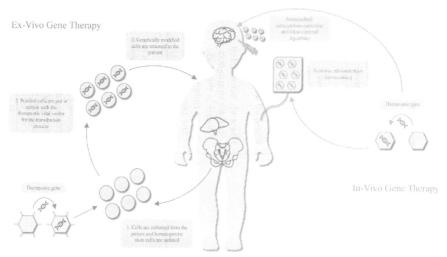

Fig. 1. Ex-vivo and in-vivo GT. Ex-vivo GT requires patient's cell collection followed by CD34+ cell isolation; subsequently, the purified cells are cultured with the therapeutic viral vector for gene delivery; finally, genetically modified stem cells are returned to the patient. Conversely, by in-vivo GT the viral vector is infused directly into the patient by either intravenous or local brain injections.

Retroviral (RV) and lentiviral (LV) vectors are generally used for ex-vivo GT, whereas adeno-associated viruses (AAV) are preferable for in-vivo gene therapy. Although RV and LV integrate into the genome of transduced cells, AAV vectors remain as episomes in the nuclei of transduced cells. Multiple serotypes of AAV are available with distinct tissue tropism. AAV8 has been used for liver-directed GT because of its higher hepatotropism,[16] whereas AAV9 has been preferred for in-vivo GT aiming at transduction of neurons after either local brain delivery or systemic iv injections.[17]

This review summarizes the most recent developments in terms of ex-vivo and in-vivo GT strategies for MPSs. The potential future clinical applications of both gene addition and gene editing approaches in MPSs are also discussed. Ongoing clinical and preclinical GT studies for MPSs are summarized in **Table 1**.

MUCOPOLYSACCHARIDOSIS TYPE I, HURLER VARIANT

Mucopolysaccharidosis type I (MPSI) is caused by defects in the gene *IDUA* encoding for the alfa-L-iduronidase that hydrolyzes dermatan sulfate and heparan sulfate. The impaired degradation of these GAGs leads to a wide range of clinical manifestations, including hepatosplenomegaly, dysostosis multiplex, coarse facial features, hearing and vision problems, cardiorespiratory impairments, hydrocephalus, and spinal cord compression. Progressive neurologic deterioration develops in patients with the most severe Hurler syndrome (MPSIH) phenotype.

In the last decade ex-vivo GT has become a developing treatment modality for LSDs characterized by extensive CNS and peripheral nervous system involvement, as treated early onset metachromatic leukodystrophy (MLD) patients[18,19] showed preserved cognitive function and motor development in most cases , leading to recent market approval in the European Union (EU).[20]

Building on this experience and on preclinical works using LV-based HSPC-GT in MPSI mice, which demonstrated correction of MPSI phenotype and long-term safety and efficacy,[21,22] a first-in-human phase I/II clinical trial (NCT00243023) of HSPC-GT

Table 1
Ongoing ex-vivo and in-vivo clinical and preclinical GT studies for MPSs

	Sponsor and Trial Number	Vector	Administration Route and Dose[c]	Status
MPSI	Orchard Therapeutics NCT0024303[a]	LV-IDUA (human PGK gene promoter)	Ex vivo CD34+ cells (IV) (minimum dose of $\geq 4 \times 10^6$ CD34+ cells/Kg and maximum dose of 35×10^6 CD34+ cells/Kg)	Phase I/II, active, not recruiting
	Masonic Cancer Center, University of Minnesota NCT04284254[a]	Sleeping Beauty transposon system	IV (dose escalation: phase 1: dose level 1: 5×10^7 cells/kg on day 0; dose level 2: 1×10^8 cells/kg on day 0; dose level 3: 1×10^8 cells/kg × 2 doses on day 0 and day 30 +/-3 days. Phase 2: Maximum Tolerated Dose established in Phase I	Phase I/II active, not recruiting
	Regenxbio RGX-111 NCT03580083[a]	AAV9-IDUA	IC (dose escalation: dose 1: 1×10^{10} GC/g brain mass; dose 2: 5×10^{10} GC/g brain mass)	Phase I/II active recruiting
	Sangamo SB-318 NCT02702115[a]	AAV6-ZFN	IV (ascending dose)	Phase I/II, terminated (All three subjects dosed in the study have rolled over to the Long-Term Follow-up Study IVPRP-LT01)
MPSII	University of Manchester	LV-IDS LV-IDS/APOEII (human CD11b myeloid-specific promoter)	Ex vivo CD34+ cells (IV)	Not approved yet Grants for GMP vector production obtained in 2019
	Sangamo SB-913 NCT03041324[a]	AAV6-ZFN	IV (ascending dose)	Phase I/II, terminated (subjects rolled-over to the Long-Term Follow-up Study IVPRP-LT01)
	Regenxbio RGX-121 NCT03566043[a]	AAV9-hIDS	IC (6.5×10^{10} GC/g brain mass)	Phase I/II, active recruiting

MPSIIIA	University of Manchester NCT04201405[a]	LVV-CD11b-SGSH (human CD11b myeloid-specific promoter)	Ex vivo CD34+ cells (IV)	Phase I/II, active, not recruiting
	Lysogene SAF-302 NCT03612869[a]	AAVrh10-hSGSH	IC	Phase II/III, active, not recruiting
	Abeona ABO-102 NCT02716246[a]	scAAV9-U1a.hSGSH (U1a promoter)	IV (dose escalation: cohort 1: 0.5×10^{13} vg/kg; cohort 2: 1×10^{13} vg/kg cohort 3: 3×10^{13} vg/kg)	Phase I/II, active recruiting
	Esteve EGT-101 2015-000359-26[b]	AAV9-hSGSH	ICV	Phase I/II, not recruiting
MPSIIIB	UniQure Biopharma B.V. NCT03300453[a]	AAV5-hNAGLU	intra-cerebral (4×10^{12} vg in total)	Phase I/II, completed
	Abeona NCT03315182[a]	AAV9-CMV-hNAGLU (CMV enhancer/promoter)	IV (dose escalation: cohort 1: 2×10^{13} vg/kg; cohort 2: 5×10^{13} vg/kg cohort 3: 1×10^{14} vg/kg)	Phase I/II, active, not recruiting
MPSIVA	Regenxbio and Dupont hospital	AAV8-TBG-hGALNS and AAV8-TBG-D8-hGALNS (liver specific TBG)	IV	Research/preclinical (murine model)
	Universitat Autònoma de Barcelona	AAV9-GALNS	IV	Research/preclinical (rat model)
	Nemours/Alfred I. duPont Hospital for Children, University of Manchester	LV-GALNS-D8 LV-GALNS (CD11b promoter) LV-GALNS (COL2A promoter)	Ex vivo CD34+ cells (IV)	Research/preclinical (murine model)
MPSVI	Fondazione Telethon NCT03173521[a]	AAV8-TBG-hARSB (liver specific TBG)	IV (starting dose: 6×10^{11} GC/kg, high dose 2×10^{12} GC/kg, very high dose 6×10^{12} GC/kg, low dose 2×10^{11} GC/kg)	Phase I/II, active not recruiting

Abbreviations, AAV, adeno-associated virus; IC, intracisternal; ICV, intracerebroventricular; IV, intravenous; LV, lentiviral.
[a] National Clinical Trial number
[b] EudraCTnumber
[c] *where known*
Data from https://clinicaltrials.gov/; last accessed on December 27th, 2021.

was conducted at SR-TIGET on 8 MPSIH patients. Autologous HSPC were collected by leukapheresis following mobilization, transduced with LV vector encoding the human *IDUA* under the control of the human phosphoglycerate kinase promoter, and infused back after a myeloablative conditioning regimen based on busulfan, which is instrumental in inducing microglia reconstitution by donor cells,[23] fludarabine and rituximab. After a median follow-up of 24 months, the treatment seemed to be safe and all patients showed prompt hematological reconstitution with sustained engraftment of gene-modified CD34+ cells, supraphysiologic IDUA activities in peripheral blood, and rapid normalization of urinary GAG excretion at 1 year after GT. Previously undetectable IDUA activity in cerebrospinal fluid (CSF) at baseline became detectable after HSPC-GT, whereas GAG concentrations in the CSF decreased over time, suggesting correction of the biochemical defect in the CNS. Although the follow-up period is still limited, patients showed progressive gain of cognitive and motor skills and early skeletal response, as shown by reduced joint stiffness and normal growth.[24] These data suggest that the supraphysiological enzyme activity allows for cross-correction of non-hematopoietic cells, including neurons and possibly skeletal cells.

Preclinical and clinical studies showed that ex-vivo GT for LSDs needs to be performed before the onset of disease manifestations to maximize efficacy. Unfortunately, this is often not an option because patients are typically diagnosed after the onset of manifestations. Several studies have focused on in-vivo GT to address the need of these patients. ICV administration of an AAV8 expressing IDUA in *Idua*−/− newborn mice resulted in supra-physiological enzyme levels in different brain regions, normalization of lysosomal storage, and amelioration of the neurocognitive impairment.[25] Studies in larger disease animal models including cats and dogs showed high and widespread brain expression with correction of lysosomal storage after a single intracisternal administration of an AAV9 vector.[26,27] When performed in nonhuman primates, AAV9 delivered by intracisternal administration did not result in procedure-related toxicity or adverse events, although minimal to moderate asymptomatic degeneration of dorsal root ganglia neurons and associated axons was observed.[28] Based on these studies a phase I clinical trial is currently open for in-vivo brain-directed GT of MPSI patients (NCT#03580083).

Loss of transgene expression due to cell division is a limitation of AAV vectors that are mostly episomal vectors. Strategies based on genome editing have the potential to overcome this obstacle by providing stable integration of the transgene at a desired locus. These approaches aim either at direct correction of the genetic defect in its chromatin locus or at inducing integration of the therapeutic gene into specific loci (eg, the albumin locus). For example, AAV vectors carrying a zinc-finger nuclease (ZFN) targeting the first intron of the hepatic albumin locus has been administered together with another vector expressing a donor sequence (ie, the therapeutic gene), and as a result of the double-strand break induced by the ZFN, the donor sequence integrated in the albumin locus and expressed the therapeutic gene at high level under the control of the albumin promoter.[29] Gene editing approaches have been shown to be effective preclinically in noncell autonomous disorders, including hemophilia and LSDs,[29] whereas initial results from clinical studies in MPSI and MPSII with ZFN showed low transgene expression (NCT02702115 and NCT03041324).[30,31]

MUCOPOLYSACCHARIDOSIS TYPE II, HUNTER SYNDROME

Mucopolysaccharidosis type II (MPSII), also known as Hunter syndrome, is an X-linked disorder caused by mutations of the *IDS* gene encoding the iduronate-2-sulfatase enzyme.

In MPSII mice, a brain-targeted HSPC-GT strategy using lentiviral vector encoding IDS fused to ApoEII , which increases the ability of IDS enzyme to cross the BBB, has been compared with a lentivirus expressing normal IDS or with a normal bone marrow transplant. In contrast to the partial amelioration observed with the LV encoding IDS, complete correction of brain pathology and behavior was obtained with the LV expressing the IDS fused with ApoEII (LV.IDS.ApoEII). Moreover, LV.IDS.ApoEII increased plasma enzyme activities and cell uptake, together with transcytosis across brain endothelial cells via both heparan sulfate/ApoE-dependent and mannose-6-phosphate receptors. In summary, brain-targeted HSPC-GT represents a promising therapy for MPSII patients and the development of a phase I/II clinical trial is ongoing at the University of Manchester.[32]

In vivo applications with AAV9 vectors have been investigated in MPSII mice for brain-directed GT by different routes, such as ICV or intracisternal injections . These studies have shown that AAV9 vectors result in high levels of cerebral transduction, correction of the lysosomal storage, and prevention of neurobehavioral deficits, as well as correction of peripheral tissues as consequence of systemic dissemination of the vector through the subarachnoid spaces.[33–35] These preclinical results are leading to a phase I/II GT clinical trial to investigate the efficacy of AAV9 encoding the human *IDS* by CNS delivery in MPSII patients (NCT#03566043).

MUCOPOLYSACCHARIDOSIS TYPE III, SANFILIPPO SYNDROME

Mucopolysaccharidosis type III (MPSIII) or Sanfilippo syndrome comprises four autosomal recessive disease subtypes caused by defects of enzymes involved in degradation of heparan sulfate: MPSIIIA due to deficiency of N-sulfoglucosamine sulfohydrolase enzyme encoded by *SGSH* gene; MPSIIIB due to deficiency of the N-α-acetyl-glucosaminidase enzyme encoded by the *NAGLU* gene; MPSIIIC due to deficiency of the heparan α-glucosaminide N-acetyltransferase enzyme encoded by the *HGSNAT* gene; and MPSIIID due to deficiency of the N-acetylglucosamine-6-sulfatase enzyme encoded by the *GNS* gene.

A phase I/II clinical trial of ex-vivo GT is under investigation (NCT04201405) at Manchester University for MPSIIIA in patients between 3 and 24 months of age with preserved neurocognitive function. In this trial, autologous HSPCs, collected after mobilization, are transduced ex-vivo with an LV encoding for the human *SGSH* gene under the CD11b promoter, cryopreserved and infused back after myeloablative conditioning with busulfan. Safety and tolerability of the drug product and expression of SGSH activity in leukocytes at 12 months post-treatment are the primary endpoints, whereas neurocognitive outcome is a secondary endpoint. Although the study is still ongoing, preliminary data from the first patients recruited show supraphysiological enzyme expression in multiple lineages and substrate reduction in plasma, CSF, and urine.[36]

Two AAV-mediated brain-directed GT trials in MPSIIIA and IIIB have been concluded and the published results have reported clinical improvement particularly in younger patients.[37,38] The MPSIIIA trial was based on comparable efficiency of AAVrh10 in transducing the CNS after systemic administration and a lower prevalence of preexisting immunity compared with AAV9.[39] SGSH is a sulfatase activated by a post-translational modification by the enzyme encoded by *SUMF1*.[40,41] Delivery of an AAV vector expressing both SGSH and SUMF1 by ICV injection in MPSIIIA mice resulted in higher SGSH activities, reduction of lysosomal storage and neuroinflammation, and improvement of memory and motor functions.[42] However, gene delivery resulted in enzyme expression and correction only in brain regions near the injection site,[43] underlying the need of multiple injections to achieve widespread brain correction. This same vector was delivered in a phase I/II, open-label, clinical trial on MPSIIIA patients (NCT#01474343) by a neurosurgical procedure entailing 12 simultaneous intraparenchymal injections in both sides of the brain[37]; the surgical procedure was well tolerated with acceptable safety throughout 1 year of follow-up. Motor and cognitive skills remained stable and the youngest subject enrolled showed some improvement in motor abilities and stable language and cognition.

In MPSIIIB an AAV5 vector encoding NAGLU was injected in 16 intraparenchymal deposits that were well tolerated. Compared with the natural history, neurocognitive progression improved in all treated patients, with the youngest patient having function close to that in healthy children.[38]

Compared with iv administration, AAV9 intracisternal injections resulted in better correction of GAG storage in brain and correction of peripheral organs, as a consequence of vector systemic dissemination.[44] Based on these preclinical data, two clinical trials with AAV9 are under development to investigate the safety and efficacy of these two routes of administration (ie, iv and ICV injections) in MPSIIIA subjects (NCT#02716246; NCT04088734).

AAV8 vectors transduce predominantly the liver but supraphysiological plasma activities of the enzyme also reduced brain GAG accumulation, likely as consequence of enzyme crossing the BBB.[45] However, to improve enzyme penetration across the BBB, bioengineered SGSH conjugated with a peptide favoring brain targeting was delivered to the liver by AAV8.[46] In this study, SGSH was fused with the signal peptide from the highly secreted IDS and the BBB-binding domain from apolipoprotein B. Importantly, besides MPSIIIA, this approach has potential to achieve brain correction also in other MPSs.

MUCOPOLYSACCHARIDOSIS TYPE IV, MORQUIO A SYNDROME

Mucopolysaccharidosis type IV (MPSIV) or Morquio A syndrome is an autosomal recessive LSD caused by mutations in the *GALNS* gene encoding the enzyme N-acetylgalactosamine-6-sulfatase (GALNS).

Treatment of MPSIVA mice with liver-directed AAV-based GT resulted in increased secretion of GALNS and normalization of keratan sulfate concentrations in plasma and tissues.[47] More recently, efficacy of an intravenous AAV9 vector administration resulting in correction of not only peripheral organs but also bone and cartilage was confirmed in MPSIVA rat model that fully recapitulated the skeletal and nonskeletal features of human MPSIVA patients.[48]

MUCOPOLYSACCHARIDOSIS TYPE VI, MAROTEAUX-LAMY SYNDROME

Mucopolysaccharidosis type VI (MPSIV) or Maroteaux-Lamy syndrome is an autosomal recessive lysosomal storage disease due to mutations in the *ARSB* gene encoding arylsulfatase B, deficiency of which results in multisystem accumulation of GAGs sparing the CNS.

Preclinical studies in rodent and feline models have shown that AAV8-mediated liver expression and secretion of ARSB resulted in increased blood ARSB activities, reduction of GAG storage, and improvement of heart and skeletal disease.[49,50] Therefore, liver-directed GT can provide sustained expression of ARSB at therapeutic levels and overcome the need of repeated iv infusions.[51,52] Given the encouraging results, a clinical trial for MPSVI (NCT#03173521) is currently ongoing.

OTHER MUCOPOLYSACCHARIDOSES

Other MPSs have also been targets of GT in preclinical studies but they have not yet matured for clinical applications. For example, brain-directed GT has been investigated in MPSIIIC and MPSIIID mouse models, resulting in phenotype correction.[53,54] GT for MPS type VII has been investigated by both systemic and intracisternal administrations of AAV9 and AAVrh10 in small and large disease animal models. However, there are no ongoing GT clinical trials for these disorders.

MPS type IX and MPS type X have been recently identified, and we need to learn more about the pathogenesis and the natural history of the diseases before GT studies can be performed.

SUMMARY

Available treatment options for MPSs have important limitations mainly related to the limited efficacy in the skeletal and CNS manifestations, highlighting the need for improved therapeutic approaches. The potential for GT to transduce cell types that can cross-correct distant body districts is very attractive. The high levels of enzyme activity achieved by GT can correct the CNS and bone, either by engrafted gene-modified HSPC or by direct infusion of the viral vector in-vivo.

In the past few years, substantial progress has been made in ex-vivo and in-vivo GT for LSDs to the point that the demonstration of the long-term clinical efficacy of HSPC-GT for MLD[20] has led to the marketing authorization in the EU of the medicinal product Libmeldy.

Taking advantage of the experience with MLD and the promising results of preclinical studies of ex-vivo HSPC-GT in mouse models,[21,22,36] phase I/II clinical trials have been developed for MPSIH and MPSIIIA. Despite the limited follow-up, data from the clinical trial of HSPC-GT for MPSIH have shown promising biological and clinical outcomes, especially at CNS and skeletal levels,[21] which are likely dependent on enzyme overexpression and efficient tissue cross-correction. Indeed, the supraphysiological levels of IDUA enzyme by gene-corrected HSPC derived cells, circulating or resident in a specific tissue, cross-correct cells of nonhematopoietic origins, including neurons and possibly skeletal cells. Therefore, osteoclasts derived from genetically corrected myeloid precursors may release high levels of enzyme in the bone microenvironment, mediating cross-correction of neighboring untransduced cells. The potential efficacy on skeletal manifestations could be a significant advantage of GT over allogeneic (allo-HSCT), which fails to correct MPS-related skeletal pathology.[55–57] Similarly, the ongoing ex-vivo GT clinical trial for MPSIIIA has generated encouraging even though very preliminary results.[36] Nevertheless, longer follow-up is necessary to demonstrate the long-term impact of HSPC-GT on clinical manifestations and to what extent previously established bone or brain damage may be reversible. Of note, significant advantages of HSPC-GT over HSCT are the reduced TRM and mortality and the absent risk of GVHD due to the autologous procedure.[10,58,59]

For correction of the brain disorder, in-vivo GT by direct administration of vectors into the CNS has the advantage to provide long-term expression of the transgene avoiding repeated administrations. Other strategies under investigation include enzyme delivery to the brain following systemic administration using AAV serotypes that can cross the BBB and transduce the CNS. Systemic administration of AAV9 for transduction of both the CNS and peripheral tissues is less invasive than IC delivery, which requires neurosurgical procedures. However, this approach results in variable levels of enzyme activity in the brain and requires higher vector doses potentially associated with higher risks of acute toxicity.[60] In addition, good manufacturing practice production for high vector doses remains a challenge.

Alternatively, the liver can be converted into a "factory organ" for production and systemic delivery of the enzyme to other tissues. This strategy seems particularly suitable for MPSs that lack of primary CNS involvement, but it could also be combined with liver-directed gene transfer of bioengineered enzymes fused with proteins that bind to a receptor on the BBB and allow enzyme transport by receptor-mediated transcytosis.[46,61]

In conclusion, this review summarizes novel GT strategies that are being developed to treat MPSs. Currently, data available from ex-vivo GT clinical and preclinical trials, and from in-vivo GT trials, even though based mostly on preclinical and limited clinical experience, are promising. Moreover, both ex-vivo and in-vivo GT approaches are compared favorably with allo-HSCT in terms of safety and biological and clinical efficacy. Although longer follow-up is needed to confirm these data, preliminary results support further clinical development of GT for several type of MPSs, and they may pave the way toward GT for other ultrarare LSDs with unmet medical needs. Expanded newborn screening is being considered for several LSDs, including MPSs.[62] Early recognition of MPSs might allow presymptomatic treatments,[18] leading to better neurologic and skeletal outcomes.

CONFLICT OF INTERESTS

A. Aiuti is PI or co-PI of clinical trials sponsored by Orchard Therapeutics. M.E. Bernardo is PI of a clinical trial sponsored by Orchard Therapeutics. N. Brunetti-Pierri has no conflicts of interests. G. Consiglieri has no conflicts of interests.

ACKNOWLEDGEMENT

A. Aiuti, M.E. Bernardo and N. Brunetti-Pierri receive funding from Fondazione Telethon. A. Aiuti is the recipient of the Else Kröner Fresenius Prize for Medical Research 2020.

REFERENCES

1. National organization for rare disorders rare disease database. Mucopolysaccharidoses. Available at: https://rarediseases.org/rare-diseases/mucopolysaccharidoses/. Accessed October 10, 2021.

2. Neufeld EF, Muenzer J. The mucopolysaccaridoses. In: Scriver C, Beaudet A, Sly W, et al, editors. The metabolic and molecular basis of inherited disease. New York: McGraw Hill; 2001. p. 3421–52.

3. Muenzer J. Overview of the mucopolysaccharidoses. Rheumatology (Oxford) 2011;50(5):v4–12.

4. Safary A, Moghaddas-Sani H, Akbarzadeh-Khiavi M, et al. Enzyme replacement combinational therapy: effective treatments for mucopolysaccharidoses. Expert Opin Biol Ther 2021;21(9):1181.

5. Valayannopoulos V, Wijburg FA. Therapy for the mucopolysaccharidoses. Rheumatology (Oxford) 2011;50:v49–59.

6. Noh H, Lee JI. Current and potential therapeutic strategies for mucopolysaccharidoses. J Clin Pharm Ther 2014;39:215–24.

7. Muenzer J, Hendriksz C, Fan Z, et al. A phase I/II study of intrathecal idursulfase-IT in children with severe mucopolysaccharidosis II. Genet Med 2016;18(1): 73–81.

8. Jones SA, Breen C, Heap F, et al. A phase 1/2 study of intrathecal heparan-N-sulfatase in patients with mucopolysaccharidosis IIIA. Mol Genet Metab 2016; 118(3):198–205.

9. Dickson PI, Kaitila I, Harmatz P, et al. Safety of laronidase delivered into the spinal canal for treatment of cervical stenosis in mucopolysaccharidosis I. Mol Genet Metab 2015;116(1–2):69–74.

10. Aldenhoven M, Jones SA, Bonney D, et al. Hematopoietic cell transplantation for mucopolysaccharidosis patients is safe and effective: results after implementation of international guidelines. Biol Blood Marrow Transplant 2015;21:1106–9.

11. Aldenhoven M, Boelens JJ, de Koning TJ. The clinical outcome of hurler syndrome after stem cell transplantation. Biol Blood Marrow Transpl 2008;14:485–98.

12. Tomatsu S, Azario I, Sawamoto K, et al. Neonatal cellular and gene therapies for mucopolysaccharidoses: the earlier the better? J Inherit Metab Dis 2016;39: 189–202.

13. Ferrari G, Thrasher AJ, Aiuti A. Gene therapy using haematopoietic stem and progenitor cells. Nat Rev Genet 2021;22(4):216–34.

14. High KA, Roncarolo MG. Gene therapy. N Engl J Med 2019;381(5):455–64.

15. Mendell JR, Al-Zaidy SA, Rodino-Klapac LR, et al. Current clinical applications of in vivo gene therapy with AAVs. Mol Ther 2021;29(2):464–88.

16. Gao GP, Alvira MR, Wang L, et al. Novel adeno-associated viruses from rhesus monkeys as vectors for human gene therapy. Proc Natl Acad Sci U S A 2002; 99(18):11854–9.

17. Fu H, McCarty DM. Crossing the blood-brain-barrier with viral vectors. Curr Opin Virol 2016;21:87–92.

18. Biffi A, Montini E, Lorioli L, et al. Lentiviral hematopoietic stem cell gene therapy benefits metachromatic leukodystrophy. Science 2013;341:1233158.

19. Sessa M, Lorioli L, Fumagalli F, et al. Lentiviral haemopoietic stem-cell gene therapy in early-onset metachromatic leukodystrophy: an ad-hoc analysis of a non-randomised, open-label, phase 1/2 trial. Lancet 2016;388:476–87.

20. Fumagalli F, Calbi V, Natali Sora MG, et al. Lentiviral haematopoietic stem-cell gene therapy for early-onset metachromatic leukodystrophy: long-term results from a non-randomised, open-label, phase 1/2 trial and expanded access. Lancet 2022;399(10322):372–83.

21. Visigalli I, Delai S, Politi LS, et al. Gene therapy augments the efficacy of hematopoietic cell transplantation and fully corrects mucopolysaccharidosis type I phenotype in the mouse model. Blood 2010;116:5130–9.

22. Visigalli I, Delai S, Ferro F, et al. Preclinical testing of the safety and tolerability of lentiviral vector–mediated above-normal alpha-l-iduronidase expression in murine and human hematopoietic cells using toxicology and biodistribution good laboratory practice studies. Hum Gene Ther 2016;27(10):813–29.

23. Capotondo A, Milazzo R, Politi LS, et al. Brain conditioning is instrumental for successful microglia reconstitution following hematopoietic stem cell transplantation. Proc Natl Acad Sci U S A 2012;109(37):15018–23.

24. Gentner B, Tucci F, Galimberti S, et al. Hematopoietic Stem- and Progenitor-Cell Gene Therapy for Hurler Syndrome. N Engl J Med 2021;385(21):1929–40.

25. Wolf DA, Lenander AW, Nan Z, et al. Direct gene transfer to the CNS prevents emergence of neurologic disease in a murine model of mucopolysaccharidosis type I. Neurobiol Dis 2011;43(1):123–33.

26. Hinderer C, Bell P, Gurda BL, et al. Intrathecal gene therapy corrects CNS pathology in a feline model of mucopolysaccharidosis I. Mol Ther 2014;22(12):2018–27.

27. Hinderer C, Bell P, Louboutin JP, et al. Neonatal tolerance induction enables accurate evaluation of gene therapy for MPS I in a canine model. Mol Genet Metab 2016;119(1–2):124–30.

28. Hordeaux J, Hinderer C, Goode T, et al. Toxicology Study of Intra-Cisterna Magna Adeno-Associated Virus 9 Expressing Human Alpha-L-Iduronidase in Rhesus Macaques. Mol Ther Methods Clin Dev 2018;10:79–88.

29. Sharma R, Anguela XM, Doyon Y, et al. In vivo genome editing of the albumin locus as a platform for protein replacement therapy. Blood 2015;126(15): 1777–84.

30. Muenzer J, Prada CE, Burton B, et al. CHAMPIONS: A Phase 1/2 clinical trial with dose escalation of SB-913 ZFN-mediated in vivo human genome editing for treatment of MPSII (Hunter syndrome). Mol Genet Metab 2019;126(2):S104.

31. First in vivo human genome editing trial. Nat Biotechnol 2018;36:5.

32. Gleitz HFR, Liao AY, Cook JR, et al. Brain-targeted stem cell gene therapy corrects mucopolysaccharidosis type II via multiple mechanisms. Mol Med 2018; 10(7):e8730.

33. Laoharawee K, Podetz-Pedersen KM, Nguyen TT, et al. Prevention of neurocognitive deficiency in mucopolysaccharidosis type II mice by central nervous system-directed, AAV9-mediated iduronate sulfatase gene transfer. Hum Gene Ther 2017;28(8):626–38.

34. Motas S, Haurigot V, Garcia M, et al. CNS-directed gene therapy for the treatment of neurologic and somatic mucopolysaccharidosis type II (Hunter syndrome). JCI Insight 2016;1(9):e86696.

35. Hinderer C, Katz N, Louboutin JP, et al. Delivery of an Adeno-Associated Virus Vector into Cerebrospinal Fluid Attenuates Central Nervous System Disease in Mucopolysaccharidosis Type II Mice. Hum Gene Ther 2016;27(11): 906–15.

36. Kinsella J, Buckland K, Church H, et al. Preliminary outcomes of haematopoietic stem cell gene therapy in a patient with mucopolysaccharidosis IIIA. Mol Ther 2020;28(4S1):231.

37. Tardieu M, Zérah M, Husson B, et al. Intracerebral administration of adeno-associated viral vector serotype rh.10 carrying human SGSH and SUMF1 cDNAs in children with mucopolysaccharidosis type IIIA disease: results of a phase I/II trial. Hum Gene Ther 2014;25(6):506–16.

38. Tardieu M, Zérah M, Gougeon ML, et al. Intracerebral gene therapy in children with mucopolysaccharidosis type IIIB syndrome: an uncontrolled phase 1/2 clinical trial. Lancet Neurol 2017;16(9):712–20.

39. Tanguy Y, Biferi MG, Besse A, et al. Systemic AAVrh10 provides higher transgene expression than AAV9 in the brain and the spinal cord of neonatal mice. Front Mol Neurosci 2015;8:36.

40. Cosma MP, Pepe S, Annunziata I, et al. The multiple sulfatase deficiency gene encodes an essential and limiting factor for the activity of sulfatases. Cell 2003; 113(4):445–56.

41. Dierks T, Schmidt B, Borissenko L, et al. Multiple sulfatase deficiency is caused by mutations in the gene encoding the human C(alpha)-formylglycine generating enzyme. Cell 2003;113(4):435–44.

42. Fraldi A, Hemsley K, Crawley A, et al. Functional correction of CNS lesions in an MPS-IIIA mouse model by intracerebral AAV-mediated delivery of sulfamidase and SUMF1 genes. Hum Mol Genet 2007;16(22):2693–702.

43. Winner LK, Beard H, Hassiotis S, et al. A Preclinical Study Evaluating AAVrh10-Based Gene Therapy for Sanfilippo Syndrome. Hum Gene Ther 2016;27(5): 363–75.

44. Haurigot V, Marcò S, Ribera A, et al. Whole body correction of mucopolysacchar-idosis IIIA by intracerebrospinal fluid gene therapy. J Clin Invest 2013;123(8): 3254–71.

45. Ruzo A, Garcia M, Ribera A, et al. Liver production of sulfamidase reverses pe-ripheral and ameliorates CNS pathology in mucopolysaccharidosis IIIA mice. Mol Ther 2012;20(2):254–66.

46. Sorrentino NC, D'Orsi L, Sambri I, et al. A highly secreted sulphamidase en-gineered to cross the blood-brain barrier corrects brain lesions of mice with mucopolysaccharidoses type IIIA. EMBO Mol Med 2013;5(5):675–90.

47. Sawamoto K, Karumuthil-Melethil S, Khan S, et al. Liver-targeted AAV8 gene ther-apy ameliorates skeletal and cardiovascular pathology in a mucopolysaccharido-sis IVA murine model. Mol Ther Methods Clin Dev 2020;18:50–61.

48. Bertolin J, Sànchez V, Ribera A, et al. Treatment of skeletal and non-skeletal alter-ations of Mucopolysaccharidosis type IVA by AAV-mediated gene therapy. Nat Commun 2021;12(1):5343.

49. Cotugno G, Annunziata P, Tessitore A, et al. Long-term amelioration of feline Mu-copolysaccharidosis VI after AAV-mediated liver gene transfer. Mol Ther 2011; 19(3):461–9.

50. Ferla R, O'Malley T, Calcedo R, et al. Gene therapy for mucopolysaccharidosis type VI is effective in cats without pre-existing immunity to AAV8. Hum Gene Ther 2013;24(2):163–9.

51. Ferla R, Claudiani P, Cotugno G, et al. Similar therapeutic efficacy between a sin-gle administration of gene therapy and multiple administrations of recombinant enzyme in a mouse model of lysosomal storage disease. Hum Gene Ther 2014;25(7):609–18.

52. Ferla R, Alliegro M, Marteau JB, et al. Non-clinical Safety and Efficacy of an AAV2/8 Vector Administered Intravenously for Treatment of Mucopolysaccharidosis Type VI. Mol Ther Methods Clin Dev 2017;6:143–58.

53. Tordo J, O'Leary C, Antunes ASL, et al. A novel adeno-associated virus capsid with enhanced neurotropism corrects a lysosomal transmembrane enzyme defi-ciency. Brain 2018;141(7):2014–31.

54. Roca C, Motas S, Marcò S, et al. Disease correction by AAV-mediated gene ther-apy in a new mouse model of mucopolysaccharidosis type IIID. Hum Mol Genet 2017;26(8):1535–51.

55. Aldenhoven M, Wynn RF, Orchard PJ, et al. Long-term outcome of Hurler syn-drome patients after hematopoietic cell transplantation: an international multi-center study. Blood 2015;125(13):2164–72.

56. Gardner CJ, Robinson N, Meadows T, et al. Growth, final height and endocrine sequelae in a UK population of patients with Hurler syndrome (MPS1H). J Inherit Metab Dis 2011;34(2):489–97.

57. Langereis EJ, Borgo A, Crushell E, et al. Treatment of hip dysplasia in patients with mucopolysaccharidosis type I after hematopoietic stem cell transplanta-tion: results of an international consensus procedure. Orphanet J Rare Dis 2013;8:155.

58. Lum SH, Miller WP, Jones S, et al. Changes in the incidence, patterns and out-comes of graft failure following hematopoietic stem cell transplantation for Hurler syndrome. Bone Marrow Transpl 2017;52(6):846–53.

59. Boelens JJ, Aldenhoven M, Purtill D, et al. Outcomes of transplantation using various hematopoietic cell sources in children with Hurler syndrome after myeloa-blative conditioning. Blood 2013;121(19):3981–7.

60. Hinderer C, Katz N, Buza EL, et al. Severe Toxicity in Nonhuman Primates and Piglets Following High-Dose Intravenous Administration of an Adeno-Associated Virus Vector Expressing Human SMN. Hum Gene Ther 2018;29(3): 285–98.
61. Scarpa M, Orchard PJ, Schulz A, et al. Treatment of brain disease in the mucopolysaccharidoses. Mol Genet Metab 2017;122S:25–34.
62. Matern D, Gavrilov D, Oglesbee D, et al. Newborn screening for lysosomal storage disorders. Semin Perinatol 2015;39(3):206–16.

Moving?

Make sure your subscription moves with you!

To notify us of your new address, find your **Clinics Account Number** (located on your mailing label above your name), and contact customer service at:

Email: journalscustomerservice-usa@elsevier.com

800-654-2452 (subscribers in the U.S. & Canada)
314-447-8871 (subscribers outside of the U.S. & Canada)

Fax number: 314-447-8029

Elsevier Health Sciences Division
Subscription Customer Service
3251 Riverport Lane
Maryland Heights, MO 63043

*To ensure uninterrupted delivery of your subscription, please notify us at least 4 weeks in advance of move.

ELSEVIER